Yearbook of Diabetes 2026

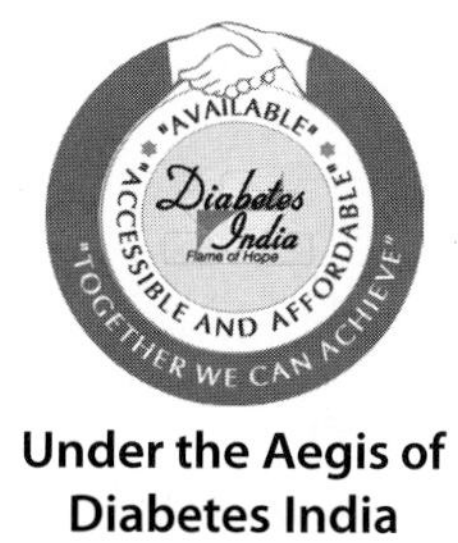

Under the Aegis of
Diabetes India

Yearbook of Diabetes 2026

Editor-in-Chief

Sujoy Ghosh
Professor
Department of Endocrinology
Institute of Post Graduate Medical Education and Research
Kolkata, West Bengal, India

Assistant Editor

Abhranil Dhar
Senior Resident
Department of Endocrinology
Institute of Post Graduate Medical Education and Research
Kolkata, West Bengal, India

SR Aravind
President, DiabetesIndia

Banshi Saboo
Secretary, DiabetesIndia

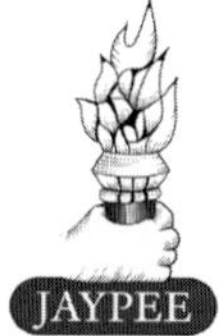

JAYPEE BROTHERS MEDICAL PUBLISHERS
The Health Sciences Publisher
New Delhi | London

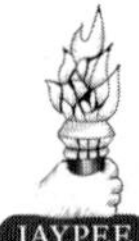

JAYPEE **Jaypee Brothers Medical Publishers (P) Ltd**

Headquarters
EMCA House, 23/23-B
Ansari Road, Daryaganj
New Delhi 110 002, India
Landline: +91-11-23272143, +91-11-23272703
+91-11-23282021, +91-11-23245672
e-mail: jaypee@jaypeebrothers.com

Corporate Office
4838/24, Ansari Road, Daryaganj
New Delhi 110 002, India
Phone: +91-11-43574357
Fax: +91-11-43574314
e-mail: jaypee@jaypeebrothers.com

Overseas Office
JP Medical Ltd.
83, Victoria Street, London
SW1H 0HW (UK)
Phone: +44-20 3170 8910
e-mail: info@jpmedpub.com

EU GPSR Authorised Representative
Logos Europe, 9 rue Nicolas Poussin
17000, La Rochelle, France
Phone: +33 (0) 6 67 93 73 78
e-mail: contact@logoseurope.eu

Website: www.jaypeebrothers.com
Website: www.jaypeedigital.com

Inquiries for bulk sales may be solicited at: jaypee@jaypeebrothers.com

Yearbook of Diabetes 2026 / Sujoy Ghosh

First Edition: **2026**

ISBN: 978-93-7545-533-2

Printed at: Samrat Offset Pvt. Ltd.

Contributors

SECTION EDITORS

Section 1: Basic Science

Arijit Singha
Assistant Professor
Department of Endocrinology
Institute of Post Graduate Medical Education and Research
Kolkata, West Bengal, India

Section 2: Epidemiology

Soham Tarafdar
Consultant Endocrinologist
Manipal Hospitals – Dhakuria
Kolkata, West Bengal, India

Section 3: Complications

Abhranil Dhar
Senior Resident
Department of Endocrinology
Institute of Post Graduate Medical Education and Research
Kolkata, West Bengal, India

Section 4: Drugs and Therapeutics (Part 1)

Sunetra Mondal
Assistant Professor
Department of Endocrinology
Nil Ratan Sircar Medical College and Hospital
Kolkata, West Bengal, India

Section 5: Drugs and Therapeutics (Part 2)

Pritam Biswas
Senior Resident
Department of Endocrinology
Nil Ratan Sircar Medical College and Hospital
Kolkata, West Bengal, India

Section 6: Type 1 Diabetes

Sumit Kumar Chakrabarti
Consultant Endocrinologist
Disease Area Expert, Type 1 Diabetes Project
Institute of Post Graduate Medical Education and Research
Kolkata, West Bengal, India

Section 7: Diabetes in Pregnancy

Indira Maisnam
Assistant Professor
Department of Endocrinology
Institute of Post Graduate Medical Education and Research
Kolkata, West Bengal, India

Section 8: Newer Technologies in Diabetes

Mainak Banerjee
Consultant Endocrinologist
Narayana Health Rabindranath Tagore International Institute of Cardiac Sciences
Kolkata, West Bengal, India

Section 9: Miscellaneous

Nisha Batra
Assistant Professor
Department of Medicine/Endocrinology
Himalayan Institute of Medical Sciences
Dehradun, Uttarakhand, India

Message from the Desk of DiabetesIndia

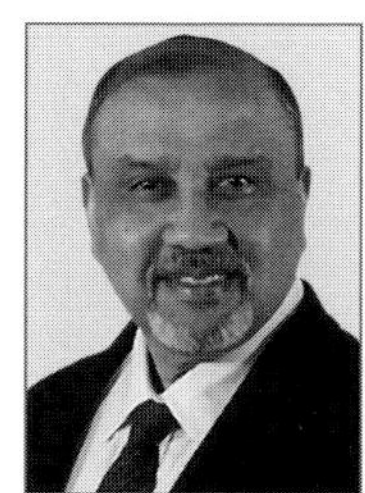

SR Aravind
President, DiabetesIndia

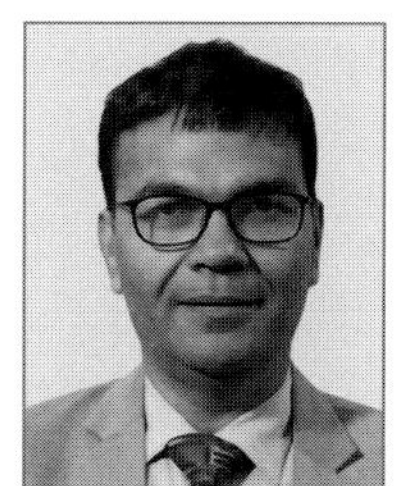

Banshi Saboo
Secretary, DiabetesIndia

The "*Yearbook of Diabetes 2026*" presents a curated collection of abstracts highlighting recent and breakthrough developments in diabetes reported between January 1, 2025, and December 31, 2025, selected from leading journals across the globe. Each abstract is accompanied by expert commentary, offering critical appraisal of clinical relevance and facilitating translation of evidence into everyday practice. This format enables readers to rapidly identify and assimilate and apply key advances in diabetes care. The goals of the Yearbook are to remain current, concise, accessible, and comprehensible, catering to learners and practitioners of medicine across all stages of their careers.

The book is structured into Nine thematic sections, clustering closely related subjects and spanning the full spectrum of diabetes—from basic science and epidemiology to contemporary clinical practice and emerging future directions.

We together extend our sincere appreciation and gratitude to the Editor-in-Chief, Dr Sujoy Ghosh, for his visionary leadership, scholarly insight, and unwavering commitment to upholding the highest editorial standards. His guidance has been central to the thoughtful shaping, integration, and academic rigor of this edition.

We are deeply thankful to the distinguished editorial team, whose expertise and support have been invaluable throughout the development of this volume.

We also gratefully acknowledge the significant contributions of Drs Arijit Singha, Soham Tarafdar, Abhranil Dhar, Sunetra Mondal, Pritam Biswas, Sumit Kumar Chakrabarti, Indira Maisnam, Mainak Banerjee, and Nisha Batra, whose scholarly input has greatly enriched the content of this Yearbook.

Special recognition is extended to Assistant Editor Dr Abhranil Dhar, whose meticulous coordination, and editorial support were instrumental in compiling and harmonizing this extensive work.

We take immense pride in presenting this edition of the Diabetes Yearbook that readers will agree that the clarity of writing, academic depth, and clinical relevance of the contributions establish it as a durable and valuable resource for education, teaching, and clinical practice in diabetes.

Message from The President, International Diabetes Federation

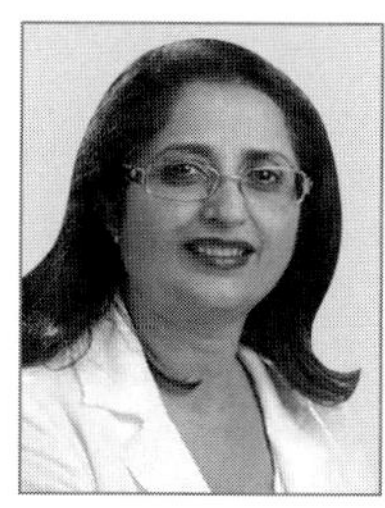

Niti Pall
President-Elect
International Diabetes Federation (IDF)

It is indeed a matter of great pride that DiabetesIndia is publishing the *"Yearbook of Diabetes 2026"*.

One of the core objectives of DiabetesIndia has been to actively promote research, education, and academic excellence in the field of diabetes in India. A yearbook—curating significant research articles in diabetes and allied disciplines published over the preceding year, serves as a valuable and comprehensive resource that captures recent advances and evolving concepts in diabetes care.

This compilation will provide physicians, postgraduate students, and researchers with a concise overview of contemporary developments, facilitating evidence-based clinical practice. It is expected that this initiative will further stimulate original research in diabetes and ultimately contribute to improved patient outcomes.

I am personally delighted to be associated with this important educational endeavor. I extend my sincere compliments to Dr Sujoy Ghosh, the editor of the book.

I congratulate President Dr SR Aravind and Secretary Dr Banshi Saboo along with the entire editorial team for their commendable efforts and convey my best wishes for the success of the Yearbook of Diabetes 2026.

Preface

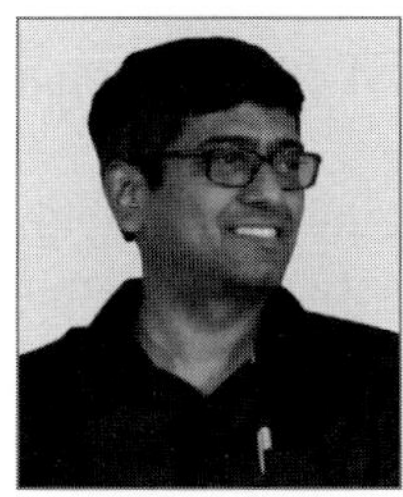

Sujoy Ghosh
Professor
Department of Endocrinology
Institute of Post Graduate Medical Education and Research
Kolkata, West Bengal, India

Yearbooks are available across most specialties and subspecialties of medical science. Given that more than 70,000 diabetes-related articles were published on PubMed in 2025 alone, it is hardly surprising that few have ventured to undertake the herculean task of compiling a comprehensive yearbook in diabetology.

As a teacher, I am frequently asked by students which studies are most important to read and how to interpret them. Practicing clinicians—both in primary care and in specialty practice—often attend conferences and scientific meetings with the aim of updating their understanding of diabetes. However, the demands of routine clinical service make it extremely difficult to keep pace with the rapidly expanding literature. Additionally, many physicians have expressed challenges in critically interpreting clinical studies and, at times, have been influenced by deliberate or inadvertent bias in the interpretation of evidence, whether from industry or opinion leaders.

It is therefore imperative that a yearbook summarizing the most important publications in diabetes be made available in a concise, readable, and critically appraised format for the physician. *DiabetesIndia*, being one of the largest and most influential organizations in diabetology worldwide, is uniquely positioned to shoulder this responsibility.

Why then did I agree to take on this challenge? As we embarked on this journey with our editorial team and authors, I was reminded of Arthur Conan Doyle's words in *The Hound of the Baskervilles*: *"The boldest, or it may be the most drunken, rode forward."*

For this edition, we systematically screened major diabetes-related publications from leading journals worldwide published between January 1, 2025, and December 31, 2025. From nearly 15,000 original research articles, a carefully selected set was identified, organized into Nine thematic sections, and subjected to detailed critical appraisal. Each unstructured summary aims to provide context regarding what was known prior to the study, highlight what the study adds to existing medical knowledge, outline the key take-home messages for clinicians, and discuss strengths, limitations, and potential directions for future research.

I was privileged to work with an exceptional team of dedicated clinicians and academicians, comprising physicians, diabetologists, and endocrinologists. I would like to place on record my sincere appreciation for the efforts of my Assistant Editor, Dr Abhranil Dhar, and also Dr Ananya Chakravorty, whose scientific support was invaluable. The entire writing team deserves special commendation for their scholarly contributions, delivered within a demanding timeframe.

This book would not have seen the light of day without the unwavering support, guidance, and encouragement of Mr Sabyasachi Hazra of Jaypee Brothers Medical Publishers (P) Ltd., whose commitment was instrumental in bringing this work to success.

Finally, I extend my heartfelt gratitude to my colleagues and to my family, who have been a constant source of motivation and support throughout this endeavor.

I dedicate this book to all healthcare professionals involved in the care of people with diabetes, with the hope that it will contribute meaningfully to improved understanding, better clinical decision-making, and ultimately enhanced patient outcomes.

Contents

SECTION 1: BASIC SCIENCE

Section Editor: Arijit Singha

SECTION 2: EPIDEMIOLOGY

Section Editor: Soham Tarafdar

SECTION 3: COMPLICATIONS

Section Editor: Abhranil Dhar

SECTION 5: DRUGS AND THERAPEUTICS (PART 2)

Section Editor: Pritam Biswas

SECTION 6: TYPE 1 DIABETES

Section Editor: Sumit Kumar Chakrabarti

SECTION 9: MISCELLANEOUS

Section Editor: Nisha Batra

Section 1: BASIC SCIENCE

Section Editor: Arijit Singha

1. Comparison of Serum Creatinine- and Cystatin C-based eGFR at Baseline and their Prediction of Incident Moderate Albuminuria in Individuals with Type 1 Diabetes

Ref: Harjutsalo V, Thorn LM, Groop PH. Comparison of Serum Creatinine- and Cystatin C-Based eGFR at Baseline and Their Prediction of Incident Moderate Albuminuria in Individuals With Type 1 Diabetes. Diabetes Care. 2025;48:1204-12.

ABSTRACT

Objective: In people with type 1 diabetes (T1D) at various stages of albuminuria, evaluate the concordance between serum creatinine (sCr) and serum cystatin C (sCysC)-based estimated glomerular filtration rate (eGFR); determine the factors associated with the discordance; and investigate the relationship between sCysC, eGFR on creatinine (eGFRcr), and eGFR on cystatin C (eGFRcys) with incident moderate albuminuria.

Research design and methods: 3,769 participants from FinnDiane study (51.8% men) with T1D without renal insufficiency and with available sCr and sCysC data were included. The median duration of diabetes was 19.5 [interquartile range (IQR) = 10.9–29.2] years, and the median age was 36.6 (IQR = 27.7–46.4) years. The Chronic Kidney Disease Epidemiology Collaboration equations were used to determine eGFRcys and eGFRcr. The following three groups were evaluated for concordance and discordance rates—(1) $-15 \leq$ eGFRdiff < 15, (2) eGFRdiff < -15, and (3) eGFRdiff ≥ 15 mL/min/1.73 m^2 (where eGFRdiff = eGFRcys minus eGFRcr). We also evaluated the variables that led to the discordance. Additionally, the relationship between the incidence of mild albuminuria and CysC, eGFRcr, and eGFRcys was assessed.

Results: The absolute eGFRdiff mean (±sD) was 14.0 ± 12.2 mL/min/1.73 m^2. Overall, there was 62.9% concordance, 20.4% negative discordance, and 16.7% positive discordance. The discordance was caused by a number of factors, including sex, albuminuria status, smoking, retinal laser photocoagulation, HbA1c, HDL cholesterol, high-sensitivity C-reactive protein, and insulin dosage per kilogram. While eGFRcr was not linked to the occurrence of mild albuminuria, sCysC and eGFRcys were. People with T1D frequently have discordant eGFRcys and eGFRcr levels.

Conclusion: These results imply that sCysC may help identify people at risk for albuminuria early.

CRITICAL APPRAISAL

What was Known Prior to this Study?

Prior research has established that, despite advancements in diabetes management, a significant residual risk of diabetic kidney disease (DKD) continues to exist. Approximately, one-third of individuals diagnosed with type 1 diabetes (T1D) are expected to develop moderate albuminuria within three decades. The presence of early albuminuria greatly heightens the risk of cardiovascular complications and kidney failure. Conventional assessments of DKD primarily utilize serum creatinine-based estimated glomerular filtration rate (eGFR) (eGFRcr), which presents several limitations. Creatinine levels can be affected by various factors, including muscle mass, age, and dietary habits, and tend to elevate only after considerable kidney damage has occurred. Conversely, cystatin C-based eGFR (eGFRcys) offers a more accurate estimation, as it remains independent of muscle mass. While previous studies have indicated that eGFRcys may more effectively predict early kidney dysfunction and cardiovascular outcomes, findings have been inconsistent. Additionally, there is a notable lack of large-scale prospective data that compare eGFRcr and eGFRcys, especially with regards to their discrepancies and predictive value for the onset of albuminuria in individuals with T1D.

What this Study Adds?

This study presents compelling evidence that the cystatin C-based eGFRcys serves as a more robust predictor of early diabetic kidney disease (DKD) compared to the traditional eGFRcr in individuals with T1D. Utilizing data from over 3,700 participants in the FinnDiane cohort, the analysis found that discrepancies between eGFRcys and eGFRcr occur in nearly 40% of patients. These discrepancies have been associated with various clinical and metabolic factors, including sex, HbA1c levels, inflammation (as indicated by C-reactive protein or CRP), and smoking. Significantly, both serum cystatin C (sCysC) and eGFRcys demonstrated a strong correlation with the future development of moderate albuminuria, whereas eGFRcr did not show such an association. These findings underscore the potential of cystatin C-based estimates to detect early kidney dysfunction and assess DKD risk prior to changes being evident through traditional markers. This evidence supports the integration of cystatin C into clinical risk assessments for individuals with T1D, thereby enhancing patient care and outcomes.

Limitations of the Study

The primary limitations of this study are the absence of directly measured GFR values and the lack of serial measurements of cystatin C, which impede the assessment of temporal changes in kidney function. Furthermore, the follow-up data on new cases of albuminuria were incomplete for participants with normal baseline urinary albumin excretion, potentially introducing bias into the results. Lastly, the authors highlight the necessity for further validation before cystatin C can be routinely implemented in clinical practice for the assessment of DKD risk.

Impact on Clinical Practice

This study advocates for the integration of sCysC into clinical practice for the early detection of kidney dysfunction in individuals with T1D. The use of sCysC may provide valuable insights prior to the appearance of albuminuria or a decline in eGFRcr.

2. Mind the Gap: Discordance between Cystatin C and Creatinine eGFR and Diabetes Complications

Ref: MacIsaac RJ. Mind the Gap: Discordance Between Cystatin C and Creatinine eGFR and Diabetes Complications. Diabetes Care. 2025;48:1158-60.

ABSTRACT

Estimation of glomerular filtration rate (GFR) using estimated GFR on serum creatinine (eGFRcr), eGFR on cystatin C (eGFRcys), or a combination of both biomarkers is a well-established method for assessing kidney function. Recently, the discrepancy between eGFRcr and eGFRcys—referred to as eGFRdiff—has gained attention as a valuable indicator of overall health status and a predictor of adverse outcomes in individuals with diabetes, as reported by Harjutsalo et al.

More than four decades ago, Grubb and colleagues proposed serum cystatin C as an alternative marker of GFR, suggesting that it is less affected by nonrenal factors compared with serum creatinine.

Cystatin C is a 13.3-kDa low-molecular-weight protein produced at a constant rate by all nucleated cells. It is freely filtered at the glomerulus and subsequently metabolized in the proximal tubule. However, growing evidence indicates that cystatin C levels, like creatinine, are also influenced by factors unrelated to GFR.

Serum creatinine is well known to be affected by age, sex, dietary protein intake, physical activity, and conditions influencing tubular secretion. In contrast, cystatin C concentrations are influenced by adiposity, systemic inflammation, thyroid dysfunction, and corticosteroid use. The limitations of eGFRcr in certain clinical settings, particularly among patients with diabetes, are well documented.

Overall, eGFRcys demonstrates superior performance compared with eGFRcr when evaluated against measured GFR, especially at higher normal GFR levels. Consequently, recent clinical guidelines recommend greater utilization of cystatin C in GFR estimation, either alone or in combination with serum creatinine.

CRITICAL APPRAISAL

What was Known Prior to this Commentary?

Estimated GFR based on serum creatinine (eGFRcr) has long been the standard method for assessing kidney function but it can be influenced by muscle mass, age, sex, diet, and physical activity. Cystatin C–based eGFR (eGFRcys) was known to correlate better with measured GFR in certain settings, especially at higher or near-normal GFR ranges. Prior studies in the general population had shown that discordance between eGFRcr and eGFRcys is common. In diabetes, limitations of creatinine-based eGFR were recognized, but the prognostic significance of eGFR discordance for microvascular complications was not fully established. KDIGO guideline has started to recommend broader use of cystatin C, but its routine clinical role in diabetes care remained uncertain.

What this Commentary Adds?

This commentary synthesizes emerging evidence showing that discordance between eGFRcr and eGFRcys is not merely a measurement artifact but a clinically meaningful risk marker in diabetes. It highlights robust data from FinnDiane study (among patients with type 1 diabetes), which showed that eGFRcys predicts incident albuminuria better than eGFRcr. UK Biobank and multinational cohorts showed that negative discordance (eGFRcys < eGFRcr) predicts higher risk of microvascular complications, cardiovascular events, and mortality in patients with type 2 diabetes. The commentary also introduces the concept that eGFR discordance may reflect underlying systemic pathology such as sarcopenia, inflammation, and metabolic ill-health rather than kidney disease alone. It reinforces the idea that cystatin C–based assessment may reclassify risk in patients with apparently "normal" kidney function.

Limitation of this Study

As this is a commentary, conclusions are dependent on the quality and heterogeneity of cited studies. Definitions of discordance (absolute vs. relative differences) vary across studies, reducing uniform applicability. Most supporting data are observational, limiting causal inference. There is limited discussion on cost, availability, and standardization of cystatin C assays, especially in low- and middle-income countries. Mechanistic explanations of "shrunken pore syndrome" remain largely speculative and not proven.

Impact on Clinical Practice

The commentary encourages clinicians to view eGFR discordance as a red flag for heightened cardiometabolic and microvascular risk, even when creatinine-based eGFR appears normal. It supports selective use of cystatin C in people with diabetes who have disproportionate complications, sarcopenia or low BMI, and high inflammatory burden. But it does not yet justify routine cystatin C testing in all patients with diabetes, but strengthens the case for targeted implementation.

Scope for Future Research

Prospective studies are required to determine whether acting on eGFR discordance improves clinical outcomes. Exploration of mechanistic pathways (inflammation, sarcopenia, endothelial dysfunction, and shrunken pore syndrome) is much needed. Need for development of standardized thresholds for clinically meaningful eGFR discordance. Need cost-effectiveness analyses and implementation studies, particularly in resource-limited settings.

3. One-hour Plasma Glucose Predicts the Progression from Normal Glucose Tolerance to Prediabetes

Ref: Abdul-Ghani M, Abu-Farha M, Abdul-Ghani T, Chavez-Velazquez A, Merovci A, DeFronzo RA, et al. One-Hour Plasma Glucose Predicts the Progression From Normal Glucose Tolerance to Prediabetes. Diabetes Care. 2025;48(7):1273-79.

ABSTRACT

Objective: To determine if the 1-hour plasma glucose (1-h PG) concentration during the oral glucose tolerance test (OGTT) can predict the likelihood that people with normal glucose tolerance (NGT) will develop prediabetes.

Research design and methods: A total of 1,557 San Antonio Heart Study individuals, who had a baseline and who were free of type 2 diabetes, and had a follow-up OGTT after 7.5 years were assessed. Based on American Diabetes Association (ADA) criteria, the capacity of 1-h PG concentration to forecast the onset of prediabetes was assessed.

Results: At 7.5 years, about 25% of individuals with NGT (24.7%) developed prediabetes (22.5% with 1-h PG < 155 mg/dL and 42.5% with 1-h PG > 155 mg/dL). A 1-hour cut point of 120 mg/dL exhibited 61% sensitivity and 67% specificity in identifying those with NGT who were at high risk of developing prediabetes. Severe insulin resistance and metabolic abnormalities typical of the insulin resistance syndrome were present in participants with a 1-h PG of 120–155 mg/dL and a decline in glucose tolerance (progression to prediabetes) at follow-up.

To highlight this group's substantial future risk of declining glucose tolerance, we propose the name pre-prediabetes.

Conclusion: Individuals with a 1-h PG of 120–155 mg/dL are at a higher risk of developing prediabetes, and an increase in 1-h PG concentration precedes the onset of prediabetes. For this population with a higher risk of declining glucose tolerance, we propose the term pre-prediabetes.

CRITICAL APPRAISAL

What was Known Prior to this Study

Before this study, the American Diabetes Association (ADA) defined prediabetes based on fasting plasma glucose (FPG), 2-hour plasma glucose (2-h PG), and HbA1c levels. However, research has shown that up to 40% of individuals who later develop type 2 diabetes (T2D) present with normal glucose tolerance (NGT) according to these criteria, suggesting that current thresholds may overlook many at-risk individuals. Recent findings indicate that 1-hour plasma glucose (1-h PG) levels during an oral glucose tolerance test (OGTT) are more reliable predictors of future T2D than FPG or 2-h PG levels. A 1-h PG cutoff of >155 mg/dL can identify individuals at a risk comparable to those diagnosed with prediabetes. Additionally, individuals with NGT but elevated 1-h PG may show early impairments in insulin sensitivity and β-cell function. Recognizing this, the International Diabetes Federation (IDF) proposed 1-h PG > 155 mg/dL as a potential diagnostic marker for increased diabetes risk. However, limited long-term prospective studies validating 1-h PG as a predictor of progression from NGT to prediabetes highlight the importance of the present investigation.

What this Study Adds?

This study provides strong longitudinal evidence that measuring 1-h PG during an OGTT is a highly effective early indicator of the progression from NGT to prediabetes. Compared to conventional measures such as FPG, 2-h PG, and HbA1c, 1-h PG shows superior predictive performance. The results indicate that individuals with NGT but elevated 1-h PG levels (above 155 mg/dL) already exhibit decreased insulin sensitivity and impaired β-cell function, even before traditional markers of dysglycemia show abnormal results. Over a 7.5-year follow-up period, participants with higher 1-h PG levels were significantly more likely to progress to prediabetes, highlighting its importance in detecting metabolic changes earlier than current ADA criteria allow. These findings provide strong support for incorporating 1-h PG testing into standard risk assessment and screening practices, enabling earlier identification and prevention of T2D.

Limitations of the Study

The current study has several limitations. The OGTT performed at follow-up did not measure the 1-h PG concentration. As a result, it is not clear that how many participants with NGT and elevated 1-hour PG at baseline reverted to normal levels at follow-up. Additionally, the analysis was focused on a subgroup of participants from the San Antonio Heart Study, of whom 70% are Mexican American. Therefore, it is important to confirm these findings in other ethnic groups before generalizing the results.

Impact on Clinical Practice

This study suggests that monitoring 1-h PG could enable earlier detection and intervention in diabetes risk. Incorporating 1-h PG testing into routine screening may help clinicians prevent or delay diabetes through timely lifestyle or therapeutic measures.

4. Large-scale Proteomics Improve Risk Prediction for Type 2 Diabetes

Ref: Xie R, Vlaski T, Trares K, Herder C, Holleczek B, Brenner H, et al. Large-Scale Proteomics Improve Risk Prediction for Type 2 Diabetes. Diabetes Care. 2025;48:922-6.

ABSTRACT

Objective: When proteomic indicators were introduced to the clinical Cambridge Diabetes Risk Score (CDRS), this study assessed their incremental predictive usefulness in determining 10-year type 2 diabetes (T2D) risk.

Research design and methods: For model derivation and internal validation, data from 21,898 UK Biobank participants were utilized; for external validation, data from 4,454 participants in the

Epidemiological Study to Chancen der Verhütung, Früherkennung und optimierten Therapie chronischer Erkrankungen in der älteren Bevöolkerung (ESTHER) cohort (Germany) were utilized. The Olink Target 96 Inflammation panel (73 proteins) and Olink Explore (2,085 proteins) were used in proteomic profiling.

Results: In internal validation, adding 15 proteins from Olink Explore or 6 proteins from the Olink Inflammation panel increased the CDRS's C-index by 0.029 or 0.016, respectively, with net reclassification of 23.0% and 29.0%. Only the six-protein-extended model underwent external validation, and the C-index increased by 0.014.

Conclusion: The CDRS model performance was most improved by the Olink Explore-based 15-protein model, and this promising prediction model needs external validation. This is a promising attempt, as demonstrated by our successful external validation of the Olink Inflammation panel-based six-protein model.

CRITICAL APPRAISAL

What was Known Prior to this Study?

Type 2 diabetes (T2D) represents a significant global health challenge, associated with elevated mortality rates, diminished quality of life, and escalating healthcare expenditures. The early identification of high-risk individuals is critical for effective prevention; however, existing prediction models frequently exhibit limited accuracy and do not adequately encompass the wide array of contributing factors. Given that proteins are directly involved in the mechanisms of disease, proteomics has emerged as a promising avenue for enhancing risk prediction. While high-throughput studies have identified various protein biomarkers related to diabetes risk, inconsistencies in findings have restricted their clinical implementation. This study aims to investigate whether proteomic biomarkers can improve the prediction of T2D risk across two large, independent cohorts in Europe.

What this Study Adds?

This study presents compelling evidence that the integration of proteomic profiling with traditional risk factors significantly enhances the prediction of T2D development. By analyzing two large, independent cohorts from Europe, the researchers identified specific protein signatures indicative of inflammatory activity, lipid regulation, and insulin resistance, which provide valuable biological insights that extend beyond standard clinical predictors. Notably, the study established that these proteomic-based models retain their accuracy across diverse populations, addressing a significant limitation observed in prior research. The findings indicate that incorporating proteomic biomarkers into routine risk assessments could enable healthcare professionals to identify individuals at high risk earlier, tailor prevention strategies, and progress toward a precision medicine approach in diabetes care.

Limitations of the Study

The study has several limitations. The UK Biobank showed a lower incidence of T2D than the ESTHER cohort, likely due to differences in age and more thorough case identification in ESTHER. The OLINK proteomic platforms used varied, lacking absolute protein concentrations, which limited direct comparisons and may have resulted in overestimating model performance. Differences in sample types, such as plasma versus serum, could also have affected protein measurements. Lastly, the findings are based on middle-aged to older European populations, which may limit their applicability to younger or non-European groups.

Impact on Clinical Practice

This study highlights the potential of integrating proteomic biomarkers into diabetes risk models for earlier and more accurate identification of individuals at high risk for T2D. By enhancing predictive precision, this approach could support personalized prevention strategies and targeted interventions. However, standardization and cost-effective implementation are necessary before routine clinical adoption.

5. Large-scale Plasma Proteomics Improves Prediction of Peripheral Artery Disease in Individuals with Type 2 Diabetes: A Prospective Cohort Study

Ref: Yu H, Zhang J, Qian F, Yao P, Xu K, Wu P, et al. Large-Scale Plasma Proteomics Improves Prediction of Peripheral Artery Disease in Individuals With Type 2 Diabetes: A Prospective Cohort Study. Diabetes Care. 2025;48:381-9.

ABSTRACT

Objective: Although peripheral arterial disease (PAD) is a serious consequence of type 2 diabetes (T2D), it is still unknown how plasma proteomics and PAD are related in T2D patients. We sought to determine whether proteomics may improve PAD risk prediction and investigate the connection between plasma proteomics and PAD in T2D patients.

Research design and methods: 1,859 T2D patients from the UK Biobank were included in this cohort study. The relationships between 2,920 plasma proteins and incident PAD were investigated using multivariable-adjusted Cox regression models. The least absolute shrinkage and selection operator (LASSO) penalty was used to further select proteins as predictors. Harrell's C-index, time-dependent area under the receiver operating characteristic curve, continuous/categorical net reclassification improvement, and integrated discrimination improvement were used to evaluate predictive performance.

Results: There were 157 incident PAD cases with a median follow-up of 13.2 years. 463 proteins were found to be linked to the risk of PAD; these proteins were mostly involved in signal transduction, inflammatory response, plasma membrane, protein binding, and cytokine-cytokine receptor interactions. According to *p* values, the top five proteins linked to a higher risk of PAD were (1) EDA2R, (2) ADM, (3) NPPB, (4) CD302, and (5) NPC2, while the top five proteins linked to a lower risk of PAD were (1) BCAN, (2) UMOD, (3) PLB1, (4) CA6, and (5) KLK3. Beyond clinical factors alone, the addition of 45 LASSO-selected proteins or a weighted protein risk score greatly improved PAD prediction, achieving a maximum C-index of 0.835.

Conclusion: This study found plasma proteins linked to the incidence of PAD in T2D patients. PAD prediction was greatly enhanced by incorporating proteomic data into the clinical model.

CRITICAL APPRAISAL

What was Known Prior to this Study?

Prior to this study, it was well established that diabetes significantly heightens the risk of peripheral artery disease (PAD), a condition that is a major contributor to morbidity, mortality, and lower-limb amputation. Individuals with diabetes are two to four times more likely to develop PAD and experience markedly elevated risks of amputation and death compared to those without diabetes. The early identification of high-risk patients is essential for effective prevention strategies. However, existing prediction models for PAD in diabetic patients primarily rely on clinical factors and often lack biological specificity. Recent advancements have highlighted the potential of proteins as key mediators in biological processes, positioning them as promising biomarkers for vascular complications. Nevertheless, previous research examining the relationship between plasma proteomics and PAD has been constrained by small sample sizes, cross-sectional study designs, and limited protein panels. Only a handful of circulating proteins have been linked to PAD, which leaves the wider proteomic landscape and its predictive potential largely unexplored. Consequently, there is a pressing need for large-scale, prospective studies to determine whether proteomic profiling can enhance our understanding and improve the prediction of PAD risk in individuals with type 2 diabetes (T2D).

What this Study Adds?

The study offers significant insights into the role of plasma proteomic profiling in enhancing risk prediction for peripheral artery disease (PAD) in individuals with T2D. By examining data from >8,000 participants over an extended follow-up period, researchers identified 42 circulating proteins that are primarily linked to inflammation, endothelial dysfunction, and lipid metabolism, which significantly predict future PAD events. The integration of these proteins into clinical predictive models has been shown to improve accuracy, with an increase in the C-index of +0.021 and a net reclassification improvement of +18% over traditional risk factors. These findings highlight the promising potential of proteomics-based risk assessment in facilitating earlier detection and fostering personalized prevention strategies for PAD in patients with T2D.

Limitations of the Study

Firstly, the findings from the predictive model lack external validation due to the absence of an independent dataset. However, the internal validation demonstrated that the 45 proteins selected through the LASSO method, along with a weighted polygenic risk score (PRS), significantly enhanced the prediction of PAD beyond traditional clinical variables. Future research involving large-scale proteomic and clinical datasets will be essential for further validation. Secondly, it is important to note that the majority of participants in the UK Biobank are of European ancestry, which necessitates caution when generalizing these findings to other populations. Thirdly, undiagnosed PAD at baseline may introduce potential reverse causation bias. Finally, the identification of PAD cases through hospital admissions and death registries using ICD codes may result in the underreporting of mild or asymptomatic cases.

Impact on Clinical Practice

This comprehensive proteomics study identified plasma proteins linked to PAD in individuals with T2D. The proteomics data significantly enhanced the prediction of PAD. However, standardization and cost-effective implementation are necessary before routine clinical adoption.

Section 2: EPIDEMIOLOGY

Section Editor: Soham Tarafdar

1. Comparative Efficacy of Glucagon-like Peptide 1 Receptor Agonists for Cardiovascular Outcomes in Asian versus White Populations: Systematic Review and Meta-analysis of Randomized Trials of Populations with or without Type 2 Diabetes and/or Overweight or Obesity

Ref: Lee MMY, Ghouri N, Misra A, Kang YM, Rutter MK, Gerstein HC, et al. Comparative Efficacy of Glucagon-Like Peptide 1 Receptor Agonists for Cardiovascular Outcomes in Asian Versus White Populations: Systematic Review and Meta-analysis of Randomized Trials of Populations With or Without Type 2 Diabetes and/or Overweight or Obesity. Diabetes Care. 2025;48(3): 489-93.

ABSTRACT

Background: According to cardiovascular outcome trials (CVOTs), Asian people get more CV benefit from glucagon-like peptide 1 receptor agonists (GLP-1RAs) than do White people.

Goals: Compare the CV effectiveness of GLP-1 RAs in white and Asian people.

Sources of data: PubMed and ClinicalTrials.gov were systematically reviewed between January 1, 2015 and November 1, 2024.

Selection of study: GLP-1RA CVOTs that are randomized and placebo-controlled. Bias risk was evaluated (RoB 2).

Data extraction: Hazard ratios (HRs) for major adverse cardiovascular events (MACE) according to ethnicity.

Data synthesis: Eight trials (5,909 Asian and 55,855 White) were included in random effects meta-analyses conducted in accordance with the Preferred Reporting Items for Systematic Reviews and Meta-Analyses (PRISMA) guidelines. The GLP-1RA-associated MACE HR was 0.85 (95% CI 0.79, 0.91) in White individuals and 0.69 (95% CI 0.58, 0.83) in Asian individuals ($P_{interaction}$ = 0.045). Asian individuals had an absolute MACE risk reduction of 2.9% (95% CI 1.5, 4.2) compared to 1.4% (0.9, 1.9) for White individuals.

Limitations: The Asian group could not be thoroughly subclassified due to a lack of individual patient-level data.

Conclusion: When compared to White people, Asian people get more CV benefit from GLP-1RAs in terms of MACE reductions.

CRITICAL APPRAISAL

Introduction and Study Rationale

The global burden of type 2 diabetes (T2D) has shifted dramatically toward Asia, characterized by a distinct "Asian phenotype" of visceral adiposity and early β-cell dysfunction occurring at lower body mass indices (BMIs) than in White populations.[1,2] This phenotype carries a heightened risk of atherosclerotic cardiovascular disease (ASCVD). Glucagon-like peptide 1 receptor agonists (GLP-1RAs) have established cardiovascular benefits in major cardiovascular outcome trials (CVOTs). However, Asian participants have been historically underrepresented in these global trials, often comprising <10% of cohorts.[1]

Prior meta-analyses suggested a potential "Asian advantage" with GLP-1RAs. For instance, Kang et al. (2019) reported a hazard ratio (HR) for major adverse cardiovascular events (MACE) of 0.35 in Asians, though with wide confidence intervals and borderline statistical interaction.[3,4] This signal of enhanced efficacy appeared specific to GLP-1RAs, as sodium-glucose cotransporter-2 (SGLT-2) inhibitors showed no such racial divergence.[5] Crucially, previous knowledge was limited by a focus on relative risk rather than absolute risk reduction (ARR), borderline statistical significance, and the exclusion of nondiabetic cohorts (e.g., obesity with ASCVD), leaving the pharmacoeconomic value and mechanism in Asian populations uncertain.

What this Study Adds to Preexisting Knowledge

The 2025 systematic review and meta-analysis by Lee et al. provides the most definitive evidence to date, synthesizing data from eight major placebo-controlled trials: LEADER, SUSTAIN-6, EXSCEL, Harmony Outcomes, REWIND, PIONEER 6, AMPLITUDE-O, and SELECT.[1] This study adds:

- *Definitive statistical confirmation*: By pooling 5,909 Asian and 55,855 White participants, the study confirmed a statistically significant racial interaction ($P_{interaction}$ = 0.045). The HR for MACE was *0.69 (95% CI 0.58–0.83)* in Asians versus *0.85 (95% CI 0.79–0.91)* in Whites, confirming a 31% relative risk reduction in Asians compared to 15% in Whites.[1]
- *Absolute risk metrics*: Crucially, the study calculated the ARR as *2.9% (95% CI 1.5–4.2)* for Asians, more than double the *1.4% (95% CI 0.9–1.9)* observed in Whites.[1,2]
- *Pharmacoeconomic clarity*: The number needed to treat (NNT) to prevent one MACE event was established at *35 (95% CI 24–66)* for Asians, compared to *73 (95% CI 54–112)* for Whites, demonstrating superior efficiency.[1]
- *Inclusion of nondiabetic obesity*: By incorporating the SELECT trial, the study demonstrated that this racial disparity persists in individuals with overweight/obesity and ASCVD *without* diabetes ($P_{interaction}$ = 0.345 for diabetes status), suggesting the benefit is intrinsic to the GLP-1 mechanism and not solely glucose-dependent.[1]
- *High consistency*: The study revealed remarkably low heterogeneity within the Asian subgroup (I^2 = 0%), indicating a robust class effect across different GLP-1RA molecules and delivery methods.[1,6]

Major Strengths of this Study

- *Methodological rigor*: The study adhered to PRISMA guidelines and utilized the Cochrane RoB 2 tool, confirming a low risk of bias for all eight included trials. The evidence was graded as "high certainty" using the GRADE approach.[1]
- *High statistical power*: Aggregating data from nearly 6,000 Asian participants overcame the power limitations of individual trials, enabling the detection of a significant interaction effect that smaller studies missed.[1]
- *Clinical relevance*: The focus on ARR and NNT transforms abstract statistical findings into actionable clinical metrics, allowing for direct comparison with other interventions and informing cost-effectiveness decisions.[1]
- *Broad generalizability*: The inclusion of diverse cohorts—ranging from secondary prevention in T2D to primary prevention risk factors and nondiabetic obesity—ensures the findings are applicable across the spectrum of metabolic cardiovascular risk.[1]

Limitations of this Study

- *Lack of individual participant data (IPD)*: The reliance on trial-level summary data prevented adjustment for potential confounders such as baseline BMI, body weight, or renal function. Consequently, it remains unclear if the "Asian advantage" is a biological difference or a pharmacokinetic artifact (e.g., higher drug exposure due to lower body weight in Asians).[1,6]

- *Monolithic "Asian" category*: The study groups diverse populations (East Asians, South Asians) into a single category. This obscures potential differences between phenotypes, such as the β-cell dysfunction of East Asians versus the insulin resistance of South Asians.[1,6]
- *Marginal significance*: The interaction *p*-value (0.045) is close to the significance threshold. While the directional consistency across trials supports the finding, the statistical fragility warrants cautious interpretation.[6]
- *Exclusion of specific trials*: Trials such as ELIXA and FREEDOM-CVO were excluded due to missing racial subgroup data or unique delivery mechanisms, meaning the analysis does not capture the absolute entirety of the GLP-1RA landscape.[1]

Implication of Findings on Clinical Practice

- *Guideline revision*: The findings challenge "race-neutral" guidelines. For Asian patients with T2D and ASCVD risk, GLP-1RAs demonstrate superior efficacy compared to White populations and should arguably be prioritized over SGLT-2 inhibitors (which show racial neutrality) for MACE reduction.[1,5]
- *Earlier initiation*: The robust absolute benefit (NNT 35) supports earlier and more aggressive use of GLP-1RAs in Asian treatment algorithms, potentially even in those with lower ASCVD risk burdens than typically required for White patients.[1]
- *Pharmacoeconomic justification*: In resource-constrained Asian healthcare systems, the significantly lower NNT provides a strong economic argument for reimbursement and access. The data indicates that investment in GLP-1RAs yields double the "event prevention" return in Asian populations compared to Western ones.[1]
- *Obesity management*: For Asian individuals with obesity and ASCVD but without diabetes, GLP-1RAs are confirmed as high-value preventive agents. Clinicians should consider these therapies at lower BMI thresholds (e.g., BMI $\geq$ 23 or 25 kg/m^2 consistent with Asian-specific obesity definitions.[1]

Knowledge Gaps Identified and Future Scope for Research

- *IPD meta-analysis*: A collaborative IPD analysis is urgently needed to adjust for baseline body weight and determine if the enhanced efficacy is driven by exposure (dose/kg) or intrinsic biology.[1,6]
- *Phenotypic granularity*: Future research must disaggregate "Asian" data to compare East versus South Asian responses, tailoring precision medicine to specific metabolic defects (β-cell failure vs. insulin resistance).[6]
- *Mechanistic studies*: Translational research comparing pharmacokinetics (PK)/pharmacodynamics (PD) profiles, incretin receptor sensitivity, and gastric emptying rates between races is required to elucidate the biological drivers of this disparity.[1]
- *Region-specific trials*: Dedicated CVOTs conducted exclusively in Asia or with stratified, powered Asian cohorts are necessary to validate these findings and move beyond post-hoc subgroup analyses.[4]
- *Broader outcomes*: Similar race-stratified analyses should be conducted for renal outcomes and heart failure to provide a comprehensive picture of GLP-1RA efficacy in Asian populations.[1]

2. Differential Treatment Effects on β-cell Function Using Model-based Parameters in Type 2 Diabetes: Results from the Glycemia Reduction Approaches in Diabetes: A Comparative Effectiveness Study (GRADE)

Ref: Utzschneider KM, Tripputi M, Butera NM, Mari A, Rosin SP, Banerji MA, et al. Differential Treatment Effects on β-Cell Function Using Model-Based Parameters in Type 2 Diabetes: Results From the Glycemia Reduction Approaches in Diabetes: A Comparative Effectiveness Study (GRADE). Diabetes Care. 2025;48(4):623-31.

ABSTRACT

Objective: To assess the relationship between glycemic worsening in people with type 2 diabetes (T2D) and model-based measures of b-cell function that alter with glucose-lowering therapy.

Research design and methods: B-cell function parameters obtained from mathematical modeling of oral glucose tolerance tests were measured at baseline (*n* = 4,712) and at 1, 3 and 5 years after randomization to insulin glargine, glimepiride, liraglutide, or sitagliptin, added to baseline metformin, in the Glycemia Reduction Approaches in Diabetes: A Comparative Effectiveness Study (GRADE). Insulin secretion rate (ISR), rate sensitivity (early insulin response), glucose sensitivity (insulin reaction to glucose), and potentiation were among the parameters. Changes between treatments were compared using linear mixed-effects models. We assessed relationships between model parameters and glycemic failure (HbA1c >7.5%; 58.5 mmol/mol) using Cox proportional hazards and Classification and Regression Tree (CART) analyses.

Results: At the 1st year, B-cell function characteristics varied among treatments, but they later decreased for every therapy. Changes that were statistically significant were observed. The biggest gains in ISR, glucose sensitivity, and potentiation were caused by liraglutide, which continued to be above baseline at the end of the study. With only slight impacts on other metrics, sitagliptin increased glucose sensitivity. While glimepiride slightly improved glucose sensitivity or potentiation, it momentarily raised ISR and rate sensitivity. Glargine caused the greatest increase in rate sensitivity. Although therapy did not change the association between these parameters and glycemic outcomes, higher B-cell function indicators were protective against glycemic worsening.

Conclusion: Several physiological aspects of B-cell function in T2D are impacted by common glucose-lowering drugs. Lower B-cell function was linked to early glycemic failure regardless of the type of treatment, and B-cell function gradually decreased following initial recovery.

CRITICAL APPRAISAL

Introduction and Study Rationale

Type 2 diabetes (T2D) is a chronic, progressive metabolic disorder driven by two primary pathophysiological defects: Peripheral insulin resistance and pancreatic beta-cell dysfunction.[7] While insulin resistance is often the earliest detectable abnormality, the transition from prediabetes to overt diabetes and the subsequent failure to maintain glycemic control are fundamentally caused by the progressive failure of beta-cells to secrete sufficient insulin to compensate for the prevailing resistance.[8]

Historical data from landmark trials, such as the United Kingdom Prospective Diabetes Study (UKPDS), established that beta-cell function declines by approximately 5–10% annually, regardless of whether patients are treated with diet, sulfonylureas, or insulin.[7] This relentless deterioration necessitates the sequential intensification of therapy over time.

Prior to the current study, the understanding of how specific glucose-lowering medications influence beta-cell physiology was limited. Previous research often relied on small, short-term studies or used static surrogate markers such as homeostatic model assessment of insulin resistance (HOMA-IR) or simple C-peptide indices.[9] While useful, these static measures fail to capture the dynamic nature of insulin secretion, which involves sensitivity to glucose concentration (dose-response), responsiveness to the rate of change in glucose (rate sensitivity), and augmentation by gut hormones (potentiation).[10] Furthermore, there was a lack of large-scale, long-term head-to-head comparisons of modern drug classes—specifically glucagon-like peptide-1 receptor agonists (GLP-1 RAs) and dipeptidyl peptidase-4 (DPP-4) inhibitors—against older agents like sulfonylureas and basal insulin regarding their specific effects on these dynamic physiological parameters.[11]

What this Study Adds to the Preexisting Knowledge

This study by Utzschneider et al. (2025) presents a secondary analysis of the GRADE (Glycemia Reduction Approaches in Diabetes: A Comparative Effectiveness Study) trial, providing the most comprehensive characterization to date of how four major classes of diabetes medications affect dynamic beta-cell function over a 5-year period.[12] By applying sophisticated mathematical modeling (the Mari model) to oral glucose tolerance test (OGTT) data from 4,712 participants, the study delineates distinct "physiological fingerprints" for each drug class:

- *Liraglutide (GLP-1 RA):* Demonstrated the most robust and durable enhancement of beta-cell function. It significantly increased *glucose sensitivity* (the slope of the dose-response curve) and *potentiation* (the augmentation of secretion by nonglucose factors). Notably, liraglutide was the only agent to maintain total insulin secretion and glucose sensitivity above baseline levels at the end of the 5-year study.[12]
- *Sitagliptin (DPP-4i)*: Improved glucose sensitivity but had a more modest effect on potentiation compared to liraglutide. Uniquely, it significantly increased *rate sensitivity* (the dynamic response to the rate of glucose rise), likely mediated by the modest preservation of endogenous GIP and GLP-1 levels.[12]
- *Glimepiride (sulfonylurea)*: Acts primarily by increasing the *insulin secretion rate (ISR) at a fixed glucose concentration* (ISR@8mM) and transiently improving rate sensitivity. However, it failed to sustain improvements in glucose sensitivity or potentiation, leading to a rapid decline in efficacy after the 1st year.[12]
- *Insulin glargine*: Surprisingly resulted in the most pronounced and sustained increase in *rate sensitivity* (early phase response). This suggests that effective lowering of fasting glucose with basal insulin may induce "beta-cell rest," restoring the cell's ability to respond rapidly to glucose excursions, a mechanism distinct from the direct stimulation seen with secretagogues.[12]

Crucially, the study identified that *glucose sensitivity* was the strongest predictor of glycemic failure across all groups. Despite the distinct mechanisms of action, the study confirmed that beta-cell function parameters declined progressively after the 1st year in *all* treatment arms, reinforcing the concept that current pharmacotherapies generally fail to arrest the underlying disease process.[12]

Major Strengths of this Study

The primary strength of this study is its *scale and duration*. Analyzing model-derived physiological parameters in over 4,700 participants with up to 5 years of follow-up is unprecedented in diabetes research and provides high-certainty evidence regarding the durability of treatment effects that smaller mechanistic studies cannot offer.[12]

Secondly, the use of *mathematical modeling (the Mari model)* transforms standard clinical trial data (OGTTs) into deep physiological insights. By dissecting insulin secretion into components—glucose sensitivity, rate sensitivity, and potentiation—the authors moved beyond simple "high versus low" insulin levels to explain *how* the beta-cell is responding. This allowed for the novel finding that basal insulin improves early phase secretory dynamics (rate sensitivity), a finding that would be invisible to standard HOMA-beta analysis.[10,12]

Thirdly, the *comparative effectiveness design* is a significant asset. Randomizing patients to four distinct medication classes added to metformin allowed for a direct, unconfounded comparison of their physiological impacts. The analysis was rigorous, adjusting for potential confounders such as baseline BMI, age, and insulin sensitivity, ensuring that the observed differences were attributable to the specific pharmacological mechanisms of the drugs.[12]

Limitations of this Study

Despite its robust design, the authors acknowledge several limitations:

- *Population homogeneity*: The study cohort was predominantly White, which limits the generalizability of the findings to other racial and ethnic groups, particularly Asian populations who are known to have a distinct phenotype characterized by primary beta-cell secretory defects rather than insulin resistance.[12,13]
- *Surrogate measures*: The study relied on HOMA2-%S as a surrogate for insulin sensitivity. In the insulin glargine group, the presence of exogenous insulin complicates the measurement of fasting endogenous insulin/C-peptide, potentially confounding the adjustment of beta-cell parameters for prevailing insulin sensitivity.[12]
- *Precision of rate sensitivity*: The authors note that estimating rate sensitivity (early secretion) from OGTT data is less precise than from intravenous glucose tolerance tests (IVGTT). While the OGTT is more physiological, it may miss subtle defects in first-phase secretion that are critical in early diabetes.[12]
- *Absence of newer classes*: The GRADE trial was designed before the widespread adoption of SGLT-2 inhibitors and dual GIP/GLP-1 agonists (e.g., tirzepatide). Consequently, the study does not provide data on these potent newer agents, which are now central to modern treatment guidelines.[12,14]

Implication of Findings on Clinical Practice

These findings have immediate relevance for the personalized management of type 2 diabetes:

- *Targeting the physiological defect*: For patients where the primary defect is a loss of glucose sensitivity (a flat dose-response curve), *GLP-1 RAs (liraglutide)* appear to be the most physiologically targeted therapy, offering the greatest enhancement of this specific parameter.[12]
- *Understanding "failure":* The study underscores that "glycemic failure" is synonymous with "beta-cell failure." The universal decline in function after year 1 suggests that clinicians should anticipate this deterioration. The current "fail-first" paradigm of sequential monotherapy may be physiologically flawed; earlier combination therapy might be required to maintain beta-cell function.[12]
- *Role of basal insulin*: The finding that glargine improves rate sensitivity challenges the dogma that insulin is merely replacement therapy for late-stage disease. By resting the beta-cell and reducing glucotoxicity, early basal insulin may have a functional restorative role, supporting its use earlier in the treatment algorithm for patients with severe hyperglycemia.[12]
- *Prognostic value*: Since model-derived glucose sensitivity was a strong independent predictor of glycemic failure, markers of secretory capacity could theoretically be used to stratify high-risk patients who require more aggressive early intervention.[12]

Knowledge Gaps Identified and Future Scope for Research

The study highlights the inability of current therapies to permanently arrest beta-cell decline, identifying critical gaps for future research:

- *Reversing dysfunction*: Future research must focus on identifying the molecular drivers of the inexorable decline in glucose sensitivity observed after year 1 in all groups. Is this driven by dedifferentiation, amyloid deposition, or oxidative stress? Therapies targeting these specific pathways are urgently needed.[12,15]
- *Newer classes*: There is an urgent need to apply this sophisticated modeling approach to *SGLT-2 inhibitors* and *Tirzepatide*. Given Tirzepatide's potent weight loss and GIP activity, it is hypothesized that it might sustain glucose sensitivity longer than GLP-1RAs alone.[12]
- *Precision medicine*: The heterogeneity in response suggests future trials should test whether assigning treatment based on a patient's baseline physiological profile (e.g., low potentiation vs. low rate sensitivity) yields better long-term durability than standard guidelines.[16]
- *Mechanisms of "rest"*: The mechanism by which glargine improves rate sensitivity warrants further investigation. If "beta-cell rest" can be optimized or mimicked pharmacologically without the risk of hypoglycemia associated with insulin, it could offer a new pathway for preserving function.[12]

3. Analysis of Long-term Follow-up of a Randomized Clinical Trial with Departures from Assigned Treatments: Estimation of Metformin Effects on Diabetes and Its Complications in the Diabetes Prevention Program Outcomes Study

Ref: Knowler WC, Pan Q, Shu S, Tripputi MT, Dabelea D, Edelstein SL, et al. Analysis of Long-term Follow-up of a Randomized Clinical Trial With Departures From Assigned Treatments: Estimation of Metformin Effects on Diabetes and Its Complications in the Diabetes Prevention Program Outcomes Study. Diabetes Care. 2025;48(10):1668-75.

ABSTRACT

In order to prevent diabetes in high-risk adults, the Diabetes Prevention Program (DPP) was a 3-year randomized clinical trial (RCT) that compared metformin and lifestyle treatments with a placebo. The long-term Diabetes Prevention Program Outcomes Study (DPPOS) was planned to evaluate the development of diabetes and its sequelae over a 22-year period after both therapies dramatically decreased the incidence of diabetes. Deviations from the initial metformin or placebo assignment during follow-up were mostly caused by patients developing diabetes with HbA1c ≥7.0%, which was, according to protocol, treated by clinicians outside the study. The emergence of diabetes resulted in modifications to metformin therapy and the addition of additional glucose-lowering medications. Despite these variations, we consistently discovered that metformin decreased the incidence of diabetes using statistical techniques intended to evaluate intervention effects. The results of the more straightforward intention-to-treat analysis, which did not take treatment modifications into consideration, were not significantly altered by employing these techniques to assess whether metformin use for prediabetes provides ongoing advantages following diabetes diagnosis. With the exception of diabetes incidence, all analytical techniques produced comparable metformin effect estimates with 95% CIs for hazard ratios, including 1.0 (no effect) for all outcomes. Beyond its benefits on diabetes prevention, it is difficult to understand metformin's long-term significance in reducing diabetes-related complications.

CRITICAL APPRAISAL

Introduction and Study Rationale

Randomized clinical trials (RCTs) are considered the gold standard for establishing causal relationships between medical interventions and outcomes because randomization eliminates baseline confounding. The standard analytic approach for RCTs is the "Intention-to-Treat" (ITT) analysis, which compares groups based on their original random assignment regardless of whether they actually received or adhered to the intervention. While ITT preserves the benefits of randomization and answers the pragmatic question of treatment policy effectiveness, it may underestimate the true biological efficacy of a drug if participants stop taking it or if the control group starts taking it (contamination).

This issue is particularly pronounced in long-term prevention trials like the Diabetes Prevention Program (DPP) and its extension, the Diabetes Prevention Program Outcomes Study (DPPOS). Previous reports from the DPP/DPPOS established that metformin significantly reduces the incidence of type 2 diabetes compared to placebo.[17] However, over the 22-year follow-up, many participants originally assigned to placebo developed diabetes and subsequently initiated metformin treatment as part of routine clinical care.[18] Conversely, adherence in the original metformin group varied over time. This "departure from assigned treatments" complicates the assessment of metformin's long-term effects on slowly developing outcomes such as cancer, cardiovascular disease (CVD), and mortality, as the clear distinction between "treated" and "untreated" groups blurs over decades.

What this Study Adds to the Preexisting Knowledge

The study by Knowler et al. (2025) systematically applies and compares four distinct statistical methods to estimate the long-term causal effects of metformin on diabetes incidence and major complications [cancer, nephropathy, major adverse cardiovascular events (MACE), and mortality] in the face of significant treatment switching.[19] The methods evaluated were:

- *Intention-to-treat (ITT)*: The standard comparison of randomized groups
- *As-treated (AT)*: A time-dependent analysis comparing periods of actual metformin use versus non-use, adjusting for covariates
- *Instrumental variable (IV)*: A method using randomization as an "instrument" to predict exposure, designed to account for unmeasured confounding
- *Inverse probability of censoring weighting (IPCW)*: A technique that censors data upon treatment deviation and reweights remaining participants to maintain balance

Key Findings

- *Diabetes prevention*: All four methods consistently demonstrated that metformin significantly reduced diabetes incidence (hazard ratios ranging from 0.70 to 0.82).[19] The consistency across methods reinforces the robustness of metformin's preventive efficacy.
- *Complications:* For long-term outcomes (cancer, MACE, nephropathy, and mortality), the results were largely consistent across methods in showing *no statistically significant benefit* of metformin, with 95% confidence intervals (CIs) crossing 1.0.[19]
- *Impact on disease progression*: The study highlights a critical analytical challenge: once participants developed diabetes (specifically reaching HbA1c ≥7.0%), the protocol mandated referral to community care. This led to widespread initiation of open-label metformin and other glucose-lowering agents in the placebo group. The study shows that after this "diabetes management change," the ability to estimate metformin's specific effect is severely compromised because the comparator is no longer "placebo" but a variable mix of other therapies.

Major Strengths of this Study

The primary strength of this research is the *unprecedented duration of follow-up* (median 22 years) in a large, well-characterized randomized cohort. It represents one of the most rigorous attempts to grapple with the "real-world" messiness of long-term clinical trials.

Analytically, the study is strong because it moves beyond the binary ITT versus Per-Protocol debate. By employing *Instrumental Variable (IV)* and *IPCW* analyses, the authors attempt to reconstruct the counterfactual scenario—what would have happened if adherence had been perfect. The IV method is particularly sophisticated as it theoretically controls for unmeasured confounders, a feat impossible with standard multivariable regression (AT analysis).

Furthermore, the stratification of analyses by the "diabetes management change" time-point (before vs. after HbA1c ≥7.0%) provides crucial insight. It disentangles the period where the trial intervention (metformin vs. placebo) was distinct from the period where clinical necessity dictated treatment, thereby exposing the specific mechanism by which the clear treatment signal is diluted over time.

Limitations of this Study

The most significant limitation is that despite advanced statistical techniques, *the confounding caused by protocol-driven treatment changes could not be fully overcome.* Once a participant develops diabetes and requires treatment, they are fundamentally different from a participant who remains disease-free. The drugs used after diabetes onset (e.g., SGLT-2 inhibitors, statins) act as time-varying confounders that may independently affect cardiovascular and renal outcomes, masking any specific benefit of metformin.

Secondly, the study suffers from *statistical power limitations* regarding complications. Although the cohort was large (over 2,000 participants in the analyzed groups), the number of specific events (e.g., cancers and MACE) may still be too low to detect modest risk reductions, especially when using complex methods like IPCW which inevitably widen confidence intervals.[19]

Thirdly, the *generalizability* of the "As-Treated" findings is limited by the fact that metformin use in the placebo group was not random; it was driven by worsening health (diabetes diagnosis). While the authors adjusted for this, residual confounding by indication (where sicker patients take the drug) likely persists, potentially biasing estimates toward the null or even harm (e.g., the slight increase in mortality risk seen in the AT analysis).[19]

Implication of Findings on Clinical Practice

For clinicians, this study reinforces the pivotal role of metformin in diabetes prevention. The finding that metformin reduces diabetes incidence is consistent regardless of the data analysis method employed. The ITT analysis remains the most pertinent for the policy question: "Should we prescribe metformin to individuals with prediabetes?" The answer is unequivocally affirmative for prevention.[19]

However, the study suggests *caution in expecting metformin to independently prevent downstream complications* (like cancer or CVD) solely through early initiation in prediabetes. The data do not support the hypothesis that starting metformin early (in prediabetes) confers a "legacy effect" of cardiovascular protection distinguishable from the effects of standard diabetes care initiated later. This implies that while metformin prevents the *diagnosis* of diabetes, its specific long-term protection against organ damage in this population may be less than previously hoped.

Knowledge Gaps Identified and Future Scope for Research

The study identifies a critical gap in *methodology for long-term trials.* It demonstrates that current statistical tools (even IV and IPCW) struggle to provide precise estimates when the "departure from assigned treatment" is not random but a structural feature of disease progression management. Future research needs to develop study designs or analytic frameworks that can better handle "treatment switching" driven by the primary outcome (diabetes) itself.

Biologically, a gap remains regarding *metformin's nonglycemic effects*. Since the study could not definitively rule out benefits for cancer or CVD (due to wide CIs), larger studies or meta-analyses of individual participant data (IPD) are needed to determine if metformin has pleiotropic protective effects in specific subgroups (e.g., those with high baseline CVD risk) that were diluted in the broad DPPOS cohort. The potential signal for cancer reduction, while not significant here, warrants continued investigation in dedicated oncology trials.

4. Long-term Effects and Effect Heterogeneity of Lifestyle and Metformin Interventions on Type 2 diabetes Incidence Over 21 Years in the US Diabetes Prevention Program Randomized Clinical Trial

Ref: Knowler WC, Doherty L, Edelstein SL, Bennett PH, Dabelea D, Hoskin M, et al. Long-term effects and effect heterogeneity of lifestyle and metformin interventions on type 2 diabetes incidence over 21 years in the US Diabetes Prevention Program randomised clinical trial. Lancet Diabetes Endocrinol. 2025;13(6):469-81.

ABSTRACT

Background: Type 2 diabetes incidence was lowered by 58% with intensive lifestyle intervention (ILS) and by 31% with metformin when compared to a placebo in the US Diabetes Prevention Program (DPP), a 3-year randomized clinical trial involving 3,234 persons with prediabetes. Over the course of almost 21 years of follow-up, we aimed to evaluate the long-term consequences and potential heterogeneity of treatment results.

Methods: The DPP Outcomes Study (DPPOS) was a continuation of the DPP study with protocol adjustments. In the DPPOS, the ILS group received group-based booster intervention classes twice a year, the placebo was stopped, metformin (850 mg twice a day as tolerated) was continued after unmasking, and all participants received group-based lifestyle intervention four times a year. Diabetes incidence, as defined by American Diabetes Association standards, was the predetermined primary endpoint during DPP and DPPOS. Since COVID-19 caused a significant disruptions in clinic visits and longitudinal data analysis, February 23, 2020 was chosen as the closing date of the analysis. The DPPOS protocol defined ongoing diabetes incidence as an endpoint. We evaluated the variability of effects in subgroups identified by baseline diabetes risk variables as well as the long-term persistence of intervention effects on diabetes incidence. The combined study's follow-up is provided from July 31, 1996 to February 23, 2020. Analysis was done using intention to treat. The trial is registered with ClinicalTrials.gov under the numbers NCT00004992 (DPP) and NCT00038727 (DPPOS); enrollment is closed save for former DPP participants, although follow-up is still ongoing.

Findings: The current analysis included 3,195 individuals who were first recruited in the DPP. This population had a mean baseline age of 50.6 years (SD 10.7), with 2,171 (67.9%) female participants and 1024 (32.1%) male individuals. Individual follow-up periods varied from 0–2 to 23–2 years [median 8–0 years (IQR 3–0 to 18–0)]; administrative censorship caused the remaining numbers at risk to drastically decline after 21 years, hence follow-up was deemed to cover a 21-year period. The original ILS group [hazard ratio (HR) 0.76 (95% CI 0.68–0.85), rate difference (RD) −1.59 cases (95% CI −2.25 to −0.93] per 100 person-years] and the original metformin group [HR 0.83 (0.74–0.93), RD −1·17

(−1.85 to −0.49)] experienced corresponding increases in median diabetes-free survival. The metformin and ILS groups had lower incidence rates than the placebo group, and the diabetes cumulative incidence curves split early, particularly in the first 3 years. With prolonged follow-up, the metformin and ILS curves gradually converged. Large early impacts during the DPP seemed to be the cause of the overall treatment effects. Participants with higher baseline fasting glucose, HbA1c, and multivariable clinical and physiological risk index values had stronger absolute intervention benefits (measured as RDs vs. placebo) with ILS, and younger participants with metformin.

Interpretation: After the DPP trial's significant early intervention results, cumulative diabetes incidence continued to decline for 21 years. Based on a few baseline factors, the results of the intervention varied. The current type 2 diabetes epidemic may be addressed with precision therapies based on these findings.

CRITICAL APPRAISAL

Introduction and Study Rationale

Before the publication of this 21-year follow-up, the efficacy of lifestyle and pharmacological interventions in preventing type 2 diabetes (T2D) had been established primarily through short-to-medium-term randomized clinical trials (RCTs). The original Diabetes Prevention Program (DPP), concluded in 2001, demonstrated that over a mean follow-up of 2.8 years, an intensive lifestyle intervention (ILS) reduced the incidence of diabetes by 58%, while metformin reduced it by 31% compared to placebo in adults with impaired glucose tolerance.[17] Similar findings were reported in the Finnish Diabetes Prevention Study and the Da Qing Diabetes Prevention Study.[20,21]

However, knowledge regarding the durability of these effects over decades was limited. While the Da Qing study provided evidence of long-term benefits (up to 30 years) from a 6-year lifestyle intervention, there was a paucity of data comparing the long-term sustainability of lifestyle modification versus pharmacological intervention (metformin) in a diverse US population.[21] It remained unclear whether the delay in diabetes onset observed in the initial years would translate into a sustained reduction in cumulative incidence over a lifetime, or if the effects would wane completely once the intensity of the interventions was reduced.

What this Study Adds to the Preexisting Knowledge

The study by Knowler et al. (2025) extends the follow-up of the DPP cohort to a median of 21 years, providing critical insights into the long-term trajectory of diabetes prevention.[22]

- *Sustained cumulative benefit*: The study confirms that the initial period of intensive intervention confers a long-lasting benefit. Despite the attenuation of the interventions over time, the cumulative incidence of diabetes remained significantly lower in the original ILS group [hazard ratio (HR) 0.76] and the metformin group (HR 0.83) compared to placebo after 21 years. This translated to a median delay in diabetes onset of 3.5 years for ILS and 2.5 years for metformin.[22]
- *Convergence of incidence rates*: A key physiological insight is that while cumulative incidence remained lower, the *annual* incidence rates in the intervention groups eventually converged with the placebo group. This suggests that the long-term differences are largely driven by the profound risk reduction achieved in the first few years of the trial, rather than a continued divergence in risk late in the course.[22]
- *Effect heterogeneity*: The study provides granular data on *who* benefits most. It established that metformin's absolute efficacy was significantly heterogeneous by

age, being robust in younger participants (25–44 years) but ineffective in those aged >60 years. Conversely, the absolute benefit of ILS was greatest in participants with the highest baseline risk (e.g., higher fasting glucose, HbA1c, or physiological risk scores), although it remained effective across all age groups.[22]

Major Strengths of this Study

- *Study design and duration*: This is one of the longest-running RCTs in the field of metabolic disease. Following a large cohort (n = 3,195) for over two decades with high retention rates allows for the assessment of outcomes that evolve slowly, which shorter trials cannot capture.[22]
- *Rigorous phenotyping*: The study utilized gold-standard diagnostic methods, including annual oral glucose tolerance tests (OGTTs), rather than relying solely on medical records or HbA1c. This ensures highly accurate ascertainment of the primary outcome.[22]
- *Diversity*: The cohort included a substantial proportion (45%) of participants from US minority racial and ethnic groups, enhancing the generalizability of the findings to populations disproportionately affected by T2D.[22]
- *Statistical robustness*: The use of both relative (hazard ratio) and absolute (rate difference) measures, along with detailed subgroup analyses using composite risk indices, provides a nuanced understanding of intervention effects that goes beyond simple averages.[22]

Limitations of this Study

- *Protocol changes and contamination*: The transition from the blinded DPP phase to the open-label DPPOS phase introduced significant confounding. The placebo group was discontinued, and a group-based lifestyle intervention was offered to *all* participants. This likely diluted the observed differences between groups, making the results a conservative estimate of the true biological efficacy of the original interventions.[22]
- *Survivor bias*: The analysis of incidence rates over time is complicated by the fact that the most susceptible individuals developed diabetes early and were removed from the "at-risk" pool. This "depletion of susceptibles" can make incidence rates appear to decrease artificially in the placebo group over time.[22]
- *Generalizability of eligibility*: The strict inclusion criteria (requiring both impaired fasting glucose and impaired glucose tolerance) identify a very high-risk phenotype. The results may not fully apply to individuals with isolated prediabetes phenotypes (e.g., isolated impaired fasting glucose), which are more common in the general population but carry lower conversion risks.[22]

Implication of Findings on Clinical Practice

- *Start early and hit hard*: The finding that long-term benefits are driven by early risk reduction supports an aggressive approach to identifying and treating prediabetes immediately. Clinicians should not wait for glycemic parameters to worsen before initiating prevention strategies.
- *Personalized prevention*: The heterogeneity data supports a precision medicine approach. Metformin should be strongly considered for *younger adults* (25–44 years) with prediabetes, a group often overlooked for pharmacological prevention but who derive the greatest absolute benefit. In contrast, older adults (>60 years) should primarily be targeted with lifestyle interventions, as metformin showed no significant benefit in this demographic.[22]
- *Resource allocation*: Since the absolute benefit of lifestyle intervention was greatest in those with the highest physiological risk, public health programs with limited resources might prioritize intensive lifestyle coaching for individuals with the highest combined risk factors (e.g., highest BMI and glucose levels).

Knowledge Gaps Identified and Future Scope for Research

- *Comparison with newer agents*: The study highlights that metformin and lifestyle are effective, but it did not compare these established interventions with modern, potent therapies like GLP-1 receptor agonists (e.g., semaglutide, tirzepatide). Future research must determine if these newer agents can produce even greater or more durable delays in diabetes onset, particularly in those who fail metformin or lifestyle modification.[22]
- *Maintenance of weight loss*: The waning of the lifestyle effect correlates with weight regain. Future research needs to focus on novel behavioral or pharmacological strategies to maintain weight loss over decades, which could potentially prevent the convergence of incidence rates seen in this study.
- *Mechanisms of age-related metformin failure*: The biological reasons why metformin is less effective in older adults remain unclear and warrant mechanistic investigation to optimize pharmacotherapy in the aging population.

5. Associations between Long-term Metformin Use, the Risk of Vitamin B12 Deficiency, and Neuropathy: An All of Us Research Program Study

Ref: Sepassi A, Wang J, Yankowski S, Enkoji A, Okenwa M, Morello CM, et al. Associations between long-term metformin use, the risk of vitamin B12 deficiency, and neuropathy: An All of Us research Program study. Diabetes Res Clin Pract. 2025;228: 112424.

ABSTRACT

Aim: After the Diabetes Prevention Program (DPP) trial's significant early intervention results, cumulative diabetes incidence continued to decline for 21 years. Based on a few baseline factors, the results of the intervention varied. The current type 2 diabetes epidemic may be addressed with precision therapies based on these findings.

Methods: NIH's All of Us database was used for a retrospective observational cross-sectional analysis. Peripheral neuropathy and vitamin B12 deficiency were examined between long-term (≥4 years) and short-term (<0.001) metformin users. Long-term users had a 39% greater prevalence of peripheral neuropathy than short-term users ($p < 0.001$), although this difference was not statistically significant when compared to nonusers.

Conclusion: In those with type 2 diabetes, long-term metformin use is linked to a higher risk of peripheral neuropathy and vitamin B12 insufficiency. When evaluating the symptoms of peripheral neuropathy, providers should consider about regularly assessing the vitamin B12 status of long-term users.

CRITICAL APPRAISAL

Introduction and Study Rationale

Metformin is the cornerstone first-line pharmacotherapy for the management of type 2 diabetes mellitus (T2DM) worldwide due to its efficacy, safety profile, and cardiovascular benefits.[23] However, the association between long-term metformin use and vitamin B12 (cobalamin) deficiency has been recognized for decades, first described in the 1970s.[24] The mechanism is thought to involve metformin-induced alteration of calcium-dependent absorption of the vitamin B12-intrinsic factor complex in the terminal ileum.[25] Vitamin B12 deficiency is clinically significant because it can lead to hematological abnormalities (megaloblastic anemia) and neurological damage, specifically peripheral neuropathy.[26]

This presents a unique clinical challenge in diabetes care because peripheral neuropathy is also a common microvascular complication of diabetes itself (diabetic peripheral neuropathy or DPN). Distinguishing between DPN caused by hyperglycemia and neuropathy caused by iatrogenic vitamin B12 deficiency is difficult as the symptoms—paresthesia, numbness, and sensory loss—often overlap.[27] While previous studies, including the Diabetes Prevention Program Outcomes Study (DPPOS), confirmed the risk of deficiency increases with duration of use,[28] data regarding the direct translation of this biochemical deficiency into clinical neuropathy in diverse, real-world populations has been inconsistent. Furthermore, most prior studies lacked the racial and ethnic diversity necessary to generalize findings across the broad demographic spectrum of patients with T2DM in the United States.[23]

What this Study Adds to the Preexisting Knowledge

The study by Sepassi et al. (2025) utilizes the National Institutes of Health's (NIH's) "All of Us" database to provide one of the largest and most diverse investigations into this triad of metformin, vitamin B12, and neuropathy.[23] By analyzing 14,808 adults with T2DM, the authors move beyond simple associations to examine the impact of *duration* of use on clinical outcomes.

Key findings that expand current knowledge include:

- *Quantification of risk by duration:* The study establishes a clear temporal link, finding that long-term metformin users (≥4 years) have a *67% higher likelihood* of vitamin B12 deficiency compared to nonusers (adjusted odds ratio 1.67) and a *38% higher likelihood* compared to short-term users.[23] This reinforces that the risk is cumulative and time-dependent.
- *Link to neuropathy*: Crucially, the study provides evidence linking this usage pattern to clinical neuropathy. Long-term users had a *39% higher prevalence* of peripheral neuropathy compared to short-term users ($p < 0.001$).[23] This suggests that a subset of "diabetic neuropathy" cases in long-standing patients may actually be driven or exacerbated by medication-induced nutritional deficiency.
- *Interaction with disease duration*: The authors performed a nuanced interaction analysis, finding that while long-term use generally increases neuropathy risk, this specific medication-associated risk appears to diminish relative to other factors as the duration of diabetes increases.[23] This highlights the complex interplay between neurotoxicity from hyperglycemia and vitamin deficiency over time.

Major Strengths of this Study

The most significant strength of this study is the use of the *"All of Us" research program database*, which ensures a high degree of racial and ethnic diversity (approximately 45% non-White participants).[23] This addresses a major limitation in biomedical research where minority populations—who often bear a disproportionate burden of T2DM—are underrepresented. This enhances the generalizability of the findings to a broader population.

Secondly, the *study design rigor* regarding exclusion criteria strengthens the internal validity. By excluding participants with a history of vitamin B12 deficiency or neuropathy *prior* to the index date, the authors minimized reverse causality bias, ensuring that the observed outcomes likely developed during the exposure period.[23]

Thirdly, the *multivariable adjustment* was comprehensive. The analysis controlled for key confounders such as proton pump inhibitor (PPI) use (known to impair B12 absorption), vitamin B12 supplementation history, sociodemographic factors, and the Charlson comorbidity index (CCI).[23] This allows for a more isolated assessment of metformin's independent contribution to the outcomes.

Limitations of this Study

Despite its scale, the study has inherent limitations typical of *retrospective observational designs* using electronic health records (EHR). First, causality cannot be definitively established. While the study shows a strong association, it cannot prove that metformin caused the neuropathy, particularly because glycemic control (e.g., HbA1c history over time) was not fully accounted for as a continuous variable in all models due to data limitations. Poor glycemic control is the primary driver of DPN, and if long-term metformin users had worse historical control, this could confound the neuropathy findings.[23]

Secondly, the classification of *"Non-Users"* relies on the absence of prescription records. It is possible that some patients in this group were taking metformin prescribed outside the participating health systems or obtained it via other means, potentially diluting the differences observed.[23]

Thirdly, the definition of *neuropathy* relied on ICD-10 codes. This introduces the risk of misclassification or underreporting, as coding depends on provider documentation practices. Asymptomatic neuropathy or cases not formally coded during visits would be missed, potentially underestimating the true prevalence.[23]

Implication of Findings on Clinical Practice

The findings have immediate and actionable implications for diabetes management. The strong signal for increased risk after 4 years of therapy supports the implementation of *routine screening protocols*. Clinicians should consider measuring vitamin B12 levels annually or every 2–3 years in patients who have been on metformin for 4 years or longer, or sooner if symptoms of neuropathy develop.[23]

Furthermore, the study challenges the assumption that all neuropathy in T2DM is due to the disease itself. When a patient on long-term metformin presents with worsening paresthesia or sensory loss, providers must include B12 deficiency in the differential diagnosis. Treating this deficiency with supplementation is a low-cost, low-risk intervention that could prevent permanent neurological damage, whereas intensifying glucose control would not reverse neuropathy caused by vitamin deficiency.[27,29]

Knowledge Gaps Identified and Future Scope for Research

While this study clarifies the risk, several gaps remain that warrant future research:

- *Reversibility of neuropathy*: The study does not address whether identifying and treating the B12 deficiency results in the resolution of neuropathic symptoms in this specific population. Prospective interventional studies are needed to quantify the degree of neurological recovery possible with supplementation.[23]
- *Dietary intake*: The study could not account for dietary B12 intake (e.g., vegan/vegetarian diets). Future research should integrate nutritional data to better stratify risk.[23]
- *Interaction with GLP-1 receptor agonists*: As noted by the authors, the increasing use of GLP-1 receptor agonists in combination with metformin warrants investigation. Since GLP-1s can cause gastrointestinal side effects, it is unknown if they exacerbate malabsorption when combined with metformin.[23]
- *Optimal screening thresholds*: Research is needed to define the most cost-effective screening schedule and the specific serum B12 threshold (e.g., <200 pg/mL vs. <300 pg/mL with elevated methylmalonic acid) that should trigger intervention in metformin users.[28,30]

6. Non-pharmacological Management Strategies for Type 2 Diabetes in Children and Young Adults: A Systematic Review

Ref: Carino M, New RH, Nguyen J, Kirkham R, Maple-Brown L, Titmuss A, et al. Non-pharmacological management strategies for type 2 diabetes in children and young adults: A systematic review. Diabetes Res Clin Pract. 2025;222:112045.

ABSTRACT

Purpose: There is little proof that type 2 diabetes in children and young people can be effectively managed without medication. The purpose of this systematic review is to explore the evidence that is currently available for nonpharmacological therapies in the management of type 2 diabetes in children and young people.

Techniques: Up until March 2024, OVID MEDLINE, Ovid Emcare, EMBASE, CINAHL, Cochrane, APA PsycINFO, Joanna Briggs, ACP Journal Club, Global Health, Scopus databases, INFORMIT, Circumpolar Health, Native Health Database, Indigenous Studies Portal, Open Grey, and Clinicaltrials.gov were all thoroughly searched. Three reviewers independently extracted data on the author, year, study design, setting and population, characteristics of the intervention, and outcomes.

Results: The inclusion criteria were met by seven studies. A very low-energy diet (VLED) has been linked to lower body mass index (BMI), weight, and glycated hemoglobin (HbA1c). HbA1c was not improved by any other interventions, including peer support programs, occupational therapist-led support programs, or intensive group-based lifestyle programs. Interventions had a favorable effect on cardiometabolic outcomes, mental health, and overall well-being.

Discussion: There is little evidence to support the nonpharmacological treatment of type 2 diabetes in young people. This study shows that VLED is linked to better glycemia and weight loss. There are conflicting findings about the role of social support from family, friends, and medical experts.

CRITICAL APPRAISAL

Introduction and Study Rationale

Type 2 diabetes (T2D) in children and adolescents is an escalating global health crisis, distinct from the adult-onset form of the disease. It is characterized by a more aggressive phenotype, rapid deterioration of beta-cell function, and a higher rate of treatment failure.[31] The landmark Treatment Options for Type 2 Diabetes in Adolescents and Youth (TODAY) trial demonstrated that approximately half of youth with T2D fail to maintain glycemic control with metformin monotherapy or metformin plus lifestyle intervention.[32] This aggressive pathophysiology places young people at high risk for early onset complications, including nephropathy and cardiovascular disease.

Historically, management guidelines have relied heavily on pharmacotherapy, extrapolated largely from adult data. While lifestyle modification is universally recommended as a cornerstone of management, the evidence base supporting specific nonpharmacological interventions—such as dietary regimens, physical activity programs, or psychosocial support—has been fragmented and inconclusive for this specific age group.[33] Previous systematic reviews have predominantly focused on the *prevention* of T2D in youth or the management of T2D in *adults*. Consequently, clinicians have lacked a synthesized evidence base to guide nonpharmacological strategies for managing established T2D in the pediatric and young adult population.[31]

What this Study Adds to the Preexisting Knowledge

The study by Carino et al. (2025) provides the first systematic review specifically evaluating the effectiveness of nonpharmacological interventions for managing T2D in children and young adults (aged 5–25 years).[31] By synthesizing data from seven studies involving diverse interventions, the review offers several novel insights:

- *Efficacy of very low-energy diets (VLED)*: The review identifies VLED as the only nonpharmacological intervention currently supported by evidence to significantly reduce HbA1c and body mass index (BMI) in this population.[31] In the included studies, VLED was associated with the normalization of HbA1c and discontinuation of insulin in adherent participants, suggesting that the "remission" potential observed in adults may translate to youth.
- *Limitations of standard lifestyle/support programs*: Conversely, the study reveals that other studied interventions—including intensive group-based lifestyle modification, occupational therapy support, and peer mentorship ("Buddy Study")—did not yield statistically significant improvements in glycemic control (HbA1c).[31]
- *Psychosocial benefits*: Despite the lack of glycemic benefit, the review highlights that these supportive interventions had positive impacts on secondary outcomes, including quality of life, mental well-being, and specific health behaviors (e.g., label reading, physical activity).[31]
- *Targeting high-risk populations*: The review highlights that the available evidence is derived almost exclusively from minority ethnic groups (First Nations, Hispanic, African American), who bear the disproportionate burden of youth-onset T2D. This adds crucial context regarding the applicability of interventions across different cultural settings.[31]

Major Strengths of this Study

- *Comprehensive search strategy*: A significant strength is the authors' exhaustive search strategy. Recognizing that youth-onset T2D disproportionately affects Indigenous and minority populations, they searched specialized databases such as the Native Health Database, Circumpolar Health, and Indigenous Studies Portal, in addition to standard medical databases.[31] This ensures the review captures culturally specific gray literature that traditional reviews might miss.
- *Focus on a neglected population*: By explicitly targeting the 5–25 year age range, the study addresses a critical "evidence-practice gap". This transition age group is often lost between pediatric and adult care models, and analyzing them specifically is vital for developing age-appropriate care standards.[31]
- *Rigorous methodology*: The review adheres to PRISMA guidelines and employed the Cochrane risk of bias tool (RoB 2) and Joanna Briggs Institute tools for quality assessment. The authors transparently acknowledge the low quality and high risk of bias in the primary studies, preventing the generation of misleading pooled effect estimates.[31]
- *Holistic outcome assessment*: The review did not limit its scope to glycemic markers. By extracting data on mental health, well-being, and cardiometabolic outcomes, the authors provide a more rounded picture of therapeutic success, acknowledging that in chronic disease management, psychological engagement is often a precursor to physiological improvement.[31]

Limitations of this Study

- *Paucity of high-quality data*: The primary limitation is inherent to the field rather than the review methodology itself—the scarcity of data. Only seven studies met the inclusion criteria, and most had very small sample sizes (ranging from a single case study to 20 participants).[31] This severely limits the statistical power and generalizability of the findings.
- *Heterogeneity preventing meta-analysis*: Due to the wide variation in study designs

(RCTs, pre-post studies, mixed-methods), interventions (diet vs. peer support vs. exercise), and reported outcomes, a quantitative meta-analysis was not possible. This forces a narrative synthesis which, while descriptive, cannot provide precise estimates of treatment effect sizes.[31]

- *Risk of bias in primary studies*: Most included studies were assessed as having a high risk of bias, particularly attrition bias. High dropout rates (e.g., 62.5% in one VLED study and 40% in a peer support study) suggest that these interventions may be difficult to sustain in real-world settings, potentially inflating the reported benefits if only "super-responders" remained.[31]
- *Short duration*: The follow-up periods in the included studies were relatively short (8 weeks to 2 years). Given the lifelong nature of T2D, the long-term sustainability of VLED-induced remission or the long-term impact of peer support remains unknown.[31]

Implication of Findings on Clinical Practice

- *Re-evaluating dietary management*: Clinicians managing youth with T2D and obesity should consider VLEDs as a potent, short-term therapeutic option for inducing rapid weight loss and glycemic improvement, potentially to "reset" metabolic health or induce remission.[31] However, the high attrition rates suggest this must be implemented with robust support systems.
- *Holistic endpoints*: The lack of glycemic benefit from peer support and lifestyle programs should not lead to their abandonment. Since these interventions improve mental health and quality of life, they should be viewed as *complementary* therapies to support the psychosocial burden of diabetes, rather than standalone tools for glycemic control.[31]
- *Culturally safe care*: The predominance of minority participants in these studies underscores the need for culturally safe clinical practices. Interventions must be co-designed with communities to ensure they are acceptable and sustainable for the populations most at risk.[31]

Knowledge Gaps Identified and Future Scope for Research

- *Feasibility of VLED*: While VLEDs show promise, research is needed to determine how to improve adherence and safe implementation in growing children. Future studies must assess the long-term impacts of severe caloric restriction on growth, bone health, and eating disorder risk in adolescents.[31]
- *Role of technology*: The review notes a lack of studies utilizing modern diabetes technology. Future research should investigate whether continuous glucose monitoring (CGM) or digital health apps can enhance engagement and outcomes in nonpharmacological interventions.[31]
- *Family and peer dynamics*: The mixed results regarding social support highlight a gap in understanding *how* to effectively leverage family and peer networks. Future research should rigorously test family-centered interventions that move beyond simple "buddy" systems to address complex family dynamics.[31]
- *Large-scale RCTs*: There is an urgent need for adequately powered, multi-center randomized controlled trials to provide high-certainty evidence. These trials should be co-designed with patients to minimize attrition and ensure the interventions are relevant to the lived experience of young people with T2D.[31]

7. The Effect of Vitamin D3 Supplementation on the Incidence of Type 2 Diabetes in Healthy Older Adults Not at High Risk for Diabetes (FIND): A Randomized Controlled Trial

Ref: Virtanen JK, Hantunen S, Kallio N, Lamberg-Allardt C, Manson JE, Nurmi T, et al. The effect of vitamin D3 supplementation on the incidence of type 2 diabetes in healthy older adults not at high risk for diabetes (FIND): a randomised controlled trial. Diabetologia. 2025;68(4):715-26.

ABSTRACT

Aim/Hypothesis: Although vitamin D deficiency is linked to an increased risk of type 2 diabetes, there is little data from randomized trials regarding the advantages of vitamin D supplementation, particularly for people at average risk. In a cohort of usually healthy older adults, the Finnish Vitamin D Trial (FIND) examined the impact of vitamin D3 supplementation at two different levels on the prevalence of type 2 diabetes.

Methods: FIND was a 5-year, parallel-arm, randomized, placebo-controlled study that included 2,271 male and female volunteers from the general Finnish community who were at least 60 and 65 years old, respectively, and did not have diabetes or cancer. There were three arms in the study: a placebo, 1,600 IU/day of vitamin D3, or 3,200 IU/day of vitamin D3. A non-study group statistician used computerized random number generation to perform sex-stratified simple randomization in a 1:1:1 ratio. The group assignment was concealed from the participants, researchers, and study personnel. Event data was gathered from national health registries. At months 0, 6, 12, and 24, a representative sub-cohort of 505 participants underwent more thorough in-person investigations.

Results: 38 (5.0%), 31 (4.2%), and 36 (4.7%) type 2 diabetes events occurred in the placebo ($n = 760$), 1,600 IU/day vitamin D3 ($n = 744$; vs. placebo: HR 0.81; 95% CI 0.50, 1.30), and 3,200 IU/day vitamin D3 ($n = 767$; vs. placebo: HR 0.92, 95% CI 0.58, 1.45) arms, respectively (p-trend = 0.73). The HR was 0.86 (95% CI 0.58, 1.29) when the two vitamin D3 arms were combined and contrasted with the placebo arm. The HRs in the combined vitamin D3 arms compared to the placebo were 0.43 (95% CI 0.14, 1.34), 0.97 (0.50, 1.91), and 1.00 (0.57, 1.75), respectively, in the analyses stratified by BMI [<25 kg/m^2 ($n = 813$, number of type 2 diabetes events = 12), 25–30 kg/m^2 ($n = 1{,}032$, number of events = 38), and 54]. In the sub-cohort, mean (SD) baseline 25-(OH) vitamin D was 74.5 (18.1) nmol/L. Following a year, the concentrations in the placebo, 1,600 IU/day vitamin D3, and 3,200 IU/day vitamin D3 arms were 72.6 (17.7), 99.3 (20.8), and 120.9 (22.1) nmol/L, respectively. During the 24-month follow-up, there were no differences in the sub-cohort's waist circumference, BMI, or plasma glucose or insulin concentrations (p values ≥0.19).

Conclusion/Interpretation: Vitamin D3 supplementation did not significantly lower the chance of acquiring diabetes in generally healthy older persons who are not at high risk for the disease and whose serum 25(OH)D3 levels are adequate for bone health.

CRITICAL APPRAISAL

Introduction and Study Rationale

The relationship between vitamin D status and type 2 diabetes (T2D) has been a subject of intense scrutiny over the last decade. Observational epidemiological studies have consistently demonstrated an inverse association between serum 25-hydroxyvitamin D concentrations and the risk of developing T2D.[34] Biologically, vitamin D receptors are present in pancreatic beta-cells, and the active metabolite 1,25-dihydroxyvitamin D is thought to enhance insulin secretion and improve insulin sensitivity by reducing systemic inflammation.[35]

However, translating these observational associations into interventional benefits has proven challenging. Major randomized controlled trials (RCTs) specifically designed to test diabetes prevention, such as the *vitamin D and type 2 diabetes (D2d)* study in the USA and the *Diabetes Prevention with active Vitamin D (DPVD)* study in Japan, focused on high-risk individuals with prediabetes.[36,37] These trials generally showed a modest (10–13%) reduction in diabetes risk that often fell short of statistical significance in primary analyses, though meta-analyses of these trials suggest a significant benefit restricted to those with prediabetes.[38] Crucially, there has been a paucity of long-term data regarding the preventive effect of vitamin D supplementation in the *general, average-risk older population* who do not necessarily have prediabetes or vitamin D deficiency.

What this Study Adds to the Preexisting Knowledge

The FIND study by Virtanen et al. (2025) addresses this specific evidence gap by evaluating the effect of vitamin D3 supplementation on T2D incidence in a generally healthy older population *not* selected for high diabetes risk.[39] Unlike previous trials that targeted prediabetes, FIND enrolled 2,271 Finnish men (age ≥60 years) and women (age ≥65 years) free of prevalent cardiovascular disease (CVD), cancer, or medically treated diabetes.

Key contributions include:

- *Population context*: It provides rare experimental data on "primary prevention" in an average-risk cohort.
- *Dosing regimen*: It tested two pharmacological doses (1,600 IU/day and 3,200 IU/day) against placebo, which is higher than the standard 400–800 IU often used in older bone-health trials.
- *Null result*: The study found *no statistically significant reduction* in T2D incidence over 5 years. The hazard ratios (HRs) were 0.81 (1,600 IU) and 0.92 (3,200 IU) compared to placebo (p-trend = 0.73).
- *Subgroup signal*: A notable finding was the significant interaction with body mass index (BMI) ($P_{interaction}$ <0.001). In participants with a BMI <25 kg/m^2, the combined vitamin D groups showed a substantial reduction in diabetes risk (HR 0.43), whereas no benefit was seen in overweight or obese participants.

Major Strengths of this Study

- *Study design*: The randomized, double-blind, placebo-controlled design is the gold standard for causal inference, minimizing the confounding factors (e.g., physical activity, diet) that plague observational studies.
- *Duration*: The 5-year follow-up period is significant, allowing sufficient time for the cumulative metabolic effects of vitamin D to potentially manifest, which is superior to shorter trials.
- *Dose comparison*: The inclusion of two distinct active doses (1,600 and 3,200 IU) allowed for the assessment of a dose-response relationship, rather than relying on a single treatment arm.
- *High adherence and retention*: Adherence was self-reported as excellent, with 95.4% of participants taking at least 80% of pills. The study utilized national health registries for outcome ascertainment, ensuring zero loss to follow-up for the diabetes endpoint among those who did not withdraw consent.
- *Robust vitamin D status assessment*: In the sub-cohort, serum 25(OH)D levels were measured using the gold-standard LC-MS/MS method (standardized to NIST), confirming that the intervention effectively raised vitamin D levels (to ~100–120 nmol/L) compared to placebo.

Limitations of this Study

- *Statistical power*: The study was originally designed to recruit 18,000 participants but only secured ~2,500. Consequently, the study was *severely underpowered*. The number of incident diabetes cases (n = 105) was very low (incidence ~1.1 per

100 person-years), resulting in wide confidence intervals that cannot definitively rule out a modest benefit (e.g., a 15–20% reduction).

- *Baseline sufficiency*: The study population was largely vitamin D sufficient at baseline (mean 75 nmol/L), with only 9% having levels <50 nmol/L. This "ceiling effect" is a common limitation in nutrient trials; supplementing individuals who are already replete is unlikely to yield metabolic benefit.
- *Outcome ascertainment*: Diabetes diagnosis relied on national registers (medication reimbursement and hospital codes). This likely missed cases of diet-controlled diabetes or undiagnosed asymptomatic hyperglycemia, potentially diluting the event rate further.
- *Generalizability*: The cohort consisted of White, older Northern Europeans. The results may not apply to other ethnicities (e.g., South Asians, African Americans) who have different risks for T2D and vitamin D metabolism.
- *Tertiary outcome*: T2D incidence was a tertiary endpoint (primary were CVD and cancer), meaning the study was not specifically optimized or powered for this metabolic outcome.

Implication of Findings on Clinical Practice

The FIND study reinforces the growing consensus that *universal vitamin D supplementation for the sole purpose of preventing type 2 diabetes in the general healthy population is not supported by evidence.*[39]

- *No "off-target" benefit*: Clinicians should not expect that prescribing vitamin D for bone health in older adults will confer secondary protection against diabetes, particularly if the patient is already vitamin D sufficient.
- *Weight-centric approaches*: The findings underscore that traditional risk factors (obesity) overwhelm any potential micronutrient benefit. In the BMI >30 kg/m^2 group, vitamin D had zero effect, reinforcing that weight management remains the cornerstone of prevention in obese individuals.
- *Possible lean phenotype utility*: While the subgroup finding (benefit in BMI <25) requires cautious interpretation, it suggests that in lean older adults, where insulin resistance is less dominant, vitamin D might play a role in supporting beta-cell function. However, this is not yet ready for clinical guidelines.

Knowledge Gaps Identified and Future Scope for Research

- *The "deficient" population*: A critical gap remains regarding individuals with severe vitamin D deficiency (<30 nmol/L). Ethical constraints prevent long-term placebo-controlled trials in this group, but real-world data or "treat-to-target" trials are needed to see if correcting deficiency prevents T2D.
- *Interaction with adiposity*: The strong interaction between BMI and vitamin D efficacy observed here (and in D2d post-hoc analyses) warrants mechanistic research. Does sequestration of vitamin D in adipose tissue render it metabolically inactive in obese individuals? Future trials should stratify by BMI a priori.
- *Ethnic diversity*: Given that the "Asian phenotype" of diabetes involves early beta-cell failure (which vitamin D might theoretically help), similar trials are needed in non-White populations who often have lower baseline vitamin D levels.
- *Combined interventions*: Future research should explore if vitamin D acts synergistically with lifestyle interventions or metformin, rather than as a monotherapy.

8. Genetic Determinants of Variable Anti-diabetic Therapy Responses Across Diverse Populations with Type 2 Diabetes Mellitus: A Systematic Review and Meta-analysis

Ref: Ahmad F, Abubakar S, Syed Alwi SS, Chuan NO. Genetic determinants of variable anti-diabetic therapy responses across diverse populations with type 2 diabetes mellitus: a systematic review and meta-analysis. Diabetes Res Clin Pract. 2025;226:112337.

ABSTRACT

Aim: This study determines the best treatment combinations for glycemic control and investigates the connection between gene polymorphisms and glycemic responses across ethnic population. The comparability and interpretation of pooled data may be impacted by the different definitions of glycemic response used in the included trials (e.g., HbA1c <7% or >0.5% reduction).

Methods: For binary glycemic outcomes, pooled odds ratios (ORs) with 95% CI were employed; for continuous glycemic outcomes, pooled standardized mean differences (SMDs) with 95% CI were utilized. I and Cochran Q tests were used to evaluate heterogeneity.

Results: 36 studies including 10 genes and 34 SNPs were included out of the 43 papers that were screened. SLC22A1 rs622342, SLC47A2 rs12943590, TCF7L2 rs7903146, SLC22A1 rs12208357, and ABCC8 rs757110 were found to have significant correlations with improved glycemic response ($p < 0.05$). Biguanide monotherapy significantly reduced HbA1c in Arabian, Indian, Mestizo, and Persian populations ($p < 0.05$). Biguanide-sulfonylurea combination therapy also showed notable decreases in Arabian populations.

Conclusion: Genetic variations affect how different ethnic groups respond to antidiabetic medications. These results underline the necessity of individualized, genotype-guided treatment to enhance glycemic control. To investigate larger drug classifications and demographic aspects, more research is required.

CRITICAL APPRAISAL

Introduction and Study Rationale

Type 2 diabetes mellitus (T2DM) is a global health burden managed primarily through pharmacotherapy, with metformin serving as the first-line agent, often followed by sulfonylureas.[40] Despite standardized guidelines, inter-individual variability in therapeutic response is high; a significant proportion of patients fail to achieve glycemic targets despite adherence to therapy. Pharmacogenomics has long been investigated as a source of this variability, with variants in genes regulating drug pharmacokinetics (transporters like *SLC22A1*/OCT1) and pharmacodynamics (targets like *KCNJ11* and *ABCC8*) being prime candidates.[41]

However, the existing evidence base has historically been skewed toward European and Caucasian populations. Large-scale consortia, such as the Metformin Genetics Consortium (MetGen), have provided robust data for these groups, but findings have often been inconsistent when extrapolated to other ethnicities.[18] Asian, African, and Middle Eastern populations, who bear a disproportionate burden of T2DM, have been underrepresented in pharmacogenetic meta-analyses. Furthermore, prior reviews often struggled to reconcile contradictory results due to small sample sizes and diverse study designs, leaving a gap in understanding how ethnicity-specific genetic architecture influences drug efficacy.[40]

What this Study Adds to the Preexisting Knowledge

The study by Ahmad et al. (2025) significantly expands the pharmacogenomic landscape by systematically reviewing and meta-analyzing data specifically from diverse, non-Western populations, including Arabian, Indian, Mestizo, Persian, and African cohorts. By synthesizing data from 36 studies published between 2018 and 2024, the authors provide updated evidence on the impact of 34 single nucleotide polymorphisms (SNPs) across 10 genes.[40]

Key novel contributions include:

- *Validation of specific variants*: The meta-analysis confirmed significant associations between improved glycemic responses (HbA1c reduction) and specific variants: *SLC22A1* (rs622342, rs12208357), *SLC47A2* (rs12943590), *TCF7L2* (rs7903146), and *ABCC8* (rs757110).[40] Notably, for *SLC22A1* rs622342, the study found the CC genotype was associated with better HbA1c reduction, adding clarity to previously conflicting data regarding this variant.
- *Population-specific efficacy*: The study identified distinct population-based response patterns. For instance, Arabian, Indian, Mestizo, and Persian populations showed significant HbA1c reductions with biguanide monotherapy, whereas European cohorts in this specific analysis showed inconclusive results.[40] This underscores the "ethnicity effect" in pharmacotherapy.
- *Gene-drug interactions*: It reinforces the role of *TCF7L2*—traditionally a diabetes risk gene—as a pharmacogenetic marker, showing that the CC genotype at rs7903146 significantly improves HbA1c reduction compared to risk alleles, linking disease susceptibility genes directly to treatment outcomes.[40]

Major Strengths of this Study

- *Diverse population focus*: The primary strength is the explicit focus on non-European populations. By aggregating data from Indian, Pakistani, Arabian, and Mestizo groups, the study addresses a critical equity gap in precision medicine research.[40]
- *Rigorous methodology*: The authors employed a robust search strategy across five databases and utilized the Q-Genie tool to assess the quality of genetic association studies, ensuring that only studies with moderate-to-high methodological rigor were included in the synthesis.
- *Dual analytical strategy*: The use of three distinct meta-analysis strategies (Strategy A for continuous outcomes, Strategy B for binary "responder" outcomes, and Strategy C for treatment efficacy by population) allows for a nuanced interpretation of the data. This approach helps mitigate the loss of information that occurs when continuous data (HbA1c levels) is arbitrarily dichotomized into responders/nonresponders.
- *Comprehensive gene coverage*: The review covers the complete pharmacokinetic pathway of metformin (transporters *SLC22A1*, *SLC22A2*, and *SLC47A1/2*) and key targets for sulfonylureas (*ABCC8* and *KCNJ11*), providing a holistic view of relevant pharmacogenes.

Limitations of this Study

- *Heterogeneity of definitions*: A significant limitation acknowledged by the authors is the inconsistency in defining "glycemic response" across the included studies. Some studies used an absolute HbA1c reduction (e.g., >0.5%), while others used a target threshold (e.g., HbA1c <7%). This variation introduces noise into the binary meta-analysis (Strategy B) and complicates direct comparisons.[40]
- *Statistical heterogeneity*: High I^2 values (often >90%) were observed in several analyses, particularly in the population-specific treatment efficacy analysis (Strategy C). This suggests that unmeasured factors—such as diet, baseline BMI, and duration of diabetes—vary significantly between studies and influence the results beyond genetic factors.

- *Lack of newer drug classes*: The review focuses almost exclusively on metformin and sulfonylureas. While these remain foundational therapies, the lack of data on SGLT-2 inhibitors and GLP-1 receptor agonists limits the applicability of findings to modern, multidrug regimens.
- *Geographical gaps*: Despite the focus on diversity, the authors note a lack of representation from certain regions in specific analyses, and the "European" subgroup analysis yielded nonsignificant results in this specific dataset, which contrasts with other large Western cohorts, potentially due to the specific inclusion criteria of this review.[40]

Implication of Findings on Clinical Practice

The findings provide a stronger evidentiary basis for moving away from a "one-size-fits-all" approach to diabetes management in non-Western populations.

- *Personalized prescribing*: Clinicians treating patients of Arabian or South Asian descent should be aware that standard "Western" expectations of drug efficacy may not apply. The strong efficacy of biguanides in these groups supports their continued use as first-line agents, but genetic screening for *SLC22A1* or *TCF7L2* variants could identify nonresponders earlier, preventing therapeutic inertia.[40]
- *Targeted screening*: The identification of specific risk alleles (e.g., *TCF7L2* T-allele carriers) associated with poorer response suggests that these patients might benefit from earlier initiation of combination therapy or alternative drug classes, rather than waiting for monotherapy failure.
- *Guideline adaptation*: National guidelines in the represented regions (e.g., Middle East, South Asia) should consider incorporating pharmacogenetic data into their therapeutic algorithms as testing becomes more accessible.

Knowledge Gaps Identified and Future Scope for Research

- *Standardization of outcomes*: Future pharmacogenetic studies must adopt standardized definitions of "glycemic response" to facilitate accurate meta-analyses.
- *Expansion to modern therapies*: There is an urgent need to replicate this diverse-population approach for newer drug classes, specifically SGLT-2 inhibitors and GLP-1 receptor agonists, to see if similar ethnic-specific genetic determinants exist.
- *Cost-effectiveness studies*: While the study identifies *potential* genetic markers, research is needed to determine if pre-prescription genotyping is cost-effective in resource-limited settings typical of many of the studied populations.
- *Mechanism of ethnicity interaction*: Further basic science research is required to understand *why* certain populations (e.g., Arabian) show distinct responses—whether this is purely due to allele frequency differences or interactions with environmental factors like diet and microbiome.

9. Clinical Use of Polygenic Scores in Type 2 Diabetes: Challenges and Possibilities

Ref: Prasad RB, Hakaste L, Tuomi T. Clinical use of polygenic scores in type 2 diabetes: challenges and possibilities. Diabetologia. 2025;68(7):1361-74.

ABSTRACT

The single universal characteristic of type 2 diabetes, which is caused by a confluence of hereditary and environmental variables, is chronic hyperglycemia. The disease's appearance and course vary greatly. Biomarkers and techniques for disease stratification, prevention, and treatment are still lacking despite intense efforts to clarify the pathogenetic origins and natural course of the illness. Over 1,200 variants have been linked to type 2 diabetes according to genome-wide association studies, and the lower cost of producing genetic data has made it easier to create polygenic scores, which combine the effects of most or all genetic variants to estimate a person's genetic disease risk. In this review, we explain the potential clinical importance of type 2 diabetes-related polygenic scores in various ancestries and summarize the existing understanding of these scores. We investigate how type 2 diabetes polygenic scores could be used to measure genetic susceptibility for risk assessment, screening, and prediction. We also address the difficulties with their worldwide applicability because the majority of genetic risk loci are identified from populations of European descent while other ancestries are underrepresented. Polygenic scores for type 2 diabetes have minimal clinical usefulness to date; clinical measures exceed these ratings. In the future, polygenic scores may be useful in stratifying the severity of diabetes (risk for comorbidities) and treatment response, in addition to helping to analyze the pathophysiological mechanisms involved, rather than in forecasting the risk of type 2 diabetes.

CRITICAL APPRAISAL

Introduction and Study Rationale

Type 2 diabetes (T2D) is a heterogeneous condition driven by a complex interplay of genetic and environmental factors. Historically, clinical risk prediction models have relied on phenotypic variables such as age, body mass index (BMI), family history, and glycemic markers (HbA1c).[42] While effective, these models often fail to capture the biological heterogeneity of the disease, particularly in individuals who do not fit the classic "older and obese" phenotype, such as lean individuals or those with early onset disease.

Over the past two decades, genome-wide association studies (GWAS) have identified over 1,200 genomic variants associated with T2D.[42] This wealth of data facilitated the development of polygenic scores (PGS), which aggregate the small effect sizes of thousands (or millions) of genetic variants into a single score to estimate an individual's lifetime genetic susceptibility. Early PGSs were derived primarily from populations of European ancestry, leading to significant "Eurocentric bias" and poor transferability to non-European populations, such as those of African, Asian, or Hispanic descent.[42] Furthermore, while PGSs showed statistical association with T2D risk, their added clinical value over simple, noninvasive metrics like BMI and family history has been a subject of ongoing debate. It remained unclear whether PGS could effectively guide clinical decision-making, such as screening intervals or treatment selection, or if they were merely research tools describing heritability.

What this Study Adds to the Preexisting Knowledge

The review by Prasad et al. (2025) synthesizes the latest evidence on the clinical utility of PGSs, moving beyond simple risk prediction to more nuanced applications in precision medicine.

- *Partitioned polygenic scores (pPS)*: The authors highlight the shift from global PGSs to "partitioned" or "cluster-specific" scores. By grouping genetic variants based on their association with specific physiological traits (e.g., beta-cell dysfunction, insulin resistance, and lipodystrophy), pPS can classify patients into mechanistic subtypes.[42] This adds a biological layer to the clinical diagnosis, potentially identifying patients who primarily have a secretory defect versus those with insulin resistance, independent of their clinical presentation.
- *Utility in specific subgroups*: The study clarifies *where* PGSs perform best. While global T2D-PGSs add limited value to prediction models for the general middle-aged population compared to BMI and HbA1c, the authors present evidence that

PGSs are particularly valuable for *younger individuals and lean populations* (common in Asia) where traditional risk factors are absent.[42] For example, a high T2D-PGS was shown to strongly predict diabetes in lean individuals, suggesting a distinct, genetically driven pathophysiology in this group that clinical metrics might miss.

- *Ancestry-specific insights*: The review explicitly addresses the performance of PGSs across diverse ancestries. It highlights that while European-derived scores often fail in other groups, integrating ancestry-specific variants (e.g., *PAX4* in East Asians, *HNF1A* in Latin Americans) significantly improves predictive power.[42]

Major Strengths of this Study

- *Comprehensive ancestry focus*: A major strength is the critical examination of PGS performance in non-European populations. The authors do not simply report the lack of data but actively synthesize findings from recent multi-ancestry GWAS (including the 2024 Nature study by Suzuki et al.) to demonstrate how population-specific genetic architecture influences risk prediction.[42,43] This directly addresses a major equity gap in genomic medicine.
- *Integration of clinical and genetic clustering*: The authors successfully bridge the gap between "hard" genetic clustering (based solely on genotypes) and "soft" clinical clustering (like the SIDD/SIRD subtypes). By mapping genetic pathways (e.g., the lipodystrophy cluster) to clinical outcomes (e.g., cardiovascular disease), they provide a framework for how genetics could biologically validate clinical subtypes.[42]
- *Pragmatic clinical perspective*: Unlike many genetic reviews that focus on statistical power, this paper adopts a translational lens. It evaluates PGSs against the gold standard of current clinical practice (e.g., QDiabetes score), honestly acknowledging that for the "average" patient, clinical factors currently outperform genetics. This balanced view prevents overhyping the technology while identifying its niche uses.[42]

Limitations of this Study

- *Reliance on aggregate data*: As a narrative review, the study synthesizes existing literature rather than conducting a new meta-analysis. Therefore, it is limited by the quality and heterogeneity of the primary studies available, which often use different methods to calculate and weight PGSs (e.g., LDpred vs. clumping + thresholding), making direct comparisons difficult.[42]
- *Lack of prospective trial data*: The authors acknowledge a paucity of randomized controlled trials (RCTs) testing whether disclosing PGS results actually changes clinical outcomes or patient behaviors. Most evidence cited is observational or retrospective. Consequently, the claim that PGSs *could* guide treatment selection remains largely theoretical rather than proven by interventional data.
- *Complexity of "missing heritability"*: The review notes that current known variants explain only ~50% of T2D heritability.[42] This inherent ceiling limits the maximum potential accuracy of any PGS. The review discusses this but cannot overcome the fact that a significant portion of genetic risk remains "dark matter," potentially involving rare variants or structural variations not captured in standard arrays.

Implication of Findings on Clinical Practice

- *Shift from screening to stratification*: The authors suggest the immediate future of PGS is not in mass screening for T2D risk (where HbA1c is cheaper and sufficient), but in *risk stratification* for complications. For instance, a patient with a high "lipodystrophy cluster" score might be flagged for aggressive cardiovascular monitoring regardless of their current lipid levels.[42]
- *Differentiation of diabetes types*: In clinical practice, PGSs can serve as a tool for *negative prediction* or "elimination." A low T2D-PGS in a young, lean patient with hyperglycemia might prompt a clinician

to screen for monogenic diabetes (MODY) or Latent Autoimmune Diabetes (LADA), thereby preventing misdiagnosis.[42]

- *Targeting early intervention*: For younger adults (<40 years) who have not yet developed the phenotypic markers of metabolic syndrome (high BMI, hypertension), a high PGS could justify earlier, intensive lifestyle interventions before clinical risk factors emerge. This supports a move toward "primordial prevention" in high-genetic-risk families.

Knowledge Gaps Identified and Future Scope for Research

- *Gene-environment interactions*: The review identifies a critical gap in understanding how PGSs interact with environmental factors (diet, physical activity, and pollution) across different cultures.[42] Future research must determine if high genetic risk can be completely negated by lifestyle, or if "genetic determinism" exists for certain high-risk clusters.
- *Pharmacogenomics of PGS*: While single-gene pharmacogenetics (e.g., *SLC22A1* and metformin) is studied, the utility of *polygenic* scores to predict drug response is largely unexplored. Research is needed to test if specific partitioned PGSs (e.g., beta-cell dysfunction cluster) predict better responses to specific drug classes (e.g., GLP-1 receptor agonists vs. SGLT-2 inhibitors).[42]
- *Health economics*: There is a lack of cost-effectiveness analyses. Future studies must evaluate whether the cost of genotyping and calculating PGSs yields sufficient savings in avoided complications or more efficient treatments to justify reimbursement by healthcare systems, particularly in low-resource settings where the diabetes burden is growing fastest.[42]

10. A Type 1 Diabetes Genetic Risk Score Discriminates between Type 1 Diabetes and Type 2 Diabetes in a Chinese Population

Ref: Hu J, Jiang G, Qin J, Luo S, Fan B, Xie Z, et al. A type 1 diabetes genetic risk score discriminates between type 1 diabetes and type 2 diabetes in a Chinese population. Diabetologia. 2025;68(9):1969-82.

ABSTRACT

Aim/Hypothesis: Our goal was to create a community-specific type 1 diabetes genetic risk score (GRS) and evaluate its potential to enhance the ability to distinguish between type 1 and type 2 diabetes in a Chinese population.

Techniques: We conducted a genome-wide association study on 2,236 control subjects and 1,303 subjects with type 1 diabetes. The top common variant relationships were validated using an independent replication cohort of 501 type 1 diabetics and 853 controls. Tag SNPs for DQA1-DQB1 haplotypes were found using HLA typing data. To create a Chinese type 1 diabetes GRS (C-GRS), we combined important signals. An independent validation cohort of 262 persons with type 1 diabetes, 1,080 patients with type 2 diabetes, and 208 control individuals was used to test the accuracy of the C-GRS.

Outcomes: A mutation in BMPER, rs10232170, was found to represent a potential novel type 1 diabetes locus ($p = 9.897 \times 10^{-9}$). Twelve non-DQA1-DQB1 locations and thirteen DQA1-DQB1 haplotypes had tag SNPs found. C-GRS showed good discriminative power for type 1 diabetes by integrating 33 important SNPs from HLA and non-HLA areas (AUC = 0.876). It demonstrated good discrimination when tested in a separate validation cohort (AUC 0.871 for type 1 diabetes versus control group, 0.869 for type 1 diabetes versus type 2 diabetes). The C-GRS outperformed a European-derived GRS (0.871 vs. 0.773 and 0.869 vs. 0.793, respectively).

Conclusion and interpretation: In the Chinese population, a type 1 diabetes C-GRS with 33 SNPs was highly discriminative of type 1 diabetes risk and might help distinguish between type 1 and type 2 diabetes. This study demonstrates how genetic data may help to and accurately diagnose type 1 diabetes in the Chinese population.

Data accessibility: Under accession number PRJCA023730, the raw sequencing data and summary statistics of genomic DNA obtained from human samples have been submitted to the China National Center for Bioinformation (https://ngdc.cncb.ac.cn/omix).

CRITICAL APPRAISAL

Introduction and Study Rationale

Type 1 diabetes (T1D) is an autoimmune disease characterized by the destruction of pancreatic beta-cells, resulting in absolute insulin deficiency. While traditionally considered a childhood disease, a significant proportion of T1D cases present in adulthood, where they are frequently misdiagnosed as type 2 diabetes (T2D) due to the high prevalence of T2D and overlapping clinical features such as obesity.[44] Accurately distinguishing between T1D and T2D is critical because T1D requires immediate insulin therapy to prevent diabetic ketoacidosis, whereas T2D is often managed initially with lifestyle changes and oral agents. Current diagnostic methods rely on clinical features (age and BMI) and biomarkers like islet autoantibodies and C-peptide. However, autoantibodies can be negative in a subset of T1D (idiopathic T1D) or present in T2D, and C-peptide levels can be ambiguous in early disease.[45]

Genetic risk scores (GRS) derived from genome-wide association studies (GWAS) have emerged as powerful tools to aid classification. A GRS aggregates the effects of multiple risk alleles (predominantly in the HLA region) into a single score. The T1D GRS developed for populations of European ancestry (e.g., GRS1 and GRS2) has shown excellent discrimination (AUC >0.90) and clinical utility.[46] However, genetic architecture varies significantly across ancestries. The HLA haplotypes driving T1D risk in Europeans (e.g., *DRB1*03-DQB1*02* and *DRB1*04-DQB1*03:02*) differ from those in East Asian populations, where haplotypes like *DRB1*09:01-DQB1*03:03* are prominent.[47] Consequently, European-derived GRSs perform poorly in non-European populations.[48] Prior to this study, a validated, population-specific T1D GRS for the Chinese population—who account for one-fifth of the global population—was lacking.

What this Study Adds to the Preexisting Knowledge

The study by Qin et al. (2025) addresses this gap by conducting a two-stage GWAS in a Chinese cohort to develop and validate a Chinese-specific T1D genetic risk score (C-GRS).[49]

- *Novel genetic discoveries*: The study identified a potential novel susceptibility locus, *BMPER* (rs10232170), which reached genome-wide significance in the meta-analysis ($p = 9.897 \times 10^9$), although it did not replicate in the independent cohort. This gene is involved in the BMP signaling pathway, suggesting a new mechanism potentially relevant to beta-cell regulation.[49]
- *Population-specific HLA tagging*: The authors successfully identified single nucleotide polymorphisms (SNPs) that "tag" (serve as proxies for) 13 specific HLA DQA1-DQB1 haplotypes and 12 non-DQA1-DQB1 HLA loci in the Chinese population. This allows for accurate capture of HLA risk

using simple genotyping arrays rather than expensive high-resolution HLA typing.[49]

- *Development of the C-GRS:* By integrating 33 SNPs (from both HLA and non-HLA regions), the authors constructed the C-GRS. This score demonstrated high discriminative power for T1D versus controls (AUC = 0.876).[49]
- *Improved clinical classification*: Crucially, the C-GRS significantly outperformed the European-derived GRS2 in discriminating T1D from T2D in an independent Chinese validation cohort (AUC 0.869 vs. 0.793). This confirms that ancestry-specific tailoring is essential for clinical utility.[49]
- *Phenotypic correlation*: A high C-GRS was associated with classic T1D features: earlier age of onset, lower BMI, lower C-peptide levels, and multiple autoantibody positivity, validating its biological relevance.[49]

Major Strengths of this Study

- *Rigorous study design*: The study utilized a multistage design comprising a discovery cohort, an external replication cohort (from Hong Kong), and a separate validation cohort including T2D patients. This robust structure minimizes the risk of false-positive associations and overfitting.[49]
- *Ancestry-specific optimization*: Unlike previous studies that simply applied Western scores to Asian cohorts, this study built the score *de novo* from Chinese GWAS data. This ensured that the unique linkage disequilibrium patterns of the Chinese HLA region were correctly captured.
- *Direct clinical validation*: The inclusion of a large T2D control group (n = 1,080) in the validation phase is a major strength. Demonstrating discrimination between T1D and T2D is clinically more valuable than distinguishing T1D from healthy controls, as this is the specific diagnostic dilemma clinicians face.[49]
- *Integration of HLA typing*: The use of classical HLA typing data to validate the tag SNPs ensures that the GRS accurately reflects the underlying immunogenetic risk, bridging the gap between genotype and serotype.[49]

Limitations of this Study

- *Cross-sectional design*: As acknowledged by the authors, the study is cross-sectional. Therefore, it establishes associations but cannot prospectively predict the development of T1D in at-risk individuals or determine how the GRS performs in predicting progression from autoimmunity to overt diabetes.[49]
- *Sample size*: While large for a T1D study in this specific population, the sample size (total T1D cases approximately 2,000) is relatively small compared to European consortia (often >20,000 cases). This limited power may explain why the novel *BMPER* signal failed to replicate in the second cohort and suggests other minor risk loci may have been missed.[49]
- *Generalizability within Asia*: While termed a "Chinese" GRS, the study primarily recruited Han Chinese participants. Its applicability to other East Asian populations (e.g., Japanese, Korean) or other Chinese ethnic minorities remains to be fully verified, although genetic overlap is likely high.
- *Novel locus uncertainty*: The *BMPER* variant was not replicated in the independent cohort, meaning its status as a true T1D risk gene remains provisional and requires further confirmation in larger meta-analyses.[49]

Implication of Findings on Clinical Practice

This study represents a significant step toward precision medicine for diabetes in East Asia.

- *Diagnostic adjunct*: The C-GRS can currently be used as a supportive diagnostic tool in Chinese adults with ambiguous diabetes presentations (e.g., non-obese adults who are autoantibody-negative). A high C-GRS would strongly support a diagnosis of T1D or Latent Autoimmune Diabetes in Adults (LADA), potentially justifying earlier insulin therapy.[49]

- *Re-classification of patients*: The score could help identify patients currently misdiagnosed as T2D who actually have T1D, preventing complications like diabetic ketoacidosis. The defined cut-off values (>1.211 for T1D specificity) provide a tangible metric for clinicians.[49]
- *Cost-effectiveness*: SNP genotyping is inexpensive and stable over a lifetime. This offers a potentially cost-effective alternative or add-on to autoantibody screening, particularly in resource-limited settings where comprehensive autoantibody panels may be expensive or unavailable.[46,49]

Knowledge Gaps Identified and Future Scope for Research

- *Trans-ancestry integration:* Future research should aim to combine this Chinese dataset with European and other Asian datasets to create a "trans-ancestry" GRS. Such a tool would be robust for individuals of mixed heritage, a growing demographic globally.[47]
- *Prospective prediction:* Longitudinal studies are needed to assess whether the C-GRS can predict determining which autoantibody-positive individuals will progress to clinical diabetes, similar to how GRS2 is used in European newborn screening studies.[49]
- *Functional characterization of BMPER*: The identification of *BMPER* as a potential risk locus opens a new avenue for mechanistic research. Investigating how the Bone Morphogenetic Protein pathway interacts with immune regulation or beta-cell survival could reveal novel therapeutic targets.[49]
- *Integration with clinical models*: Future studies should develop composite risk models that combine the C-GRS with clinical features (BMI and age) and biomarkers (C-peptide) to create a unified diagnostic probability score for clinicians.

11. Birthweight and Risk of Chronic Kidney Disease after a Type 2 Diabetes Diagnosis in the DD2 Cohort

Ref: Hansen AL, Christiansen CF, Brøns C, Engelhard LM, Hansen T, Nielsen JS, et al. Birthweight and risk of chronic kidney disease after a type 2 diabetes diagnosis in the DD2 cohort. Diabetologia. 2025;68(4):778-91.

ABSTRACT

Aim/Hypothesis: Among those who have recently been diagnosed with type 2 diabetes, low birthweight (LBW) is linked to younger age, lower obesity, higher HTN among people diagnosed with type 2 diabetes, and a higher risk of cardiovascular morbidity and death. Whether LBW is linked to a higher risk of incident chronic kidney disease (CKD) in individuals with type 2 diabetes is unknown.

Techniques: For 5,982 individuals with newly diagnosed type 2 diabetes who were enrolled in the Danish Center for Strategic Research in Type 2 Diabetes (DD2) cohort between 2010 and 2024, original midwife records were obtained. They were monitored until the first incidence CKD diagnosis, which was determined by two eGFR readings of 3 mg/mmol spaced 90–365 days apart. Death was taken into account as a competing risk when estimating the confounder-standardized 10-year risks of CKD. Cox and spline regression analyses were used to calculate adjusted hazard ratios (aHRs) for CKD. Differences in sex, age at enrollment, birth year, family history of diabetes, and born-at-term status were taken into account in all analyses. The trajectories of eGFR and UACR after enrollment were investigated using mixed-effects models.

Results: Over a median follow-up period of 8.3 years, there were 1,501 incident CKD endpoints, or an incidence rate of 42.4 per 1,000 person-years. aHRs for CKD gradually increased as birthweight decreased, according to spline models using birthweight as a continuous metric. People with LBW (<2,500 g) had a 10-year standardized risk of CKD of 36.0%, which was comparable to those with normal (2,500–4,000 g) (33.1% and 30.6%, respectively). This resulted in an aHR of 1.10 (95% CI 0.93, 1.29) and an RD of 2.5% (95% CI −1.6%, 6.7%). High birthweight (>4,000 g) was associated with a slightly elevated risk of CKD and had a similar 10-year standardized CKD risk compared with normal birthweight (33.1% and 30.6%, respectively). A 1-kg drop in birthweight was linked to a 6.6% (95% CI 1.9, 11.1) increase in UACR in mixed-effects models analyzing eGFR and UACR trajectories, while there was no correlation for eGFR.

Conclusion and interpretation: Although the accuracy of risk estimations was limited, a history of LBW was linked to an increased risk of CKD among individuals with a recent diagnosis of type 2 diabetes.

CRITICAL APPRAISAL

Introduction and Study Rationale

The concept of "fetal programming" or the Barker hypothesis suggests that adverse conditions during fetal development can predispose individuals to chronic diseases in adulthood.[50] Low birthweight (LBW), often used as a proxy for a restricted intrauterine environment, has been well-established as a risk factor for hypertension, cardiovascular disease (CVD), and type 2 diabetes (T2D) in the general population.[51] Specifically regarding renal health, the "Brenner hypothesis" posits that LBW is associated with a congenital deficit in nephron number (oligonephronia). This deficit leads to compensatory glomerular hyperfiltration in the remaining nephrons, eventually causing glomerulosclerosis and chronic kidney disease (CKD).[52]

While the association between LBW and CKD is recognized in the general population and those with type 1 diabetes, the evidence within the specific population of individuals with type 2 diabetes is limited. Previous research has shown that among people with T2D, those with LBW exhibit a distinct phenotype characterized by earlier disease onset, lower body mass index (BMI), and higher prevalence of hypertension and CVD.[50] However, whether LBW acts as an independent risk amplifier for incident CKD *after* a diagnosis of T2D—a condition already characterized by high renal risk—remained under-investigated prior to this study.

What this Study Adds to the Preexisting Knowledge

The study by Hansen et al. (2025) investigates the association between birthweight and the risk of incident CKD in a large cohort of 5,982 individuals recently diagnosed with T2D.[50]

- *Elevated risk profile*: The study found that individuals with LBW (<2,500 g) had a 10-year standardized risk of CKD of 36.0%, compared to 30.6% in those with normal birthweight (2,500–4,000 g). This corresponds to an adjusted hazard ratio (aHR) of 1.23, suggesting an elevated risk, although statistical precision was limited.[50]
- *Continuous association*: Using spline models, the authors demonstrated a progressive increase in CKD risk with decreasing birthweight, reinforcing the biological plausibility of the association beyond arbitrary cut-offs.
- *Albuminuria versus eGFR*: A key novel finding from the trajectory modeling is that the increased risk is primarily driven by elevated urine albumin-to-creatinine ratio (UACR) rather than a decline in estimated glomerular filtration rate (eGFR). Each 1 kg decrease in birthweight was associated with a 6.6% increase in UACR.[50] Crucially, this elevation in albuminuria was present at the time of diabetes diagnosis and did not accelerate faster than in normal birthweight individuals over time, suggesting a constitutive structural deficit rather than an accelerated degenerative process.[50]

- *High birthweight signal*: The study also noted a U-shaped relationship in men, where high birthweight (>4,000 g) was associated with a slightly elevated risk of CKD, extending the understanding of fetal programming to both extremes of fetal growth.[50]

Major Strengths of this Study

- *Data validity*: A significant strength is the use of original midwife records to ascertain birthweight, eliminating recall bias which is a common limitation in adult epidemiological studies of birth outcomes.[50]
- *Study design*: The prospective cohort design within the Danish Center for Strategic Research in Type 2 Diabetes (DD2) allowed for the analysis of *incident* CKD in a well-characterized "real-world" population of newly diagnosed T2D patients.[50]
- *Sophisticated modeling:* The use of mixed-effects models to analyze the separate trajectories of eGFR and UACR provides granular insight into the specific phenotype of kidney dysfunction (albuminuria vs. filtration failure) associated with LBW.[50]
- *Robust statistical handling*: The authors employed rigorous statistical methods, including competing risk analyses (accounting for death) and the G-formula for standardization, ensuring that the absolute risk estimates are clinically relevant and adjusted for confounding structures.[50]

Limitations of this Study

- *Statistical precision:* Despite the large cohort, the number of individuals with LBW (<2,500 g) was relatively small (n = 427), leading to wide confidence intervals for the primary hazard ratios (95% CI 0.98, 1.55), which crossed unity in some analyses. This limits the ability to definitively claim statistical significance for the binary comparison.[50]
- *Creatinine confounding*: The study relied on creatinine-based eGFR and UACR. Since LBW is associated with reduced muscle mass, creatinine generation may be lower in these individuals. This could lead to an overestimation of eGFR (masking renal decline) and an overestimation of UACR (due to lower urinary creatinine), potentially confounding the specific findings regarding the dissociation between eGFR and albuminuria.[50]
- *Generalizability*: The cohort consisted of a Danish population, which is predominantly White. The findings may not be directly generalizable to other ethnicities, such as South Asians, who have different body composition profiles and risks for LBW and T2D.[50]
- *Lack of pre-diabetes data*: As the cohort was enrolled at the time of T2D diagnosis, it is impossible to determine if the renal damage (albuminuria) began during the pre-diabetic phase or earlier in life.[50]

Implication of Findings on Clinical Practice

These findings suggest that birthweight is a relevant, albeit often overlooked, stratification factor in the management of type 2 diabetes.

- *Risk stratification:* Clinicians should consider asking about birthweight when assessing T2D patients. Patients with a history of LBW may represent a distinct "high-risk" phenotype for diabetic nephropathy, characterized by early albuminuria.[50]
- *Early intervention:* The observation that UACR is elevated from baseline suggests that renal protective therapies (e.g., ACE inhibitors/ARBs, SGLT-2 inhibitors) might need to be initiated earlier or more aggressively in LBW patients to manage intraglomerular pressure, even if their eGFR appears preserved.[50]
- *Phenotypic awareness:* The study highlights that LBW patients often present with T2D at a younger age and with lower BMI. Clinicians should not assume low renal risk in lean T2D patients, as their risk may be driven by congenital nephron deficits rather than obesity-related hyperfiltration.[50]

Knowledge Gaps Identified and Future Scope for Research

- *Muscle mass correction*: Future studies should utilize cystatin C-based eGFR measurements to validate these findings.

This would determine if the lack of association with eGFR is real or an artifact of low muscle mass in LBW individuals masking a decline in filtration function.[50]

- *Mechanistic pathways:* Further research is needed to elucidate the biological mechanisms linking LBW to albuminuria specifically. Determining whether this is purely hemodynamic (hyperfiltration in fewer nephrons) or related to podocyte structural defects is crucial for targeted therapy.[50]
- *Sex-specific differences:* The finding of a U-shaped risk curve (high risk for high birthweight) in males but not females warrants further investigation to understand the sex-specific interactions between fetal growth and adult renal health.[50]
- *Diverse populations:* Replication of this study in non-White populations with high prevalences of both LBW and T2D (e.g., South Asian cohorts) is essential to establish global applicability.[50]

REFERENCES (Epidemiology)

1. Lee MMY, Kristensen SL, Khan N, Kang YM, Rutter MK, Gerstein HC, et al. Glucagon-Like Peptide 1 Receptor Agonists and Cardiovascular Outcomes in Asian Versus White Patients: A Systematic Review and Meta-analysis of Randomized Controlled Trials. Diabetes Care. 2025;48(1): 123-32.
2. Yoon KH, Lee JH, Kim JW, Cho JH, Choi YH, Ko SH, et al. Epidemic obesity and type 2 diabetes in Asia. Lancet. 2006;368(9548):1681-8.
3. Kang J, Heo SJ, Park KS, et al. Glucagon-like peptide-1 receptor agonists and cardiovascular outcomes in patients with type 2 diabetes: A meta-analysis of Asian patients. Diabetes Metab J. 2019;43(3):368-76.
4. Kristensen SL, Rørth R, Jhund PS, Docherty KF, Sattar N, Preiss D, et al. Cardiovascular, mortality, and kidney outcomes with GLP-1 receptor agonists in patients with type 2 diabetes: a systematic review and meta-analysis of cardiovascular outcome trials. Lancet Diabetes Endocrinol. 2019;7(10):776-85.
5. McGuire DK, Shih WJ, Cosentino F, Charbonnel B, Cherney DZI, Dagogo-Jack S, et al. Association of SGLT2 Inhibitors with Cardiovascular and Kidney Outcomes in Patients with Type 2 Diabetes: A Meta-analysis. JAMA Cardiol. 2021;6(2):148-58.
6. Sattar N, Lee MMY, Kristensen SL, Branch KRH, Del Prato S, Khurmi NS, et al. Cardiovascular, mortality, and kidney outcomes with GLP-1 receptor agonists in patients with type 2 diabetes: a systematic review and meta-analysis of randomised controlled trials. Lancet Diabetes Endocrinol. 2021;9(10):653-62.
7. U.K. Prospective Diabetes Study Group. U.K. Prospective Diabetes Study 16: overview of 6 years' therapy of type II diabetes: a progressive disease. Diabetes. 1995;44: 1249-58.
8. Wajchenberg BL. Beta-cell failure in diabetes and preservation by clinical treatment. Endocr Rev. 2007;28:187-218.
9. Rasouli N, Younes N, Ghosh A, Albu J, Cohen RM, DeFronzo RA, et al. Longitudinal effects of glucose-lowering medications on beta cell responses and insulin sensitivity in type 2 diabetes: the GRADE randomized clinical trial. Diabetes Care. 2024;47:580-8.
10. Mari A, Schmitz O, Gastaldelli A, Oestergaard T, Nyholm B, Ferrannini E. Meal and oral glucose tests for assessment of beta-cell function: modeling analysis in normal subjects. Am J Physiol Endocrinol Metab. 2002;283:E1159-66.
11. Nathan DM, Buse JB, Kahn SE, Krause-Steinrauf H, Larkin ME, Staten M, et al. Rationale and design of the Glycemia Reduction Approaches in Diabetes: A Comparative Effectiveness Study (GRADE). Diabetes Care. 2013;36:2254-61.
12. Utzschneider KM, Tripputi M, Butera NM, Mari A, Rosin SP, Banerji MA, et al. Differential Treatment Effects on beta-Cell Function Using Model-Based Parameters in Type 2 Diabetes: Results From the Glycemia Reduction Approaches in Diabetes: A Comparative Effectiveness Study (GRADE). Diabetes Care. 2025;48(4):623-31.
13. Lee MMY, Ghouri N, Misra A, Kang YM, Rutter MK, Gerstein HC, et al. Comparative Efficacy of Glucagon-Like Peptide 1 Receptor Agonists for Cardiovascular Outcomes in Asian Versus White Populations. Diabetes Care. 2025;48(3): 489-93.
14. American Diabetes Association. Standards of Care in Diabetes—2025. Diabetes Care. 2025;48(Suppl 1):S27-S49.
15. Bizzotto R, Jennison C, Jones AG, Kurbasic A, Tura A, Kennedy G, et al. Processes underlying glycemic deterioration in type 2 diabetes: an IMI DIRECT study. Diabetes Care. 2021;44:511-8.
16. Ahlqvist E, Prasad RB, Groop L. Subtypes of Type 2 Diabetes Determined From Clinical Parameters. Diabetes. 2020;69(10):2086-93.
17. Knowler WC, Barrett-Connor E, Fowler SE, Hamman RF, Lachin JM, Walker EA, et al. Diabetes Prevention Program Research Group. Reduction in the incidence of type 2

diabetes with lifestyle intervention or metformin. N Engl J Med. 2002;346(6):393-403.

18. Diabetes Prevention Program Research Group. Long-term effects of lifestyle intervention or metformin on diabetes development and microvascular complications over 15-year follow-up: the Diabetes Prevention Program Outcomes Study. Lancet Diabetes Endocrinol. 2015;3(11):866-75.
19. Knowler WC, Pan Q, Shu S, Tripputi MT, Dabelea D, Edelstein SL, et al. Analysis of Long-term Follow-up of a Randomized Clinical Trial With Departures From Assigned Treatments: Estimation of Metformin Effects on Diabetes and Its Complications in the Diabetes Prevention Program Outcomes Study. Diabetes Care. 2025;48(10):1668-75.
20. Tuomilehto J, Lindström J, Eriksson JG, Valle TT, Hämäläinen H, Ilanne-Parikka P, et al. Prevention of type 2 diabetes mellitus by changes in lifestyle among subjects with impaired glucose tolerance. N Engl J Med. 2001;344(18):1343-50.
21. Gong Q, Zhang P, Wang J, Ma J, An Y, Chen Y, et al. Morbidity and mortality after lifestyle intervention for people with impaired glucose tolerance: 30-year results of the Da Qing Diabetes Prevention Outcome Study. Lancet Diabetes Endocrinol. 2019;7(6):452-61.
22. Knowler WC, Doherty L, Edelstein SL, Bennett PH, Dabelea D, Hoskin M, et al. Long-term effects and effect heterogeneity of lifestyle and metformin interventions on type 2 diabetes incidence over 21 years in the US Diabetes Prevention Program randomised clinical trial. Lancet Diabetes Endocrinol. 2025;13(6):469-81.
23. Sepassi A, Wang J, Yankowski S, Enkoji A, Okenwa M, Morello CM, et al. Associations between long-term metformin use, the risk of vitamin B12 deficiency, and neuropathy: An All of Us research Program study. Diabetes Res Clin Pract. 2025;228:112424.
24. Infante M, Leoni M, Caprio M, Fabbri A. Long-term metformin therapy and vitamin B12 deficiency: An association to bear in mind. World J Diabetes. 2021;12(7):916-31.
25. Bauman WA, Shaw S, Jayatilleke E, Spungen AM, Herbert V. Increased intake of calcium reverses vitamin B12 malabsorption induced by metformin. Diabetes Care. 2000;23(9):1227-31.
26. Langan RC, Goodbred AJ. Vitamin B12 Deficiency: Recognition and Management. Am Fam Physician. 2017;96(6):384-9.
27. Bell DSH. Metformin-induced vitamin B12 deficiency can cause or worsen distal symmetrical, autonomic and cardiac neuropathy in the patient with diabetes. Diabetes Obes Metab. 2022;24(8):1423-8.
28. Aroda VR, Edelstein SL, Goldberg RB, Knowler WC, Marcovina SM, Orchard TJ, et al. Long-term Metformin Use and Vitamin B12 Deficiency in the Diabetes Prevention Program Outcomes Study. J Clin Endocrinol Metab. 2016;101(4): 1754-61.
29. Ahmed MA, Muntingh G, Rheeder P. Vitamin B12 deficiency in metformin-treated type-2 diabetes patients, prevalence and association with peripheral neuropathy. BMC Pharmacol Toxicol. 2016;17(1):44.
30. The All of Us Research Program Investigators. The "All of Us" Research Program. N Engl J Med. 2019;381(7):668-76.
31. Carino M, New RH, Nguyen J, Kirkham R, Maple-Brown L, Titmuss A, et al. Non-pharmacological management strategies for type 2 diabetes in children and young adults: A systematic review. Diabetes Res Clin Pract. 2025;222: 112045.
32. TODAY Study Group. A clinical trial to maintain glycemic control in youth with type 2 diabetes. N Engl J Med. 2012;366(24):2247-56.
33. Copeland KC, Silverstein J, Moore KR, Prazar GE, Raymer T, Shiffman RN, et al. Management of newly diagnosed type 2 Diabetes Mellitus (T2DM) in children and adolescents. Pediatrics. 2013;131(2):364-82.
34. Song Y, Wang L, Pittas AG, Del Gobbo LC, Zhang C, Manson JE, et al. Blood 25-hydroxy vitamin D levels and incident type 2 diabetes: a meta-analysis of prospective studies. Diabetes Care. 2013;36(5):1422-8.
35. Sung CC, Liao MT, Lu KC, Wu CC. Role of Vitamin D in Insulin Resistance. J Biomed Biotechnol. 2012;2012:634195.
36. Pittas AG, Jorde R, Kawahara T, Dawson-Hughes B. Vitamin D Supplementation for Prevention of Type 2 Diabetes Mellitus: To D or Not to D? J Clin Endocrinol Metab. 2020;105(12):3721-33.
37. Kawahara T, Suzuki G, Mizuno S, Inazu T, Kasagi F, Kawahara C, et al. Effect of active vitamin D treatment on development of type 2 diabetes: DPVD randomised controlled trial in Japanese population. BMJ. 2022;377:e066222.
38. Zhang Y, Tan H, Tang J, Li J, Chong W, Hai Y, et al. Effects of Vitamin D Supplementation on Prevention of Type 2 Diabetes in Patients With Prediabetes: A Systematic Review and Meta-analysis. Diabetes Care. 2020;43(7):1650-8.
39. Virtanen JK, Hantunen S, Kallio N, Lamberg-Allardt C, Manson JE, Nurmi T, et al. The effect of vitamin D3 supplementation on the incidence of type 2 diabetes in healthy older adults not at high risk for diabetes (FIND): a randomised controlled trial. Diabetologia. 2025;68:715-26.
40. Ahmad F, Abubakar S, Alwi SSS, Chuan NO. Genetic determinants of variable anti-diabetic therapy responses across diverse populations with type 2 diabetes mellitus: a systematic review and meta-analysis. Diabetes Res Clin Pract. 2025;226:112337.
41. Pearson ER. Pharmacogenetics of the treatment of type 2 diabetes: is there a clinical application? Curr Diab Rep. 2016;16(11):110.
42. Prasad RB, Hakaste L, Tuomi T. Clinical use of polygenic scores in type 2 diabetes: challenges and possibilities. Diabetologia. 2025;68:1361-74.
43. Suzuki K, Hatzikotoulas K, Southam L, Taylor HJ, Yin X, Lorenz KM, et al. Genetic drivers of heterogeneity in type 2 diabetes pathophysiology. Nature. 2024;627:347-57.
44. Thomas NJ, Lynam AL, Hill AV, Weedon MN, Shields BM, Oram RA, et al. Type 1 diabetes defined by severe insulin deficiency occurs after 30 years of age and is commonly treated as type 2 diabetes. Diabetologia. 2019;62(7): 1167-72.

45. Hope SV, Wienand-Barnett S, Shepherd M, King SM, Fox C, Khunti K, et al. Practical Classification Guidelines for Diabetes in patients treated with insulin: a cross-sectional study of the accuracy of diabetes diagnosis. Br J Gen Pract. 2016;66(646):e315-22.
46. Sharp SA, Rich SS, Wood AR, Jones SE, Beaumont RN, Harrison JW, et al. Development and standardization of an improved type 1 diabetes genetic risk score for use in newborn screening and incident diagnosis. Diabetes Care. 2019;42(2):200-7.
47. Redondo MJ, Gignoux CR, Dabelea D, Hagopian WA, Onengut-Gumuscu S, Oram RA, et al. Type 1 diabetes in diverse ancestries and the use of genetic risk scores. Lancet Diabetes Endocrinol. 2022;10(8):597-608.
48. Perry DJ, Wasserfall CH, Oram RA, Williams MD, Posgai A, Muir AB, et al. Application of a genetic risk score to racially diverse type 1 diabetes populations demonstrates the need for diversity in risk-modeling. Sci Rep. 2018;8(1): 4529.
49. Qin J, Luo S, Fan B, Xie Z, Wan R, Li X, et al. A type 1 diabetes genetic risk score discriminates between type 1 diabetes and type 2 diabetes in a Chinese population. Diabetologia. 2025;68:1969-82.
50. Hansen AL, Christiansen CF, Brøns C, Engelhard LM, Hansen T, Nielsen JS, et al. Birthweight and risk of chronic kidney disease after a type 2 diabetes diagnosis in the DD2 cohort. Diabetologia. 2025;68:778-91.
51. Barker DJ. The developmental origins of adult disease. J Am Coll Nutr. 2004;23(6 Suppl):588S-595S.
52. Brenner BM, Garcia DL, Anderson S. Glomeruli and blood pressure. Less of one, more the other? Am J Hypertens. 1988;1(4 Pt 1):335-47.

Section 3: COMPLICATIONS

Section Editor: Abhranil Dhar

1. Effects of Sodium-glucose Cotransporter-2 Inhibitors in Myocardial Infarction Patients: A Systematic Review and Meta-analysis

Ref: Jia Q, Zuo A, Song H, Zhang C, Fu X, Hu K, et al. Effects of sodium-glucose cotransporter-2 inhibitors in myocardial infarction patients: A systematic review and meta-analysis. Diabetes Obes Metab. 2025;27(3):1276-86.

ABSTRACT

Aim: In patients with heart failure (HF), type 2 diabetes mellitus (T2DM), and chronic kidney disease (CKD), sodium-glucose cotransporter-2 (SGLT-2) inhibitors have been shown to improve cardiovascular outcomes. Their effectiveness after myocardial infarction (MI) is still unknown.

Materials and methods: PubMed, Embase, the Cochrane Library, Web of Science, and ClinicalTrials.gov were used in a thorough search. Hospitalization for heart failure (HHF), cardiovascular (CV) death, a composite of HHF or CV death, all-cause death, major cardiovascular events (MACE), recurrent MI, severe arrhythmia, renal damage, and stroke were the primary outcomes. Improvements in left ventricular ejection fraction (LVEF) and left ventricular end-diastolic volume (LVEDV) were the secondary objectives.

Results: 13 studies with 22,370 patients were included. SGLT-2i reduced HHF (RR 0.69; 95% CI 0.61–0.78; $p < 0.001$), combined HHF or CV death (RR 0.87; 95% CI 0.77–0.99; $p = 0.028$), decreased all-cause mortality (RR 0.82; 95% CI 0.73–0.93; $p = 0.002$), MACE (RR 0.68; 95% CI 0.53–0.88; $p = 0.004$), recurrent MI (RR 0.81; 95% CI 0.69–0.94; $p = 0.007$), severe arrhythmia (RR 0.69; 0.61–0.78; $p < 0.001$). The SGLT-2 inhibitor group showed significantly higher improvements in LVEF (MD 3.96%; 95% CI 2.52–5.40; $p < 0.001$) and LVEDV (MD –5.52 mL; 95% CI –10.21 to –0.83; $p = 0.021$).

Conclusion: SGLT-2 inhibitors were observed to dramatically reduce the incidence of HHF, combined CV death or HHF, all-cause mortality, MACE, recurrent MI, severe arrhythmias, and renal injury in post-MI patients. SGLT-2 inhibitors also improved LVEDV and LVEF.

CRITICAL APPRAISAL

What was Known Prior to this Study?

Large cardiovascular outcome trials (CVOTs) such as EMPA-REG OUTCOME, CANVAS demonstrated significant benefit of sodium-glucose cotransporter-2 (SGLT-2) inhibitor on heart failure (HF) and cardiovascular (CV) mortality.

Multiple randomized controlled trials (RCTs) suggested possible modest reduction in patients with myocardial infarction (MI), but there is significant heterogeneity across trials. In the recently published EMPACT-MI trial, empagliflozin did not significantly lower the risk of the composite primary endpoint—first hospitalization for heart failure (HHF) or death from any cause—compared to placebo in patients with acute myocardial infarction (AMI) and increased HF risk. However, exploratory analyses showed a reduction in the relative risk of HHF. DAPA-MI trial found that dapagliflozin significantly improved cardiometabolic outcomes but had no impact on the composite of CV death or HHF compared to placebo.

What this Study Adds?

- This study specifically focuses on the association between SGLT-2 inhibitor use and CV outcomes in patients following MI.

- This systematic review and meta-analysis showed that SGLT-2 inhibitors could lower the incidence of HHF, a composite outcome including CV death and HHF, all-cause death, major cardiovascular events (MACE), recurrent MI, severe arrhythmia, and renal injury in patients following AMI.
- Moreover, the study demonstrated that SGLT-2 inhibitors therapy caused significant improvements in left ventricular ejection fraction (LVEF) and left ventricular end-diastolic volume (LVEDV).
- Reduction in HHF rates was mostly driven by the newly published EMPACT-MI trial, it was consistent across most included studies.

Major Strengths

- This study included large sample size/ pooled data
- Adjustments were done for major confounders like age, sex, diabetes duration, and baseline CV risk.

Limitations

- This study included five RCTs and eight observational studies. Therefore, bias is inevitable, and additional RCTs will be necessary in the future to verify the conclusions.
- Definitions of MACE varied across the included studies, potentially contributing to heterogeneity.
- Despite two included RCTs indicating a significantly greater reduction in NT proB-type natriuretic peptide (NT-proBNP) levels in the SGLT-2 inhibitors group compared to the placebo group, NT-proBNP was not incorporated into statistical analysis due to data limitations.
- EMPACT-MI trial, though suggestive of potential to reduce HHF, was primarily "neutral" in its main findings.

Clinical Implications

- It reinforces the role of SGLT-2 inhibitors as cardio-protective agents beyond HF.
- It supports consideration of SGLT-2 inhibitor in individuals with prior MI for secondary prevention.

Scope for Future Research

- Dedicated prospective trials in patients with MI
- Studies exploring mechanistic pathways, such as effects on plaque stability, endothelial function
- Comparative studies between different SGLT-2 inhibitors
- Evaluation of benefits in patients without diabetes
- Long-term outcome studies focusing on MI recurrence

2. Finerenone with Empagliflozin in Chronic Kidney Disease and Type 2 Diabetes

Ref: Agarwal R, Green JB, Heerspink HJL, Mann JFE, McGill JB, Mottl AK, et al; CONFIDENCE Investigators. Finerenone with Empagliflozin in Chronic Kidney Disease and Type 2 Diabetes. N Engl J Med. 2025;393:533-43.

ABSTRACT

Background: There is little evidence to recommend starting finerenone, a nonsteroidal mineralocorticoid receptor antagonist, and sodium-glucose cotransporter-2 (SGLT-2) inhibitors simultaneously in those with type 2 diabetes and chronic renal disease.

Methods: Participants with type 2 diabetes, chronic kidney disease (CKD) [estimated glomerular filtration rate (eGFR), 30–90 mL/min/1.73 m^2 of body surface area], and albuminuria [a urinary albumin-to-creatinine ratio of 100 to ≤5,000 (with albumin measured in milligrams and creatinine measured in grams)] who were already taking a renin–angiotensin system in a 1:1:1 ratio were randomly assigned to receive either empagliflozin at a dose of 10 or 20 mg daily, or a combination of empagliflozin and finerenone. The main result was the relative change from baseline to 180 days in the log-transformed mean urine albumin-to-creatinine ratio.

Results: Participants in the three groups had similar urinary albumin-to-creatinine ratios at baseline; among those with data (265 in the combination-therapy group, 258 in the finerenone group, and 261 in the empagliflozin group), the median value was 579 (interquartile range, 292–1,092). At day 180, combination therapy reduced the urinary albumin-to-creatinine ratio by 29% compared to finerenone alone [least-squares mean ratio of the difference in the change from baseline, 0.71; 95% confidence interval (CI) 0.61–0.82; $p < 0.001$] and by 32% compared to empagliflozin alone (least-squares mean ratio of the difference in the change from baseline, 0.68; 95% CI 0.59–0.79; $p < 0.001$). Neither agent caused unanticipated adverse events when used alone or in combination. Acute kidney injury, symptomatic hypotension, and hyperkalemia that required stopping medication were rare.

Conclusion: Compared to either treatment alone, initiation with finerenone + empagliflozin reduced the urine albumin to creatinine ratio more in patients with both type 2 diabetes and chronic renal disease (Funded by Bayer; CONFIDENCE ClinicalTrials.gov number, NCT05254002).

CRITICAL APPRAISAL

What was Known Prior to this Study?

Finerenone, a nonsteroidal mineralocorticoid receptor antagonist (ns-MRA), was already shown in large trials (FIDELIO-DKD and FIGARO-DKD) to reduce progression of chronic kidney disease (CKD), lower cardiovascular events in patients with type 2 diabetes and CKD. sodium-glucose cotransporter-2 (SGLT-2) inhibitors, including empagliflozin, were well established to slow CKD progression and reduce heart failure hospitalization. Both drug classes act via distinct but complementary mechanisms. Secondary analyses of clinical trials of finerenone have shown that reductions in the urinary albumin-to-creatinine ratio with finerenone were not modified according to background use of SGLT-2 inhibitors, which suggests that finerenone may have potential additive effects for reducing the urinary albumin-to-creatinine ratio and related outcomes. Posthoc analyses have limitations and do not address the clinical effects of the simultaneous initiation of both drugs. Therefore, rigorous randomized trials are much needed to evaluate the efficacy and safety of combination therapy.

What this Study Adds?

- Evidence supported additive or synergistic renal protection. Demonstrates that renal outcomes (albuminuria reduction and eGFR slope) may improve more with combination therapy than monotherapy.
- Simultaneous initiation of the nonsteroidal ns-MRA finerenone and the SGLT-2 inhibitor empagliflozin led to a reduction in the urinary albumin-to creatinine ratio that was 32% greater than that with empagliflozin alone and 29% greater than that with finerenone alone.
- A reduction in the urinary albumin-to-creatinine ratio has been considered to be a key mediator of the effects of SGLT-2 inhibitors on composite kidney outcomes.
- Reassurance regarding safety of combination therapy. The risk of hyperkalemia may not be substantially increased when used with SGLT-2 inhibitors.

Major Strengths

- Study focuses on clinically meaningful renal endpoints, like albuminuria and CKD progression markers.
- Inclusion of real-world or trial-based subgroup data improves clinical relevance.
- High percentage of participants who completed the trial and the inclusion of persons from many countries, which improved the generalizability of the findings.

Limitations

The trial used a surrogate endpoint, and participants were not followed up for long enough to adequately measure differences among groups in cardiovascular outcomes or clinical kidney disease progression.

Clinical Implications

- Study supports the safe combined use of finerenone and empagliflozin in patients with T2DM and CKD.
- Study suggests potential for improved renal outcomes with combined finerenone and empagliflozin.

Scope for Future Research

- Prospective randomized trials with combination therapy as a primary strategy
- *Long-term studies assessing*: End-stage kidney disease (ESKD), dialysis initiation, and renal death
- Evaluation of combination therapy in patients without diabetes

3. Impact of Baseline GLP-1 Receptor Agonist Use on Albuminuria Reduction and Safety with Simultaneous Initiation of Finerenone and Empagliflozin in Type 2 Diabetes and Chronic Kidney Disease (CONFIDENCE Trial)

Ref: Agarwal R, Green JB, Heerspink HJL, Mann JFE, McGill JB, Mottl AK, et al. Impact of Baseline GLP-1 Receptor Agonist Use on Albuminuria Reduction and Safety With Simultaneous Initiation of Finerenone and Empagliflozin in Type 2 Diabetes and Chronic Kidney Disease (CONFIDENCE Trial). Diabetes Care. 2025;48(11):1904-13.

ABSTRACT

Objective: When compared to monotherapy, the CONFIDENCE trial showed that starting finerenone, a nonsteroidal mineralocorticoid receptor antagonist, and a sodium-glucose cotransporter-2 (SGLT-2) inhibitor simultaneously reduced the urine albumin-to-creatinine ratio (UACR). This predetermined analysis assessed if baseline glucagon-like peptide 1 receptor agonist (GLP-1 RA) use modifies combination therapy's safety and effectiveness.

Research design and methods: Adults with type 2 diabetes [glycated hemoglobin <11% (97 mmol/mol)] and chronic kidney disease [UACR ≥ 100 to <5,000 mg/g; estimated glomerular filtration rate (eGFR) 30–90 mL/min/1.73 m^2] were randomized (1:1:1) to receive finerenone, empagliflozin, or finerenone + empagliflozin once daily.

Results: At baseline, 182 (23%) of the 800 patients utilized a GLP-1 RA. In those utilizing a GLP-1 RA, the UACR change from baseline at day 180 was −51% (95% CI −59 to −40%) with combination treatment, −34% (−48 to −18%) with finerenone, and −36% (−48 to −21%) with empagliflozin. In those who did not use a GLP-1 RA at baseline, the corresponding outcomes were −56% (−62 to −50%), −37% (−45 to −28%), and −33% (−41 to −23%). Individuals with and without baseline GLP-1 RA usage had incidence rates of hyperkalemia with combination therapy of 9.0% and 9.5%, respectively. Both those with and without baseline GLP-1 RA usage showed similar eGFR increases. Acute renal injury was rare. Systolic blood pressure decreases were noted, and they were more noticeable when combination therapy was used.

Conclusion: Regardless of prior GLP-1 RA usage, concurrent introduction of finerenone and an SGLT-2 inhibitor was both efficacious and well tolerated in CONFIDENCE trial when compared to monotherapy.

CRITICAL APPRAISAL

What was Known Prior to this Study?

CONFIDENCE trial demonstrated that the combination of finerenone and an sodium-glucose cotransporter-2 (SGLT-2) inhibitor (empagliflozin) provided additive reductions in albuminuria in participants with chronic kidney disease (CKD) with diabetes. A 2025 Cochrane review evaluated the efficacy and safety of glucagon-like peptide 1 receptor agonists (GLP-1 RAs) in people with diabetes and CKD across all CKD stages, which showed that GLP-1 RAs are likely to provide cardiovascular benefit and reduce all-cause mortality in people with diabetes and CKD. FLOW trial demonstrated that semaglutide reduced the risk of a composite kidney outcome (kidney failure, ≥50% eGFR decline, kidney, or cardio vascular death) by 24% compared with placebo.

Whether background GLP-1 RA use altered the effects of simultaneously starting finerenone and empagliflozin on top of existing renin-angiotensin system inhibition in the CONFIDENCE trial, was not explored before.

What this Study Adds?

- GLP-1 RA use at baseline did not change the efficacy or safety of finerenone, empagliflozin, or their combination.
- Urine albumin-to-creatinine ratio (UACR) reduction with empagliflozin or finerenone as monotherapies was not modified by baseline GLP-1 RA use.
- The median GLP-1 RA use duration was 13 months, which implies that any UACR lowering would largely have occurred prior to study entry.
- Numerically lower rates of severe hyperkalemia in patients with baseline GLP-1 RA use were observed, suggesting a possible protective or mitigating effect of GLP-1 RAs on hyperkalemia risk.

Major Strengths

The novel aspect of the study was to evaluate outcomes in patients receiving the four pillars of CKD care.

Limitations

- Patients receiving GLP-1 RAs at baseline had a higher mean BMI and differences in baseline characteristics compared with those not receiving GLP-1 RAs.
- Subgroup analyses by GLP-1 RA use were observational within randomized trials or pooled data sets, as randomization was not stratified by GLP-1 RA use.
- The statistical power to detect additive or synergistic effects of GLP-1 RAs in combination with other therapies (e.g., finerenone, SGLT-2 inhibitors, and RAS inhibitors) was limited by the relatively small number of patients receiving combination therapy at baseline.
- Differences in quality of care at recruiting centers and socioeconomic disparities may have influenced both the likelihood of GLP-1 RA use and the burden or progression of CKD.
- Subgroup analysis by specific GLP-1 RA agent (e.g., dulaglutide, liraglutide, and semaglutide) was not possible due to small sample sizes, and detailed dose information for individual GLP-1 RAs at baseline was not systematically collected or available.

Clinical Implications

The study supports the benefits of combination therapy with finerenone and SGLT-2 inhibitors, regardless of baseline GLP-1 RA use, supporting the implementation of all four pillars of care.

Scope for Future Research

- *Large-scale, long-term outcome trials are needed evaluating*: End-stage kidney disease (ESKD), dialysis initiation, renal, and cardiovascular mortality.
- Studies comparing simultaneous versus sequential initiation strategies are needed.
- Evaluation of combination therapy in nondiabetic CKD and heart failure with CKD overlap
- Mechanistic studies exploring antifibrotic and inflammatory biomarkers

4. Finerenone and New-onset Diabetes in Heart Failure: A Prespecified Analysis of the FINEARTS-HF Trial

Ref: Butt JH, Jhund PS, Henderson AD, Claggett BL, Desai AS, Viswanathan P, et al. Finerenone and new-onset diabetes in heart failure: a prespecified analysis of the FINEARTS-HF trial. Lancet Diabetes Endocrinol. 2025;13:107-18.

ABSTRACT

Background: There is conflicting information regarding how mineralocorticoid receptor antagonist (MRA) medication affects new-onset diabetes and glycated hemoglobin (HbA1c) levels. In the Finerenone experiment to Investigate Efficacy and Safety Superior to Placebo in Patients with Heart Failure (FINEARTS-HF) experiment, we sought to determine the impact of oral finerenone versus placebo on incident diabetes.

Methods: 6,001 participants with heart failure who had New York Heart Association functional class II–IV, left ventricular ejection fraction 40% or higher, evidence of structural heart disease, and elevated N-terminal pro-B-type natriuretic peptide levels were randomly assigned to receive finerenone or a placebo orally in this double-blind, randomized, placebo-controlled study. Concealed allocation was used for randomization. The composite of cardiovascular death and total (first and recurring) heart failure events (such as hospitalization or urgent heart failure visit) was the trial's main endpoint. Participants having diabetes at baseline (investigator-reported history of diabetes or baseline HbA1c ≥ 6.5%) were not included in this study. A HbA1c reading of 6.5% or above on two consecutive follow-up visits or the start of new glucose-lowering medication were considered indicators of new-onset diabetes. Regardless of the therapy received (i.e., intention to treat), the full-analysis set included all participants who were randomly assigned to study treatment and analyzed based on their treatment assignment. Participants who took at least one dosage of the investigational product and were randomly allocated to study therapy made up the safety analysis set, which was analyzed based on the actual treatment received. This study is no longer accepting new participants and is registered with ClinicalTrials.gov with the number NCT04435626.

Findings: 6,001 participants were recruited between September 14, 2020, and January 10, 2023, and they were randomized to receive either finerenone or a placebo. The study population consisted of 3,222 (53.7%) individuals who did not have diabetes at baseline. 115 (7.2%) individuals in the finerenone group and 147 (9.1%) in the placebo group experienced new-onset diabetes during a median follow-up period of 31.3 months [interquartile range (IQR) 21.5–36.3]. This translates to a rate of 3.0 events per 100 person-years [95% confidence interval (CI) 2.5–3.6] in the finerenone group and 3.9 events per 100 person-years (3.3–4.6) in the placebo group. Finerenone significantly decreased the risk of new-onset diabetes by 24% when compared to placebo [hazard ratio (HR) 0.76; 95% CI 0.59–0.97; $p = 0.026$]. When the competing risk of mortality was taken into consideration, Fine-Gray competing risk analysis produced a similar result [subdistribution HR 0.75 (0.59–0.96), $p = 0.024$]. Sensitivity analyses yielded similar results when the definition of new-onset diabetes was limited to HbA1c measurements only, restricted to new initiation of glucose-lowering medications only [excluding sodium-glucose cotransporter-2 (SGLT-2) inhibitor treatment], and expanded to include initiation of SGLT-2 inhibitor treatment with diabetes as indication. When individuals who had received glucose-lowering medication at baseline were eliminated ($n = 15$), the results remained the same. Across important participant subgroups, finerenone had a consistent effect on new-onset diabetes when compared to a placebo. Seven patients experienced a novel diabetes adverse event that did not fall under any of the aforementioned categories.

Interpretation: Oral finerenone decreased the risk of new-onset diabetes in heart failure patients with modestly reduced or retained ejection fraction without diabetes, indicating a significant additional clinical benefit of this medication in these patients.

CRITICAL APPRAISAL

What was Known Prior to this Study?

Steroidal mineralocorticoid receptor antagonist (MRA) spironolactone has consistently been associated with elevations in glycated hemoglobin (HbA1c) in individuals with and without diabetes. In the EMPHASIS-HF trial, which enrolled participants with heart failure and reduced ejection fraction, the steroidal MRA eplerenone did not reduce the risk of incident diabetes. In two large clinical trials of participants with chronic kidney disease and type 2 diabetes, the nonsteroidal MRA finerenone led to a reduction in kidney and cardiovascular events, including hospitalizations for heart failure. In FINEARTS-HF, which enrolled participants with heart failure with mildly reduced or preserved ejection, with and without diabetes, finerenone reduced the hazard of the primary composite outcome of total (first and recurrent) worsening heart failure events and cardiovascular death, and improved health-related quality of life.

What this Study Adds?

- In participants with heart failure with mildly reduced or preserved ejection fraction, without diabetes, the nonsteroidal MRA finerenone reduced the hazard of new-onset diabetes [defined as a HbA1c measurement of ≥6.5% on two consecutive follow-up visits or new initiation of glucose-lowering therapy, excluding sodium-glucose cotransporter-2 (SGLT-2) inhibitor treatment] by 24%.
- Results were similar in sensitivity analyses, in which the definition of new-onset diabetes was expanded to include initiation of SGLT-2 inhibitor treatment with diabetes as indication, restricted to HbA1c measurements only, and restricted to new initiation of glucose lowering drugs only (excluding SGLT-2 inhibitor treatment).

Major Strengths

- Large, well-conducted, randomized, double-blind, placebo-controlled trial
- Prespecified exploratory endpoint
- Extensive sensitivity and subgroup analyses, all showing consistent direction of benefit

Limitations

- Participants enrolled in clinical trials are selected according to specific inclusion and exclusion criteria, and the results might not be generalizable to all individuals with heart failure in the general population.
- Because this is a heart failure with mildly reduced EF (HFmrEF) or heart failure with preserved EF (HFpEF) trial, these data cannot necessarily be extrapolated to a population without HFmrEF or HFpEF, including those with HFrEF or those without heart failure.
- Plasma insulin or glucometabolic investigations were not done that might have helped better understand the effects of finerenone on new-onset diabetes.
- Since some of the glucose lowering therapies have indications beyond diabetes [e.g., glucagon-like peptide 1 (GLP-1) receptor agonists for the treatment of obesity], some participants might have initiated these drugs during follow-up for reasons other than diabetes.
- In the analyses of the association between new-onset diabetes and outcomes, the risk of residual confounding cannot be excluded, despite comprehensive adjustment for potential confounders. In addition, the confidence interval (CI) of the point estimates in these analyses were wide, and the associations should therefore be interpreted with caution.

Clinical Implications

In participants with heart failure with mildly reduced or preserved ejection fraction, without diabetes, finerenone reduced the hazard of new-onset diabetes, representing a meaningful additional clinical benefit of this treatment in these individuals.

Scope for Future Research

- Dedicated trials evaluating finerenone specifically for diabetes prevention in high-risk HF or cardiometabolic populations.
- Mechanistic studies to clarify Insulin sensitivity, β-cell function, and inflammatory pathways.
- Comparative studies of finerenone versus SGLT-2 inhibitors or GLP-1 receptor agonists for metabolic protection in HF.
- Evaluation in HFrEF and non-HF populations.

5. Efficacy and Safety of Finerenone in Type 2 Diabetes: A Pooled Analysis of Trials of Heart Failure and Chronic Kidney Disease

Ref: Ostrominski JW, Claggett BL, Miao ZM, Filippatos G, Desai AS, Jhund PS, et al. Efficacy and Safety of Finerenone in Type 2 Diabetes: A Pooled Analysis of Trials of Heart Failure and Chronic Kidney Disease. Diabetes Care. 2025;48(5):745-55.

ABSTRACT

Objective: To assess the safety and effectiveness of finerenone, a nonsteroidal mineralocorticoid receptor antagonist, in people with type 2 diabetes (T2D) and either heart failure (HF) with preserved ejection fraction (HFpEF) or mildly reduced ejection fraction (HFmrEF) or chronic kidney disease (CKD).

Research design and methods: The safety and effectiveness of finerenone were assessed in persons with a history of T2D in this prespecified participant-level pooled analysis of all phase III clinical studies comparing finerenone against placebo carried out to date (FINE-HEART). Using stratified Cox proportional hazards models, treatment effects on the primary outcome of cardiovascular death and several secondary events were assessed based on baseline glycated hemoglobin (HbA1c) and glucose-lowering therapy (GLT) protocol.

Results: 15,365 (80.9%) of the 18,991 FINE-HEART individuals had T2D and a baseline HbA1c (mean age, 66 ± 10 years; 32% women; mean HbA1c, 7.6 ± 1.4%).Insulin alone (*n* = 2,652), insulin and metformin combination (*n* = 2,005), metformin alone (*n* = 1,616), metformin and sulfonylurea (*n* = 1,039), and "other" (*n* = 8,117), which included glucagon-like peptide 1 receptor agonist (GLP-1 RA) and sodium-glucose cotransporter-2 inhibitor (SGLT-2i). Finerenone versus placebo treatment effects on cardiovascular death were consistent across baseline HbA1c ($P_{interaction} = 0.75$) and GLT regimen ($P_{interaction} = 0.46$) over a median follow-up of 2.9 years. Regardless of baseline HbA1c and GLT treatment, finerenone consistently decreased the kidney composite outcome, HF hospitalization, major adverse cardiovascular events, and all-cause mortality. Finerenone's treatment effects were constant regardless of the quantity of background GLTs and whether concurrent SGLT-2i or GLP-1RA therapy was being administered.

Conclusion: Across a wide range of glycemia and glucose-lowering regimens, finerenone consistently decreased morbidity and mortality in people with T2D.

CRITICAL APPRAISAL

What was Known Prior to this Study?

Mineralocorticoid receptor activation is a well-recognized pathophysiological pathway to systemic inflammation and fibrosis in cardiovascular–kidney–metabolic (CKM) conditions. Finerenone, a nonsteroidal mineralocorticoid receptor antagonist (MRA), has demonstrated cardiovascular and renal benefits in type 2 diabetes (T2D) with chronic kidney disease (CKD) (FIDELIO-DKD and FIGARO-DKD), in HFpEF/HFmrEF (FINEARTS-HF). Whether the benefits of finerenone are generalizable to the wide clinical spectrum of T2D or remain uncertain. Uncertainty remained regarding consistency of benefits across different glycated hemoglobin (HbA1c) strata, interaction with varied glucose-lowering therapy (GLT) regimens, safety in the context of polypharmacy, particularly insulin use and newer agents [sodium–glucose cotransporter-2 inhibitor and glucagon-like peptide 1 receptor agonist (SGLT-2i and GLP-1RA)].

What this Study Adds?

- Finerenone reduced the risk of a wide range of adverse clinical outcomes among individuals with T2D, including heart failure hospitalization, major adverse cardiovascular events, kidney events, and all-cause mortality, irrespective of baseline HbA1c or GLT regimen.
- The safety profile of finerenone was broadly consistent with prior analyses, with an expected modestly higher incidence of hyperkalemia, but without excess serious adverse events, observed in all HbA1c and GLT subgroups.

Major Strengths

- Prespecified participant-level pooled analysis
- Inclusion of three large, global, randomized phase III trials
- Large and heterogeneous population—15,000 individuals with T2D, wide spectrum of HbA1c, CKD severity, HF phenotypes, and GLT regimens

Limitations

- Owing to sample size limitations, study was unable to rigorously evaluate the efficacy and safety of all unique GLT regimens at baseline.
- Some subgroups may have been underpowered.
- Primary endpoint of cardiovascular death (exclusive of undetermined death) was narrowly missed in the overall FINE-HEART analysis, and further subgroup analysis should be interpreted in this context.

Clinical Implications

These findings support the use of finerenone to improve clinical outcomes in people with T2D and either kidney disease or HF.

Scope for Future Research

- Studies are needed focusing on earlier CKD stages, South Asian population.
- Evaluation of long-term safety beyond 3–4 years
- Mechanistic studies exploring antifibrotic effects across organ systems
- Findings from the prospective observational FINE-REAL (a noninterventional study providing insights into the use of finerenone in a routine clinical setting) study may further help to understand the safety of finerenone in routine clinical practice.

6. Effects of Semaglutide with or without Concomitant Mineralocorticoid Receptor Antagonist Use in Participants with Type 2 Diabetes and Chronic Kidney Disease: A FLOW Trial Prespecified Secondary Analysis

Ref: Rossing P, Bakris G, Perkovic V, Pratley R, Tuttle KR, Mahaffey KW, Idorn T, et al. Effects of Semaglutide With or Without Concomitant Mineralocorticoid Receptor Antagonist Use in Participants With Type 2 Diabetes and Chronic Kidney Disease: A FLOW Trial Prespecified Secondary Analysis. Diabetes Care. 2025;48:1878-87.

ABSTRACT

Objective: Semaglutide decreased the risk of significant kidney and cardiovascular (CV) events as well as all-cause mortality in individuals with type 2 diabetes (T2D) and chronic kidney disease (CKD) in the Evaluate Renal Function With Semaglutide Once Weekly (FLOW) trial. By baseline mineralocorticoid receptor antagonist (MRA) use, this prespecified investigation evaluated the impact of semaglutide on kidney, CV, and mortality events.

Research design and methods: Subcutaneous semaglutide 1.0 mg or a placebo was administered once a week to participants at random. The time to first sustained ≥ 50% estimated glomerular filtration rate (eGFR) decline from baseline, renal failure, or death from kidney/CV causes was the primary kidney outcome. Spironolactone predominated in baseline MRA; finerenone was available after recruitment was complete.

Results: Baseline MRA use [n = 257 (136 in the semaglutide group and 121 in the placebo group)] and nonuse [n = 3,276 (1,631 in the semaglutide group and 1,645 in the placebo group)] were analyzed to examine the effects. In the MRA and non-MRA categories, semaglutide decreased the risk of the major renal outcome by 49% [59 events; hazard ratio (HR) 0.51 (95% CI 0.30, 0.86)] and 21% [682 events; HR 0.79 (95% CI 0.68, 0.92); $P_{interaction} = 0.12$] compared to placebo. Semaglutide's effects on major adverse CV events (MACE) and all-cause mortality were favorable in both MRA subgroups, with no heterogeneity ($P_{interaction} > 0.7$). Semaglutide decreased albuminuria by 15% (95% CI −41, 31) among MRA users and 33% (26, 39) in nonusers compared to placebo at 104 weeks ($P_{interaction} = 0.22$). Semaglutide also decreased the estimated drop in glomerular filtration rate ($P_{interaction} = 0.71$). Semaglutide's safety profile was similar across subgroups.

Conclusion: Regardless of baseline MRA usage, semaglutide consistently improved major renal outcomes, MACE, and all-cause mortality in individuals with T2D with CKD.

CRITICAL APPRAISAL

What was Known Prior to this Study?

Mineralocorticoid receptor antagonists (MRAs) are commonly used for the treatment of type 2 diabetes (T2D) with chronic kidney disease (CKD). Semaglutide [a glucagon-like peptide 1 receptor agonist (GLP-1 RAs) improves kidney and cardiovascular (CV) outcomes in T2D in FLOW trial. The most recent update of the American Diabetes Association (ADA) guidelines now recommends GLP-1 RAs with their proven CKD benefit for T2D with CKD.

But no dedicated trials have examined the combination of GLP-1 RAs and MRAs on major kidney and CV outcomes in participants with T2D and CKD.

What this Study Adds?

- Consistent benefits of semaglutide on kidney outcomes, major adverse CV events, and all-cause mortality were observed regardless of baseline MRA use.

- Numerically, semaglutide reduced the primary end point to a greater extent in users of MRAs than in nonusers.
- The concomitant use of semaglutide with an MRA was associated with fewer serious adverse events.
- Benefits persist across varying baseline eGFR and albuminuria strata.

Major Strengths

- Potential strengths of FLOW trial were consistent enrollment and retention during the coronavirus 2019 pandemic.
- The high adherence (adherence to the trial regimen averaged 89% of the planned time during the trial period), and the lower-than-expected number of dropouts.

Limitations

- There were differences in baseline characteristics between subgroups across the study population, although important factors such as eGFR, UACR, and SGLT-2i use were similar.
- Finerenone only became available late during the FLOW trial, and its use was very limited. Additionally, it is not known whether MRAs were used in FLOW for the treatment of hypertension, heart failure, CKD, or other conditions.
- This was a prespecified analysis but with limited statistical power based on 257 users of MRAs at baseline with 59 primary outcomes, while there were 3,276 without MRA use and 682 outcomes in total.
- This analysis should be considered exploratory, as participants included in this analysis were not stratified by baseline MRA use at study initiation.

Clinical Implications

Study suggests that semaglutide and MRAs can be combined for a larger effect, but as the MRA-treated group was small, the results should be interpreted with caution.

Scope for Future Research

- Dedicated studies evaluating combination therapy (GLP-1 RA + SGLT-2i + finerenone)
- Comparative effectiveness studies GLP-1 RA versus nonsteroidal MRA (ns-MRA) versus SGLT-2i sequencing
- Mechanistic trials exploring renal inflammation, fibrosis regression
- Real-world studies in South Asian populations, patients with lower eGFR (<25 mL/min/1.73 m^2)

7. The FLOW of Progress in Diabetic Kidney Disease: Semaglutide's Role in Combination Therapy (Commentary)

Ref: Agarwal R. The FLOW of Progress in Diabetic Kidney Disease: Semaglutide's Role in Combination Therapy. Diabetes Care. 2025;48:1875-7.

ABSTRACT

The prevalence of diabetic kidney disease (DKD), which is the primary cause of end-stage kidney disease worldwide, is similar to that of the global diabetes epidemic. The fact that DKD also significantly raises the risk of cardiovascular morbidity and mortality is less known. Adverse kidney and cardiovascular outcomes are strongly predicted by the staging of chronic kidney disease (CKD), which is based on albuminuria and estimated glomerular filtration rate (eGFR). People with CKD have a significant and ongoing residual risk of developing cardiovascular and end stage kidney disease even when traditional cardiovascular risk factors are optimally controlled. In the context of cardiovascular-kidney-metabolic syndrome, the American Heart Association and American Diabetes Association emphasize the necessity of risk reduction strategies that target lifestyle, glycemia, blood pressure, lipids, and kidney disease-specific factors. Even with the high prevalence of DKD, screening and diagnosis are still not at their best. Up to 90% of people with CKD in the United States are not aware that they have the condition, and even those with advanced disease have little awareness. Missed opportunities for early intervention and the application of evidence-based therapy are caused by this diagnostic gap. All patients with type 2 diabetes should have their eGFR and urine albumin-to-creatinine ratio assessed annually, according to the American Diabetes Association and Kidney Disease: Improving Global Outcomes, but clinical practice does not always follow these recommendations. Suboptimal results are caused by obstacles such limited CKD awareness, complicated care, and a lack of awareness of guideline-directed management.

CRITICAL APPRAISAL

What was Known Prior to this Study?

Diabetic kidney disease (DKD) is the leading cause of end-stage kidney disease worldwide and is closely linked with excess cardiovascular morbidity and mortality. Since 2019, DKD management has transformed from a single-agent approach into a multidimensional approach. It consists of four pillars—(1) angiotensin-converting enzyme inhibitor/angiotensin receptor blocker (ACEi/ARB), (2) sodium-glucose cotransporter-2 inhibitors (SGLT-2i), (3) glucagon-like peptide 1 receptor agonist (GLP-1 RA), nonsteroidal mineralocorticoid receptor antagonist (MRA). This editorial highlights FLOW trial as the first dedicated renal outcome trial of a GLP-1 RA (semaglutide) in DKD.

What this Study Adds?

- Subgroup analysis of the FLOW trial demonstrates that semaglutide confers robust kidney and cardiovascular protection in patients with type 2 diabetes and CKD, with consistent benefits regard less of baseline MRA use.
- Strengthens the concept of additive and complementary cardiorenal protection when GLP-1 RAs are used alongside RAS blockers, SGLT-2 inhibitors, and MRAs.

Major Strengths

- This editorial provides a clear, well-structured synthesis of contemporary DKD management.
- Appropriately emphasizes the cardio-vascular–kidney continuum, rather than viewing renal outcomes in isolation.

Limitations

- The subgroup analysis on MRA use includes a small proportion of participants.
- Predominantly reflects spironolactone rather than finerenone, limiting generalizability.
- Positioning GLP-1 RAs as a "fourth pillar" may be difficult in real-world settings, particularly in low- and middle-income settings.

Clinical Implications

- Reinforce the four-pillar paradigm of DKD management and support the integration of GLP-1 RAs alongside renin-angiotensin system blockers, SGLT-2i, and finerenone to maximize cardiorenal risk reduction in this vulnerable population.
- With early screening for albuminuria in those with type 2 diabetes, the use of multiple agents can confer substantial lifetime cardiovascular, kidney, and mortality benefits.

Scope for Future Research

- Randomized trials evaluating optimal sequencing versus simultaneous initiation of DKD therapies
- Dedicated studies examining GLP-1 RA use in advanced CKD stages, nonalbuminuric DKD phenotypes

- Comparative effectiveness studies between GLP-1 RAs and MRAs, different GLP-1 RA molecules on renal outcomes
- Long-term mechanistic studies on fibrosis, inflammation, and structural renal changes

8. Oral Semaglutide and Cardiovascular Outcomes in High-risk Type 2 Diabetes

Ref: McGuire DK, Marx N, Mulvagh SL, Deanfield JE, Inzucchi SE, Pop-Busui R, et al. Oral Semaglutide and Cardiovascular Outcomes in High-Risk Type 2 Diabetes. N Engl J Med. 2025;392:2001-12.

ABSTRACT

Background: Oral semaglutide, a glucagon-like peptide 1 receptor agonist, has been shown to be safe for those with type 2 diabetes and high cardiovascular risk. It is necessary to evaluate the cardiovascular effectiveness of oral semaglutide in people with type 2 diabetes who also have chronic renal disease, atherosclerotic cardiovascular disease, or both.

Methods: Participants who were 50 years of age or older, had type 2 diabetes with a glycated hemoglobin level of 6.5–10.0%, and had known atherosclerotic cardiovascular disease, chronic kidney disease, or both were randomly assigned to receive either once-daily oral semaglutide (maximum dose, 14 mg) or placebo in addition to standard care in this double-blind, placebo-controlled, event-driven, superiority trial. Using a time-to-first-event analysis, the main outcome was significant adverse cardiovascular events (a composite of death from cardiovascular causes, nonfatal myocardial infarction, or nonfatal stroke). Major renal disease events (a five-point composite outcome) were among the confirmatory secondary outcomes.

Results: The mean (±SD) follow-up of the 9,650 randomly selected individuals was 47.5 ± 10.9 months, whereas the median follow-up was 49.5 months. In contrast to 668 of the 4,825 participants (13.8%; incidence, 3.7 events per 100 person-years) in the placebo group, 579 of the 4,825 participants (12.0%; incidence, 3.1 events per 100 person-years) in the oral semaglutide group experienced a primary-outcome event (hazard ratio 0.86; 95% confidence interval 0.77–0.96; $p = 0.006$). There was no significant difference between the two groups' findings for the confirmatory secondary outcomes. The incidence of gastrointestinal disturbances was 5.0% and 4.4%, respectively, whereas the incidence of major adverse events was 47.9% in the oral semaglutide group and 50.3% in the placebo group.

Conclusion: Oral semaglutide use was linked to a significantly lower risk of major adverse cardiovascular events compared to placebo in individuals with type 2 diabetes and atherosclerotic cardiovascular disease, chronic kidney disease, or both, without an increase in the incidence of serious adverse events (Funded by Novo Nordisk; SOUL ClinicalTrials.gov number, NCT03914326).

CRITICAL APPRAISAL

What was Known Prior to this Study?

Injectable semaglutide has established cardiovascular efficacy in persons with type 2 diabetes and cardiovascular disease or a high risk of cardiovascular disease, as well as in those with type 2 diabetes and chronic kidney disease. But an assessment of cardiovascular efficacy of oral formulation of semaglutide is limited. The Oral Semaglutide Cardiovascular Outcome Trial (SOUL) was designed to assess the cardiovascular efficacy of oral semaglutide in persons with type 2 diabetes and established atherosclerotic cardiovascular disease, chronic kidney disease, or both.

What this Study Adds?

- Oral semaglutide was associated with a significantly lower risk of major adverse cardiovascular events than placebo (relative risk reduction of 14%).
- Among the three components of the primary outcome, nonfatal myocardial infarction had the largest difference in risk between the oral semaglutide group and the placebo group. This finding contrasts with results from PIONEER 6, a noninferiority trial investigating the use of oral semaglutide in persons with type 2 diabetes and high cardiovascular risk, in which a reduction in the risk of death from cardiovascular causes was the dominant beneficial effect.

Major Strengths

- Large sample size and long follow-up duration (the median follow-up was 49.5 months)
- Inclusion of high-risk T2DM population, clinically meaningful endpoints (3-point MACE).

Limitations

- Inclusion criteria of a history of cardiovascular disease, chronic kidney disease, or both, which was designed to enrich the trial population for assessing the effect of oral semaglutide, but this is not representative of the global population with type 2 diabetes, as approximately 32% of persons with type 2 diabetes have cardiovascular disease, and an estimated 25–40% have chronic kidney disease.
- Only 28.9% of enrolled participants were women and only 2.6% identified as Black.

Clinical Implications

Oral semaglutide emerges as a cardiometabolically safe option in T2DM with high CV risk.

Scope for Future Research

- Longer-term trials powered for CV superiority
- Head-to-head comparisons of oral versus injectable semaglutide
- Real-world effectiveness and adherence studies
- Exploration of higher oral doses and fixed-dose combinations

9. Combination Therapy for Chronic Kidney Disease and Type 2 Diabetes: A Promising Prelude (Editorial)

Ref: Zoccali C, Mallamaci F. Combination Therapy for Chronic Kidney Disease and Type 2 Diabetes—A Promising Prelude. N Engl J Med. 2025;393(6):601-2.

ABSTRACT

Clinicians and health systems around the world continue to face challenges due to the increasing prevalence of chronic renal disease among patients with type 2 diabetes. One renin–angiotensin system inhibitors, sodium-glucose cotransporter-2 inhibitors, glucagon-like peptide 1 (GLP-1) receptor agonists, and nonsteroidal mineralocorticoid receptor antagonists are among the approved treatments for type 2 diabetes and chronic kidney disease. The best combination and order of these treatments are yet unknown, despite the fact that using any of these medications alone has improved results. In this context, CONFIDENCE trial was carried out to investigate the effect of simultaneous initiation of finerenone and empagliflozin in patients with type 2 diabetes and chronic kidney disease.

CRITICAL APPRAISAL

What was Known Prior to this Study?

Advances have been made in the management of chronic kidney disease with type 2 diabetes with the approved use of renin-angiotensin system inhibitors, sodium-glucose cotransporter-2 inhibitors (SGLT-2i), glucagon-like peptide 1 (GLP-1) receptor agonists, and nonsteroidal mineralocorticoid receptor antagonists. most evidence was derived from monotherapy or sequential add-on approaches. There was no robust randomized evidence supporting simultaneous initiation of multiple disease-modifying therapies, and uncertainty persisted regarding optimal sequencing, incremental benefit, safety, particularly hyperkalemia, and acute kidney injury.

What this Study Adds?

- Combination therapy led to a reduction in the urinary albumin-to-creatinine ratio that was 29% greater than that with finerenone alone and 32% greater than that with empagliflozin alone.
- The magnitude and rapidity of the reduction in the urinary albumin-to-creatinine ratio, >a 30% reduction at 14 days and exceeding 40% at 90 days. These suggest additive effects of combination therapy.
- Incidence of adverse events, including hyperkalemia, acute kidney injury, and symptomatic hypotension, was not substantially higher with combination therapy.

Major Strengths

- It provides a balanced interpretation and clearly explains the rationale for using albuminuria as a surrogate endpoint, supported by prior meta-analyses.
- Appropriately, it acknowledges the rigorous trial design and prespecified statistical analysis.
- Multinational and heterogeneous patient population

Limitations

- Surrogate marker was used as the primary end point rather than a direct measure of clinical events such as kidney failure or cardiovascular outcomes.
- The trial was brief relative to the lifelong nature of chronic kidney disease and type 2 diabetes.
- The rapid decline in eGFR seen with combination therapy, although largely reversible, raises the question of whether this represents a transient hemodynamic effect or a harbinger of long-term risk.
- Patients with heart failure with a reduced ejection fraction were excluded, so the trial findings may not be generalizable to the broader population of patients with both chronic kidney disease and type 2 diabetes.
- Lack of adjustment for changes in blood pressure in the main efficacy analysis

Clinical Implications

- The editorial supports early combination therapy in high-risk DKD patients to reduce residual renal risk.
- Encourages clinicians to overcome therapeutic inertia when albuminuria persists despite standard care.

Scope for Future Research

Further trials with extended follow-up, more diverse populations, and inclusion of clinical endpoints are needed to confirm that the promise of combination therapy translates into durable kidney and cardiovascular protection.

10. Toward a New SUMMIT in Heart Failure with Preserved Ejection Fraction

Ref: Felker GM. Toward a New SUMMIT in Heart Failure with Preserved Ejection Fraction. N Engl J Med. 2025;392(5):505-6.

ABSTRACT

Historically, there have been few alternatives for treating heart failure with a preserved ejection fraction. Diuretics, fitness training, and the management of concomitant illnesses were the main therapeutic suggestions, as published in 2016. Since then, effective therapies for heart failure with maintained ejection fraction have emerged, such as nonsteroidal mineralocorticoid-receptor antagonists and sodium-glucose cotransporter-2 (SGLT-2) inhibitors. Glucagon-like peptide 1 (GLP-1) receptor agonists, which encourage weight loss and improve cardiovascular outcomes in patients with obesity, have been developed concurrently with advances in the treatment of obesity. Patients with both heart failure with maintained ejection fraction and obesity are a natural population to examine these drugs because of the high prevalence of obesity among those with this condition and the pathophysiological justification for an obese phenotype. Weight loss, quality of life, and functional capacity have all improved in individuals with and without diabetes, according to data from earlier randomized clinical trials evaluating the GLP-1 receptor agonist semaglutide in patients with heart failure with preserved ejection fraction and obesity. Although this conclusion was based on a very small number of events, these trials also showed fewer heart-failure occurrences with semaglutide compared with placebo.

CRITICAL APPRAISAL

What was Known Prior to this Editorial?

There is notable emergence of effective treatments for heart failure with preserved ejection fraction (HFpEF), including sodium-glucose cotransporter-2 (SGLT-2) inhibitors and nonsteroidal mineralocorticoid-receptor antagonists. Concurrently, developments in the treatment of obesity have included glucagon-like peptide 1 (GLP-1) receptor agonists, which promote weight loss and improve cardiovascular outcomes in patients with obesity. There is pathophysiological relationship between an obesity phenotype and patients with HFpEF.

What this Editorial Adds?

- The patients who received tirzepatide had a significantly lower risk of a composite of death from cardiovascular causes or a worsening heart-failure event among patients with HFpEF.
- Adverse events leading to discontinuation of the regimen because of GI intolerance were more common in the tirzepatide group.
- The editorial has effectively pointed out that original primary endpoints of the SUMMIT trial were changed during the trial.

Major Strengths

- The editorial effectively traces the evolution of HFpEF management from symptom-based care to disease-modifying therapies (SGLT-2 inhibitors and finerenone) and too emerging obesity-targeted therapies.
- *Balanced interpretation of SUMMIT*: The editorial appropriately highlights the reduction in HF events, improvement in quality of life [Kansas City Cardiomyopathy Questionnaire (KCCQ)].
- The editorial does not overstate mortality benefit, clearly acknowledging that the composite outcome was driven mainly by HF events.

- The editorial explicitly discussed cautions against generalization and notes the small number of events highlighting wide confidence intervals.

Limitations

- While the editorial mentions that primary endpoints were changed mid-trial, but the implications of this change are not critically explored.
- *Insufficient discussion of background therapy*: The editorial does not adequately address use of SGLT-2 inhibitors, finerenone, or ARNI in the SUMMIT population.
- There is limited discussion on lean HFpEF, metabolically unhealthy but nonobese HFpEF.
- Mechanistic explanation not fully explored

Clinical Implications

Medical therapy for HFpEF is moving toward a core group of foundational therapies that improve outcomes with inclusion of GLP-1 receptor agonists in the appropriate patients.

Scope for Future Research

- Comparison with STEP-HFpEF and semaglutide trials could have been more explicit.
- Interaction with SGLT-2 inhibitors, potential sequencing versus combination strategies
- Exploration of whether HFpEF outcomes improve proportionally to weight loss or, whether there is a threshold or pleiotropic effect.
- Sarcopenia risk with aggressive weight loss

11. Cardiovascular Outcomes with Tirzepatide versus Dulaglutide in Type 2 Diabetes

Ref: Nicholls SJ, Pavo I, Bhatt DL, Buse JB, Del Prato S, Kahn SE, et al.; SURPASS-CVOT Investigators. Cardiovascular Outcomes with Tirzepatide versus Dulaglutide in Type 2 Diabetes. N Engl J Med. 2025;393:2409-20.

ABSTRACT

Background: Glycemic management and body weight are positively impacted by tirzepatide, a dual incretin agonist of the glucagon-like peptide 1 and glucose-dependent insulinotropic polypeptide receptors. Effects of tirzepatide on CV outcome are less studied.

Methods: Patients with type 2 diabetes and atherosclerotic cardiovascular disease were randomly assigned in a 1:1 ratio to receive a weekly subcutaneous injection of tirzepatide (up to 15 mg) or dulaglutide (1.5 mg), an agent that has been demonstrated to lower the incidence of cardiovascular events, as part of an active-comparator–controlled, double-blind, noninferiority trial. Tirzepatide was assessed for noninferiority to dulaglutide using a margin of 1.05 for the upper limit of the 95.3% confidence interval for the hazard ratio. The major endpoint was a composite of death from cardiovascular causes, myocardial infarction, or stroke. Tirzepatide was considered superior than dulaglutide if the upper limit was <1.00.

Results: 13,299 patients were randomized; 134 of them were later eliminated due to noncompliance with inclusion requirements. Thus, 6,586 patients in the tirzepatide group and 6,579 in the dulaglutide group made up the adjusted intention-to-treat population. The mean body-mass index (weight in kilograms divided by the square of height in meters) was 32.6 ± 5.5, the mean glycated hemoglobin level was 8.4 ± 0.9%, the mean duration of diabetes was 14.7 ± 8.8 years, the mean age (±SD) was 64.1 ± 8.8 years, and 29.0% of the patients were female. 801 patients (12.2%) in the tirzepatide group and 862 patients (13.1%) in the dulaglutide group experienced a primary endpoint event (hazard ratio, 0.92; 95.3% confidence range, 0.83 to 1.01; $p = 0.003$ for noninferiority; $p = 0.09$ for superiority). Although there were more gastrointestinal adverse events in the tirzepatide group, the incidence of adverse events seemed to be similar in both groups.

Conclusion: Regarding a composite of death from cardiovascular causes, myocardial infarction, or stroke, tirzepatide was not inferior to dulaglutide in people with type 2 diabetes and atherosclerotic cardiovascular disease (Funded by Eli Lilly; SURPASS-CVOT ClinicalTrials.gov number, NCT04255433).

CRITICAL APPRAISAL

What was Known Prior to this Study?

Clinical trials have shown that tirzepatide leads to incremental benefits with respect to glycemic control, weight, atherogenic lipoprotein levels, blood pressure, and kidney-related outcomes as compared with selective glucagon-like peptide 1 (GLP-1) receptor agonists or other glucose-lowering agents. Further, in clinical trials, dulaglutide has been shown to reduce the incidence of cardiovascular (CV) events as compared with placebo. However, data from a randomized, clinical trial of the effect of tirzepatide on CV outcomes has been lacking.

What this Study Adds?

- Treatment with tirzepatide was noninferior to treatment with dulaglutide with respect to the primary composite endpoint—death from CV causes, myocardial infarction, or stroke at a median follow-up of 4.0 years.
- The incidence of adverse events did not appear to differ substantially between the two treatment groups, although gastrointestinal events were reported more frequently by patients assigned to the tirzepatide group.

Major Strengths

- *Robust trial design*: Randomized, double-blind, active-controlled, multinational Cardiovascular Outcomes Trial (CVOT)
- Large sample size (>13,000 patients) with long median follow-up 4 years
- Use of dulaglutide as an active comparator, an agent with proven CV benefit, strengthens clinical relevance.
- Inclusion of patients with established ASCVD, aligning with real-world high-risk populations

Limitations

- Although patients were recruited from 30 countries, the level of diversity with respect to sex and race was not fully representative of the global patient population (>80% of the patients in each treatment group were White).
- Imbalances between the treatment groups with respect to the addition of an sodium-glucose cotransporter-2 (SGLT-2) inhibitor after randomization may have affected results.

Clinical Implications

Among patients with type 2 diabetes and atherosclerotic CV disease, tirzepatide was noninferior to dulaglutide.

Scope for Future Research

- CVOT of tirzepatide in patients without type 2 diabetes who have high CV risk and overweight or obesity is currently in progress.
- Dedicated trials evaluating tirzepatide in primary CV prevention.
- Mechanistic studies to clarify why greater metabolic improvement does not translate into superior CV outcomes.
- Head-to-head CVOTs with higher-dose GLP-1 RAs (e.g., semaglutide)

12. Comparative Analysis on Renal and Cardiovascular Outcomes of Antidiabetic Treatment in Chronic Kidney Disease Patients: A Systematic Review and Network Meta-analysis

Ref: Bramlage P, Vijayan A, Varghese TP, Sadanandan DM, Lanzinger S, Rodriguez CF. Comparative analysis on renal and cardiovascular outcomes of antidiabetic treatment in chronic kidney disease patients-A systematic review and network meta-analysis. Diabetes Obes Metab. 2025;27(11):6254-63.

ABSTRACT

Aim: Chronic kidney disease (CKD) and type 2 diabetes mellitus (T2DM) are common complications that raise the risk of renal failure and cardiovascular (CV) events. Promising treatments include dipeptidyl peptidase 4 (DPP-4) inhibitors, glucagon-like peptide 1 receptor agonists (GLP-1 RA), and sodium-glucose cotransporter-2 (SGLT-2) inhibitors. There is, however, little proof of their relative efficacy in lowering renal and CV outcomes.

Materials and methods: We looked for randomized controlled trials (RCTs) published between 2014 and 2024 using electronic sources such as PubMed, Scopus, and clinical trial registries. The impact of antidiabetic medications on cardiorenal outcomes was assessed using a network meta-analysis (NMA). Major adverse CV events (MACE), composite renal outcomes, and all-cause death were the main outcomes. Heart failure (HF), stroke, macroalbuminuria, a decrease in estimated glomerular filtration rate (eGFR) > 40%, or renal replacement therapy were additional outcomes.

Results: 26 studies were included with 143,296 people who had both CKD and T2DM. SGLT-2 inhibitors were very successful in lowering the risk of CV outcomes such as MACE (0.93) and HF (1.00), followed by GLP-1 RA, as well as renal outcomes such as composite events (*P*-score: 0.94), eGFR drop > 40%, or renal replacement therapy (0.99). In contrast to SGLT-2 inhibitors, GLP-1 RA was especially successful in lowering the risk of MI (0.87), macroalbuminuria (0.86), and stroke (0.83). GLP-1 receptor agonists and SGLT-2 inhibitors both significantly lower all-cause mortality (0.83). SGLT-2 inhibitors and GLP-1 RA were more beneficial than DPP-4 inhibitors.

Conclusion: For patients with T2DM and CKD, SGLT-2 inhibitors and GLP-1 RA offer significant advantages for kidney and CV health. For HF and renal outcomes, SGLT-2 inhibitors outperform GLP-1 receptor agonists, underscoring their preferred use in these clinical situations.

CRITICAL APPRAISAL

What was Known Prior to this Study?

Coexistence of type 2 diabetes mellitus (T2DM) and chronic kidney disease (CKD) significantly increases the risk of cardiovascular (CV) events and end-stage renal disease (ESRD), contributing to increased morbidity and mortality rates. Sodium-glucose cotransporter-2 (SGLT-2) inhibitors, glucagon-like peptide 1 receptor agonists (GLP-1 RA), and dipeptidyl peptidase 4 (DPP-4) inhibitors have introduced promising therapeutic options in improving glycemic control and long-term outcomes in CKD patients.

Evidence of their comparative safety and efficacy on long-term CV and renal outcomes in CKD patients is limited. Previous systematic reviews and meta-analysis have predominantly concentrated on identifying and synthesizing data from RCTs involving patients with T2DM with limited focus on those with CKD.

What this Study Adds?

- SGLT-2 inhibitors are the most effective in improving both CV and renal outcomes, followed closely by GLP-1 RA.

- SGLT-2 inhibitors have shown 20% reduction in major adverse CV events (MACE), a 33% reduction in HF incidents, and a 29% reduction in composite renal outcomes.
- The effects of GLP-1 RA on reducing MI, stroke, and progression of macro-albuminuria were found to be more pronounced than those observed with SGLT-2 inhibitors. Specifically, GLP-1 RA demonstrated a 16% reduction in MACE and a 24% reduction in renal composite outcomes.
- DPP-4 inhibitors have no meaningful advantage over SGLT-2 inhibitors and GLP-1 RA as well as placebo.

Major Strengths

Inclusion of patients with CKD, including ESRD with albuminuria, having uncontrolled diabetes with established CV risk, allowing us to compare the efficiency of drug classes in this complex high-risk population.

Limitations

- Significant heterogeneity was observed in the studies. Therefore, random-effects model was employed and sensitivity analyses was conducted to ensure the robustness of the findings.
- Subgroup analysis was performed based on duration of follow-up.
- Furthermore, the lack of individual patient data limits adjustment for confounders such as base-line HbA1c or concomitant medications use.

Clinical Implications

- SGLT-2 inhibitors are strongly supported by large clinical trials and meta-analyses for reducing HF hospitalization and slowing CKD progression in T2DM.
- However, GLP-1 receptor agonists may be preferred in patients with predominant atherosclerotic CV disease (ASCVD) risk, as they have shown significant reductions in atherothrombotic events and stroke.

Scope for Future Research

- Trials evaluating sequencing versus combination of cardiorenal drugs
- Head-to-head comparative effectiveness studies
- Long-term outcomes beyond trial durations

13. Is Screening for Heart Failure and Peripheral Artery Disease Warranted in Asymptomatic Adults with Diabetes? A Perspective on the 2025 American Diabetes Association "Standards of Care in Diabetes"

Ref: Herman WH, Kuo S. Is Screening for Heart Failure and Peripheral Artery Disease Warranted in Asymptomatic Adults With Diabetes? A Perspective on the 2025 American Diabetes Association "Standards of Care in Diabetes". Diabetes Care 2025;48:1465-71.

ABSTRACT

Every year, the American Diabetes Association (ADA) releases the "Standards of Care in Diabetes" (SOC) to provide evidence-based guidelines for managing diabetes to physicians, patients, and payers. The 2025 SOC advises clinicians to use natriuretic peptide levels to screen asymptomatic adults with diabetes for heart failure, and to use ankle-brachial index (ABI) testing to screen asymptomatic adults with diabetes ≥ 65 years of age who have any microvascular disease, foot complications, or end-organ damage from diabetes for peripheral artery disease (PAD). This viewpoint assesses those suggestions using accepted screening guidelines and available research. There is insufficient data to support the use of natriuretic peptide in heart failure screening in a number of important areas. When used as a screening test for asymptomatic individuals, N-terminal pro-B-type natriuretic peptide, and or NT-proBNP, performs poorly. Adults with diabetes and stage B heart failure may benefit from treatment with sodium-glucose cotransporter-2 inhibitors, although there is inadequate data to support this claim. Lastly, the expenses are substantial and might not be financially feasible. Similarly, there is insufficient scientific evidence to support the recommendation to screen for PAD in persons with diabetes who do not exhibit any symptoms. The research presented has limited generalizability and combines ABI screening with other useful screening tests. There are no guidelines for interpreting ABI test findings or using the information obtained to guide treatment. Although the goal of using screening to improve healthcare is admirable, the current literature and screening principles do not sufficiently support these recommendations.

CRITICAL APPRAISAL

What was Known Prior to this Literature?

In 2025, the standard of care, American Diabetes Association (ADA) recommended that clinicians should consider screening adults with diabetes by measuring a natriuretic peptide to facilitate prevention of stage C heart failure. They have also recommended to screen for peripheral arterial disease with ankle-brachial index (ABI) in asymptomatic individuals with diabetes and age ≥ 65 years, microvascular disease in any location, or foot complications or any end-organ damage from diabetes and also in individuals with diabetes duration ≥ 10 years and high cardiovascular risk.

Evidence supporting population-wide screening in asymptomatic diabetes populations has been limited and inconsistent.

What this Literature Adds?

- This article demonstrates that NT-proBNP has low positive predictive value in asymptomatic populations.
- The article shows that ABI screening lacks robust evidence for outcome modification in asymptomatic diabetes.
- It introduces a cost-effectiveness analysis, showing extremely high costs per heart failure hospitalization prevented.

Major Strengths

- It uses Wilson–Jungner screening principles consistently and transparently.
- The article acknowledges the intent of ADA recommendations while critically examining evidence gaps.

Limitations

- The standard of care recommendations provides no information about downstream diagnostic testing for patients with abnormal screening test results.
- The recommendation fails to address the potential disadvantages of downstream diagnostic testing and the costs of screening and definitive diagnosis

Clinical Implications

- It highlights against routine, blanket screening for HF and peripheral artery disease (PAD) in asymptomatic diabetes.
- It reinforces prioritization of symptom-driven evaluation, aggressive management of traditional risk factors.

Scope for Future Research

- Randomized trials specifically testing NT-proBNP–guided initiation of sodium-glucose cotransporter-2 (SGLT-2) inhibitors in asymptomatic diabetes
- RCTs using screening-based strategies versus universal SGLT-2i use for heart failure prevention
- Evaluation of alternative PAD screening modalities in diabetes

14. Screening Natriuretic Peptide Levels Predicts Heart Failure and Death in Individuals with Type 1 and Type 2 Diabetes without Known Heart Failure

Ref: Pop-Busui R, Repetto E, Baron J, Schumacher D, Vaduganathan M, Pandey A. Screening Natriuretic Peptide Levels Predicts Heart Failure and Death in Individuals With Type 1 and Type 2 Diabetes Without Known Heart Failure. Diabetes Care. 2025;48:2145-53.

ABSTRACT

Objective: Diabetes frequently results in heart failure (HF), which may initially show no symptoms. Natriuretic peptides [NPs], which include B-type natriuretic peptide (BNP) and N-terminal pro-brain natriuretic peptide (NT-proBNP), are markers that can be utilized to identify early HF in asymptomatic people who might benefit from disease-modifying treatments. In individuals with type 1 diabetes (T1D) or type 2 diabetes (T2D) who do not have documented HF, we looked at the predictive significance of NP levels.

Research design and methods: Adults (aged ≥ 18) with T1D or T2D without known HF who underwent an outpatient NP test between 2017 and 2023 were selected from Optum's de-identified Market Clarity Data. Multivariable Cox proportional hazard models were used to evaluate associations between NP levels and incident HF or mortality.

Results: Approximately 39.6% of T1D patients and 42.3% of T2D patients had BNP ≥ 50 pg/mL or NT-proBNP ≥ 125 pg/mL among 116,466 eligible adults (*n* = 2,990 with T1D and *n* = 113,476 with T2D) followed for up to 7 years (54% female; median age 64 years; mean HbA1c 7.1% at baseline). Increased NT-proBNP levels were substantially linked to an increased risk of incident HF or death in T1D patients in adjusted Cox models [for NT-proBNP levels 125–300 pg/mL: HR (95% CI) 2.04 (1.35–3.07), for NT-proBNP levels > 300 pg/mL: 4.48 (3.11–6.47), reference: NT-proBNP 300 pg/mL: 3.58 (3.39–3.78), reference: NT-proBNP < 125 pg/mL]. For BNP, similar results were noted.

Conclusion: Elevated NP levels in patients with diabetes are a strong predictor of their future risk of HF or death. The use of NP screening for HF risk assessment in individuals with diabetes is supported by these findings.

CRITICAL APPRAISAL

What was Known Prior to this Study?

Heart failure (HF) is common in diabetes and may be asymptomatic in early stages. Natriuretic peptides (NPs), specifically B-type natriuretic peptide (BNP) and N-terminal pro-BNP (NT-proBNP), are detected in the blood in response to cardiac wall stress and have emerged as sensitive and specific biomarkers for the detection of early-stage HF. Prognostic implications of NP testing are well established in type 2 diabetes (T2D), But there is limited evidence in type 1 diabetes (T1D).

What this Study Adds?

- Approximately 42% of individuals tested had elevated NP levels. Markedly elevated NP levels were associated with significantly shorter HF-free survival compared with those with normal NP levels.
- NP testing has similar prognostic implications among individuals with T1D as in T2DM.
- Posthoc analysis of CANVAS and EXAMINE, demonstrated graded relationships between baseline NT-proBNP and subsequent risk of HF hospitalization and CV death.

Major Strengths

- This is a large, real-world data set examining NP testing with long-term follow-up.
- Multiple sensitivity analyses were done, including using stricter HF definitions and excluding early post-testing events, further support the robustness of the findings.

Limitations

- Due to observational nature of the study, exact indications for NP testing in the study cohort cannot be assessed.
- NP testing was driven by clinical decisions of the provider rather than standardized protocols, potentially introducing selection bias.
- Despite comprehensive adjustment for demographic and clinical factors, residual confounding by unmeasured variables such as functional status, socioeconomic factors, and adherence to preventive care remains possible.
- Diabetes duration was not available in the database and possibly represented an unadjusted confounder.

Clinical Implications

- Previous work has demonstrated that NT-proBNP is an important predictor of risk of HF among individuals with T2D or prediabetes. This real-world evidence extends these observations to T1D, providing robust support for current American Diabetes Association guidelines that recommend NT-proBNP screening for at-risk individuals across the diabetes spectrum.
- NT-proBNP testing helps to identify high-risk patients who would benefit from more intensive CV disease preventive strategies and more timely initiation of effective, guideline-directed medical therapies such as sodium-glucose cotransporter-2 inhibitors (SGLT-2i) or glucagon-like peptide 1 receptor glucagon-like peptide 1 receptor agonist (GLP-1 RA).

Scope for Future Research

- Prospective longitudinal studies evaluating predictive value of NPs for incident HF in T1D versus T2D
- Studies defining diabetes-specific reference ranges for NPs
- Research in diverse populations, including South Asian cohorts, where cardiometabolic risk is high.

15. Ranibizumab with Luseogliflozin in Type 2 Diabetes with Diabetic Macular Edema: A Randomized Clinical Trial

Ref: Ishibashi R, Takatsuna Y, Koshizaka M, Tatsumi T, Takahashi S, Nagashima K, et al; COMET Trial investigators. Ranibizumab with luseogliflozin in type 2 diabetes with diabetic macular oedema: A randomised clinical trial. Diabetes Obes Metab. 2025;27(5):2473-84.

ABSTRACT

Aim: The usual treatment for diabetic macular edema (DME) is antivascular endothelial growth factor (VEGF) medication, yet there are still unmet needs. The purpose of this study was to evaluate how well sodium-glucose cotransporter-2 inhibitors (SGLT-2i) work to treat DMO.

Supplies and procedures: 60 patients with DMO who qualified for anti-VEGF treatment participated in this multicenter randomized open-label trial. Patients were randomized to either glimepiride or luseogliflozin. The target eye received the first dose of ranibizumab, and subsequent doses were given in accordance with procedure. Readmission rates and the quantity of ranibizumab dosages administered up to week 48 were assessed. Assessments were also made on fellow ocular injections.

Results: There were 60 individuals, half of them had anti-VEGF medication previously and the majority of whom had diabetic retinopathy. Glycated hemoglobin, central retinal thickness (CRT), and best corrected visual acuity gains were comparable in the SGLT-2i and sulfonylurea (SU) groups. The target eye injection frequency was comparable between groups (SGLT-2i vs. SU:3.9 ± 0.7 vs. 4.7 ± 0.7 times, $p = 0.36$). The SGLT-2i group showed a substantial decrease in readministration rates following the fourth injection ($p = 0.030$, HR: 0.45; 95% CI: 0.22–0.92). Compared to the SU group, the eyes in the SGLT-2i group had significantly lower CRT and fewer injections (1.3 ± 0.6 vs. 3.4 ± 0.8, $p = 0.016$).

Conclusion: Some individuals responded well to SGLT-2i and needed fewer injections, despite the fact that the total amount of anti-VEGF injections in the target eye did not differ significantly. SGLT-2i's effectiveness in treating early-stage DMO is suggested by the decrease in fellow eye injections. Trial Registration: University Hospital Medical Information Network Clinical Trial Registry (UMIN000033961); Japan Registry of Clinical Trials (jRCTs031180210).

CRITICAL APPRAISAL

What was Known Prior to this Study?

Antivascular endothelial growth factor (VEGF) therapy is the standard of treatment for diabetic macular edema (DME). Nonclinical studies with sodium-glucose cotransporter-2 inhibitors (SGLT-2i) have elucidated mechanisms by which it improves diabetic retinopathy and DMO locally within the retina. SGLT-2i reduces microglial activation, inhibits angiopoietin-2 release, suppresses early DMO changes, and decreases VEGF expression. Prospective interventional studies combining anti-VEGF therapy and SGLT-2i have not been conducted before.

What this Study Adds?

- No overall difference was observed in treatment efficacy for severe DMO in ranibizumab with luseogliflozin combination group.
- Reduction in the rate of intravitreal ranibizumab readministration was observed in some patients, suggesting potential efficacy.
- Fellow eyes in the SGLT-2i group showed significant central retinal thickness (CRT) reduction and fewer injections compared with those in the sulfonylurea group.

Major Strengths

- This is a well-designed randomized controlled trial with standardized visual acuity endpoints.
- Objective optical coherence tomography (OCT)-based retinal thickness
- Inclusion of comparator arms (laser ± ranibizumab) enhances interpretability.
- Established safety profile with careful monitoring of ocular and systemic adverse events

Limitations

- As there is no prior study exist on DMO using SGLT-2i, the study was not strictly based on existing research.
- The observation period was short, at 1 year.
- Owing to ethical concern, the effects of SGLT-2i alone were not observed.

Clinical Implications

- The study reinforces the use of ranibizumab as a first-line therapy for center-involving DME.
- Reduction in fellow eye injections suggests SGLT-2i's efficacy in treating early-stage DMO.

Scope for Future Research

- Head-to-head comparisons with other anti-VEGF agents (aflibercept and bevacizumab)
- Studies evaluating biomarkers of response to anti-VEGF treatment
- Cost-effectiveness analyses in resource-limited settings

16. Early Worsening of Diabetic Retinopathy in Individuals with Type 2 Diabetes Treated with Tirzepatide: A Real-world Cohort Study

Ref: Buckley AJ, Tan GD, Gruszka-Goh M, Scanlon PH, Ansari I, Suliman SGI. Early worsening of diabetic retinopathy in individuals with type 2 diabetes treated with tirzepatide: a real-world cohort study. Diabetologia. 2025;68:2069-76.

ABSTRACT

Aims/Hypothesis: Treatment with glucagon-like peptide 1 receptor agonists, such as subcutaneous semaglutide, has been linked to early worsening of diabetic retinopathy (EWDR). It is unclear if EWDR happens after starting tirzepatide, a powerful glucagon-like peptide 1/gastric inhibitory polypeptide receptor agonist.

Methods: Using real-world clinical data, we matched 3,435 tirzepatide-exposed (≥180 days treatment) individuals with type 2 diabetes 1:1 with 3,434 tirzepatide-unexposed individuals for sex, diabetes duration, retinopathy status, glycated hemoglobin (HbA1c), number of retinal screening episodes, and use of glucose-lowering medications. Conditional logistic regression was used to investigate new-onset diabetic retinopathy and retinopathy progression.

Results: The study's participants had strict baseline glycemic control [mean HbA1c 56.1 ± 15.8 mmol/mol (7.28 ± 1.43%)]. 1.1% of tirzepatide-exposed people (n = 33) and 0.5% of tirzepatide-unexposed persons (n = 17) developed new-onset proliferative diabetic retinopathy (PDR) (grades R3M0 and R3M1). After controlling for known risk variables, tirzepatide was substantially linked to new-onset PDR in multivariate analysis [OR 2.15 (95% CI 1.24, 3.74), $p < 0.01$]. But in multivariate analysis, tirzepatide was also linked to lower odds of new onset of retinopathy [OR 0.73 (95% CI 0.62, 0.86), $p < 0.001$] in people without diabetic retinopathy (R0M0) at initiation, and it was not significantly linked to the progression of retinopathy in people with mild non-PDR (NPDR and grade R1M0 or R1M1).

Conclusions/Interpretation: Particularly in those with mild NPDR with maculopathy (grade R1M1) or moderate-to-severe NPDR with or without maculopathy (grade R2M0 and R2M1), tirzepatide treatment significantly enhanced the risks of incident PDR. According to the Early Treatment Diabetic Retinopathy Study (ETDRS) guidelines, the increased likelihood of progression would support a referral to a specialist ophthalmologist.

CRITICAL APPRAISAL

What was Known Prior to this Study?

Worsening of DR was reported in people with type 1 diabetes undergoing intensive glucose lowering as part of the DCCT trial and has also been described in people with type 2 diabetes in small case-control studies. Mechanism is poorly understood, although higher baseline glycated hemoglobin (HbA1c), greater HbA1c reduction, longer diabetes duration, and severity of preexisting retinopathy have been identified as risk factors in meta-analysis. It can also be associated with use of glucagon-like peptide 1 receptor agonists (GLP-1 RAs). Previous data have shown that retinopathy status was subsequently stable or improved in the majority of patients who continued treatment. Recent meta-analysis of the SURPASS clinical trials did not detect an increase in risk of early worsening of diabetic retinopathy (EWDR) related to tirzepatide treatment. But these studies did not implement additional retinal screening and their protocols excluded individuals with PDR, severe preproliferative retinopathy, or maculopathy.

What this Study Adds?

- Increased incidence of PDR in tirzepatide-exposed individuals contrasts with the low rates of PDR reported in the SURPASS 1–5 clinical trials.
- Tirzepatide exposure was not associated with progression of retinopathy in individuals with mild NPDR at baseline and appeared to reduce the odds of new retinopathy in individuals without retinopathy.
- However, tirzepatide was significantly and independently associated with new onset of PDR, with the majority of events occurring in individuals with mild NPDR with maculopathy or, moderate-to-severe NPDR with maculopathy.

Major Strength

- Large study population, enabling good quality of matching and providing sufficient endpoints for multivariate analysis.
- Comprehensive consultant-led in-house retinal screening program, and a relatively consistent 3 monthly cycle of clinic attendance.

Limitations

- Study participants had a relatively long mean diabetes duration and the majority of individuals in the treatment group were switched to tirzepatide from a GLP-1 RA, potentially reducing the applicability of our findings to GLP-1 RA naive patients being initiated on tirzepatide.
- Although this study is based on real-world data in a representative population of people with type 2 diabetes, enhancing its external validity, the improvements in HbA1c seen after introduction of tirzepatide were modest in comparison with those seen in clinical trials and may not be applicable in a population with less-optimized baseline glycemic control.

Clinical Implications

- Assess baseline retinopathy status before initiating potent glucose-lowering therapy.
- Avoid overly rapid HbA1c reduction in patients with advanced DR.

Scope for Future Research

- Dedicated, prospective studies with retinopathy as a prespecified outcome
- Analyses exploring dose-response relationships, impact of rate of glycemic improvement on retinal outcomes
- Comparative studies with other potent incretin-based therapies

17. Which Treatment Modality Offers the Best Outcomes for Diabetic Retinopathy? A Systematic Review and Network Meta-analysis

Ref: Chen KY, Chan HC, Chan CM. Which treatment modality offers the best outcomes for diabetic retinopathy? A systematic review and network meta-analysis. Diabetes Res Clin Pract. 2025;227:112379.

ABSTRACT

Background and objective: Proliferative diabetic retinopathy (PDR) and diabetic macular edema (DME) are the most vision-threatening consequences of diabetic retinopathy (DR), which is a major cause of avoidable blindness worldwide. The conventional treatment for PDR has been panretinal photocoagulation (PRP); however, antivascular endothelial growth factor (anti-VEGF) medications have shown promise. The relative effectiveness and safety of various therapies are still unknown, though. The purpose of this network meta-analysis was to assess and contrast the efficacy of PRP, anti-VEGF medications, and combination treatments in enhancing anatomical and visual outcomes in DR patients.

Methods: Up until February 2025, a thorough search of PubMed, Embase, the Cochrane Library, and clinical trial registries was carried out. RCTs were included, that compared PRP, anti-VEGF medications (ranibizumab, aflibercept, and bevacizumab), or both in DR patients. Central retinal thickness (CRT) and best-corrected visual acuity (BCVA) were the primary outcome. Neovascularization regression, rates of vision-threatening complications, and adverse events were secondary outcome. To combine direct and indirect evidence, a Bayesian network meta-analysis was carried out.

Results: There were 28 RCTs with a total of 6,450 patients. At 12 months, anti-VEGF treatments showed better BCVA improvement than PRP (mean difference +3.39 letters; 95% CI +1.85 to +4.93). Additionally, anti-VEGF drugs increased the frequencies of neovascularization regression (odds ratio: 6.15) and CRT reduction (24.50 μm; 95% CI 39.03–9.97). Additional improvements for CRT reduction (–33.10 μm at 3 months) were seen with combination therapy. Compared to PRP, anti-VEGF medicines exhibited less side effects, such as decreased rates of intraocular pressure and visual field loss.

Conclusion: Anti-VEGF treatments have better safety profiles and are more successful than PRP in enhancing visual acuity, decreasing macular thickness, and regulating neovascularization in DR patients. In certain situations, combination treatment may provide further advantages. Anti-VEGF drugs are recommended as first-line therapies for vision-threatening DR based on these findings.

CRITICAL APPRAISAL

What was Known Prior to this Study?

Antivascular endothelial growth factor (VEGF) agents have shown promising results in reducing neovascularization and improving visual acuity outcomes compared to panretinal photocoagulation (PRP). They have the advantages of less peripheral visual field loss and reduced need for vitrectomy. But, anti-VEGF therapy is associated with higher costs, frequent injections, and potential systemic side effects. Comprehensive comparison of anti-VEGF agents and PRP is essential to guide clinicians in selecting optimal treatment strategies for patients with DR.

What this Study Adds?

- Anti-VEGF therapy exceeded PRP for best-corrected visual acuity with improvements of +2.35 letters at 3 months and +3.39 letters at 12 months.
- Ranibizumab and aflibercept had slight, nonsignificant advantages over other anti-VEGF drugs.
- In terms of central retinal thickness, anti-VEGF treatments had significantly greater reductions than PRP, with combination therapy showing the most improvements.
- Anti-VEGF therapy was associated with higher neovascularization regression rates compared to PRP, with combination therapy achieving 92.7% regression versus 70.5% with PRP.
- Safety profiles showed fewer complications with anti-VEGF therapy, including lower incidences of visual field loss, vitreous hemorrhage, and need for vitrectomy.
- PRP had higher rates of increased intra-ocular pressure.
- Additionally, anti-VEGF therapy significantly reduced the risk of vision—impairing diabetic macular edema (DME) compared to PRP.

Major Strengths

- It includes objective outcomes such as visual acuity and disease progression.
- It reflects real-world challenges in DR management, including variability in response.

Limitations

- Variability among the included trials in terms of baseline characteristics, treatment methods, and outcome assessments. There was considerable variation in patient populations across studies, with differences in diabetes duration, glycemic control, and comorbidities potentially affecting treatment outcomes.

- Some studies did not provide detailed classifications of diabetic retinopathy subtypes, which might obscure the varying treatment effects based on disease severity.
- Additionally, the differing follow-up durations made it challenging to directly compare results, especially when evaluating long-term outcomes beyond the usual clinical trial timeframe.
- Geographic and demographic differences further restrict generalizability, as treatment effectiveness may vary due to healthcare systems, genetic factors, and environmental influences across different populations.

Clinical Implications

- Anti-VEGF therapy is superior to traditional PRP in managing diabetic retinopathy across various outcome measures.
- Anti-VEGF agents resulted in better visual outcomes, more significant anatomical improvements, and fewer complications than PRP.
- Combination therapy yielded promising results for specific aspects such as neovascularization regression and CRT reduction.
- However, choosing a treatment requires balancing efficacy with considerations of treatment burden, patient compliance, and individual characteristics.

Scope for Future Research

- Research on gene therapy, which offers a groundbreaking method for treating resistant diabetic retinopathy, using technologies such as CRISPR-Cas9 to correct genetic defects or control abnormal blood vessel growth.
- Stem cell therapy using retinal pigment epithelial cells and neural stem cells holds potential for repairing damaged retinal tissue and restoring vision.
- New pharmacological strategies deserve exploration, such as receptor-interacting protein kinase 1 (RIP1 kinase) inhibitors targeting necroptotic cell death pathways, sodium-glucose cotransporter-2 (SGLT-2) inhibitors for early-stage diabetic retinopathy, and hormonal therapies aimed at retinal vascular leakage.
- Advanced drug delivery systems, including nanoparticles and sustained-release formulations, might enhance bioavailability and longevity of therapeutic agents, reducing the need for frequent intravitreal injections and related complications.
- Personalized medicine approaches based on genetic and biomarker data represent another promising area for disease progression and treatment.

18. Benefit of Semaglutide in Symptomatic Peripheral Artery Disease by Baseline Type 2 Diabetes characteristics: Insights From STRIDE, a Randomized, Placebo-controlled, Double-blind Trial

Ref: Rasouli N, Arslan EG, Catarig AM, Houlind K, Ludvik B, Nordanstig J, et al. Benefit of Semaglutide in Symptomatic Peripheral Artery Disease by Baseline Type 2 Diabetes Characteristics: Insights From STRIDE, a Randomized, Placebo-Controlled, Double-Blind Trial. Diabetes Care. 2025;48(9):1529-35.

ABSTRACT

Objective: Once-weekly subcutaneous semaglutide 1.0 mg significantly improved functional outcomes, symptoms, and quality of life in people with symptomatic peripheral artery disease (PAD) and type 2 diabetes, according to the Semaglutide and Walking Capacity in People with Symptomatic Peripheral Artery Disease and Type 2 Diabetes (STRIDE) trial (NCT04560998). It is unclear whether these benefits are consistent across all diabetes related characteristics.

Methods and design of research: The ratio to baseline (ETR) in maximum walking distance (MWD) was the primary outcome and the pain-free walking distance (PFWD) was a crucial secondary endpoint. A constant load treadmill was used to test both at 52 weeks. Body mass index (BMI), glycated hemoglobin (HbA1c), duration of diabetes, and diabetic drugs were used to perform subgroup analysis. For repeated measurements, a mixed model was employed that included the treatment-by-subgroup interaction, baseline value as a covariate, and treatment, region, and subgroup as fixed factors.

Results: 35.1% of the 792 patients (median duration of diabetes: 12.2 years, HbA1c: 7.1%, BMI: 28.7 kg/m^2) used sodium-glucose cotransporter-2 inhibitors, while 31.7% used insulin. Regardless of the duration of diabetes (ETR of 1.15 vs. 1.13 for <10 vs. ≥10 years, $p = 0.80$), BMI (1.12 vs. 1.16 for <30 vs. $p = 0.58$), HbA1c (1.13 for <7% and ≥7%, $p = 0.99$), or medication use, semaglutide significantly improved MWD. Additionally, semaglutide enhanced PFWD in all subgroups ($p > 0.1$ for all interactions). BMI reduction was more noticeable in the control group with higher baseline BMI and had a slight correlation with improvements in MWD. The safety results were the same for all subgroups.

Conclusion: Walking function was enhanced with semaglutide in persons with type 2 diabetes and PAD, including those with well-controlled HbA1c and those without obesity. Benefits extended beyond weight or glycemic reduction and were consistent across BMI and HbA1c categories.

CRITICAL APPRAISAL

What was Known Prior to this Study?

Glucagon-like peptide 1 (GLP-1) receptor activation improves endothelial function, reduces arterial stiffness, enhances microvascular perfusion, and has anti-inflammatory properties, all of which may contribute to improved walking capacity in peripheral artery disease (PAD) with type 2 diabetes mellitus (T2DM). Previous posthoc analysis reported a reduced risk of amputation in people with type 2 diabetes treated with liraglutide. STRIDE trial reported significant benefits of semaglutide, a GLP-1 RA, in the functional capacity [as measured by constant load treadmill (CLT)] in individuals with symptomatic PAD and T2DM. Whether benefits are consistent in patients with varying metabolic profiles, including baseline glycemic control, body weight, and duration of diabetes, are still largely unknown.

What this Study Adds?

Semaglutide improved walking function in T2DM with PAD, including individuals without obesity and those with well-controlled glycated hemoglobin (HbA1c).

This finding support effectiveness of semaglutide beyond weight or glycemic changes.

Major Strength

- Findings are clinically relevant given the high burden of PAD in diabetes and limited therapeutic options.
- Provides insights into mechanisms linking metabolic therapy and vascular disease.

Limitations

- STRIDE trial was not designed to assess semaglutide's interaction with diabetes characteristics, making this a secondary, exploratory analysis.

- The analyses may be underpowered to detect interaction effects in smaller subgroups, such as insulin users; thus, nonsignificant interaction *p* values should not be interpreted as definitive evidence.
- As it was an exploratory analysis, no formal adjustment for multiple comparisons was applied, which increases the risk of type I error. These findings are hypothesis-generating and warrant confirmation in future adequately powered studies.

Clinical Implications

- Clinicians should not restrict the use of this therapy to patients with PAD and T2DM who have elevated HbA1c or high body mass index (BMI).
- Mechanisms underlying the observed improvements in functional capacity are likely independent of glycemic control and weight loss.

Scope for Future Research

- Dedicated trial which would provide valuable insight into mechanism of action of this therapy's effect on PAD.
- Additionally, studies should be designed to assess long-term outcomes, including PAD progression and amputation-free survival.
- Need future trials which will evaluate the potential benefits of semaglutide in combination with other PAD interventions, such as revascularization and supervised exercise therapy.

19. Use of SGLT-2i versus DPP-4i as an Add-on Therapy and the Risk of PAD-related Surgical Events (Amputation, Stent Placement, or Vascular Surgery): A Cohort Study in Veterans with Diabetes

Ref: Griffin KE, Snyder K, Javid AH, Hackstadt A, Greevy R, Grijalva CG, et al. Use of SGLT-2i Versus DPP-4i as an Add-on Therapy and the Risk of PAD-Related Surgical Events (Amputation, Stent Placement, or Vascular Surgery): A Cohort Study in Veterans with Diabetes. Diabetes Care. 2025;48:361-70.

ABSTRACT

Objective: To compare the risk of new users of dipeptidyl peptidase 4 inhibitors (DPP-4is) and sodium-glucose cotransporter-2 inhibitors (SGLT-2is) for composite peripheral artery disease (PAD) surgical outcomes, such as peripheral revascularization and amputation procedures.

Research design and methods: From October 1, 2000, to December 31, 2021, a retrospective cohort study of American veterans with diabetes who were at least 18 years old and received care from the Veterans Health Administration was conducted. Medicare, Medicaid, and the National Death Index were connected to the data. An connection between PAD surgery for peripheral revascularization and amputation and the novel use of SGLT-2i or DPP-4i drugs as an adjunct to metformin, sulfonylurea, or insulin treatment alone or in combination was assessed. In a propensity score-weighted cohort with a competing risk of mortality and a provision for events to occur up to 90 or 360 days after quitting SGLT-2is, a Cox proportional hazards model for time to-PAD event analysis compared the risk of a PAD event between SGLT-2is and DPP-4is.

Results: There were 76,072 SGLT-2i and 75,833 DPP-4i usage episodes in the weighted cohort. HbA1c was 8.4% [interquartile range (IQR) 7.5–9.4%], the median age was 69 years, and the median duration of diabetes was 10.1 (IQR 6.6–14.6) years. SGLT-2i and DPP-4i users experienced 874 and 780 PAD incidents, respectively, with event rates of 11.2 (95% CI 10.5–11.9) and 10.0 (9.4–10.6) per 1,000 person-years [adjusted hazard ratio (aHR) 1.18 (95% CI 1.08–1.29)]. The aHR was 1.16 (95% CI 1.06–1.26) when PAD episodes were permitted for 360 days following the conclusion of SGLT-2i usage.

Conclusion: Compared to DPP-4i, SGLT-2i as an additional treatment for diabetes was linked to a higher cause-specific risk of PAD operations.

CRITICAL APPRAISAL

What was Known Prior to this Study?

In the CANVAS and CANVAS-R trials, investigators reported an increased risk of amputation among sodium-glucose cotransporter-2 inhibitor (SGLT-2i) users. Later, CREDENCE study found no statistical difference in amputation among SGLT-2i users. Uncertainty remains about the use of SGLT-2is in populations with high risk for peripheral artery disease (PAD) and revascularization.

What this Study Adds?

The SGLT-2i as an add-on therapy was associated with an increased cause specific hazard of PAD surgeries compared with dipeptidyl peptidase 4 inhibitor (DPP-4i). This finding was consistent when evaluating amputations and revascularization procedures separately.

Major Strength

- Broad outcome definition that includes revascularization procedures. This serves to capture events occurring earlier in the disease process of PAD than amputation.
- Use of a trial emulation approach and real-world methodology encompassing medication use and tracking.
- Study of a high-risk cohort of veterans with long-standing diabetes, and extensive control of covariates.

Limitations

- Approximately 57% of the cohort used SGLT-2is or DPP-4is as third-line treatment, indicating a longer duration of diabetes. Recently, SGLT-2is have been used more often, including as first- and second-line therapy, given their benefit in heart failure and chronic kidney disease.
- Median follow-up for both groups was 0.7 years. This limited follow-up time could impact the number of amputations and revascularization events.
- Study population mainly consisted of white men, limiting their generalizability.

Clinical Implications

Clinicians should be cautious in adding SGLT-2i in patients with high risk of amputation.

Scope for Future Research

- Prospective randomized trials focusing on PAD-specific endpoints (limb ischemia, amputation, and walking distance)
- Head-to-head comparisons between SGLT-2 inhibitors and GLP-1 receptor agonists in PAD
- Real-world studies in diverse populations, including South Asian

20. SGLT-2 Inhibitors and Nephrolithiasis Risk in Patients with Type 2 Diabetes: A Cohort Study and Meta-analysis

Ref: Yeh JA, Liu YC, Huang AH, Peng CC, Loh CH, Munir KM, et al. SGLT-2 inhibitors and nephrolithiasis risk in patients with type 2 diabetes: A cohort study and meta-analysis. Diabetes Res Clin Pract. 2025;222:112088.

ABSTRACT

Aims: The purpose of this study was to assess the association between the usage of sodium-glucose cotransporter-2 inhibitors (SGLT-2i) and the risk of nephrolithiasis.

Techniques: We examined electronic health records from the TriNetX Analytics Network, which comprises patients from 64 US healthcare organizations, in this real-world cohort study. Included were adult patients with type 2 diabetes (T2D) who started using glucagon-like peptide 1 receptor agonists (GLP-1 RAs), dipeptidyl peptidase-4 inhibitors (DPP4is), or SGLT-2is between January 2015 and December 2023. SGLT-2is and GLP-1 RAs as well as SGLT-2is and DPP4is were compared. Patients were monitored for a maximum of 5 years. To summarize the available data, a meta-analysis was also carried out.

Results: The cohort study comprised 482,284 patients (241,142 pairs) for SGLT-2is versus GLP-1 RAs comparisons and 500,000 patients (250,000 pairs) for SGLT-2is versus DPP4is comparisons. Compared to DPP4i (HR 0.86; 95% CI 0.83–0.90) and GLP-1 RA users (HR 0.90; 95% CI 0.86–0.94), SGLT-2i users had a significantly decreased incidence of nephrolithiasis. These results were corroborated by a meta-analysis that included our research with four more real-world studies.

Conclusion: By lowering the risk of nephrolithiasis, this study implies that SGLT-2is may have advantages beyond glycemic control.

CRITICAL APPRAISAL

What was Known Before this Study?

Type 2 diabetes (T2D) is recognized as a potential risk factor for nephrolithiasis. A 2019 meta-analysis revealed no association between the use of sodium-glucose cotransporter-2 inhibitors (SGLT-2is) and reduction of nephrolithiasis. Later in 2022, posthoc analyses of clinical trials indicated a potential reduction in risk of nephrolithiasis among SGLT-2i users. Recently, two cohort studies suggested that SGLT-2is may reduce the risk of nephrolithiasis. 2024 US cohort study also showed that SGLT-2is lower the risk of nephrolithiasis in T2D, compared with both glucagon-like peptide 1 receptor agonists (GLP-1 RAs) and dipeptidyl peptidase 4 inhibitors (DPP4is).

The SGLT-2is can increase urinary flow, which dilutes lithogenic substances in the urine, reducing the risk of nephrolithiasis. Further, SGLT-2is may reduce uric acid stone formation by raising urine pH.

What this Study Adds?

- This study showed that individuals treated with SGLT-2is had a reduced risk of nephrolithiasis in T2D compared to DPP4is or GLP-1 RA.
- In subgroup analyses, the reduction in nephrolithiasis risk with SGLT-2i use was more significant in the younger subgroup (≤65 years old).
- Additionally, in our sex-stratified analysis showed that significant risk reduction was observed only in the male subgroup.

Major Strength

- Large sample size, improving statistical power for relatively uncommon events.
- Inclusion of real-world data enhances generalizability.
- Comparative approach with other antidiabetic drug classes strengthened interpretability.

Limitations

- Study outcomes were identified using diagnostic codes rather than direct clinical assessments, which may have affected the accuracy of recorded data, including missing data.
- Possibility of unmeasured or residual confounding from factors such as dietary intake and hydration status cannot be entirely ruled out.
- The study focused on epidemiological associations rather than the underlying biological mechanisms.

Clinical Implications

This study helps clinicians to take treatment decisions for patients with T2D, particularly when considering options not only for glycemic control but also nephrolithiasis risk reduction.

Scope for Future Research

- Further study is required evaluating nephrolithiasis as a primary outcome.
- Mechanistic and interventional studies are needed to better understand the potential biological association between SGLT-2 inhibitor use and the reduced risk of nephrolithiasis.

21. Impact of SGLT-2 Inhibitors on Kidney Health and Survival in Patients with Polycystic Kidney Disease and Type 2 Diabetes

Ref: Yen FS, Huang JY, Dong C, Hwu CM, Hsu CC, Wei JC. Impact of SGLT-2 inhibitors on kidney health and survival in patients with polycystic kidney disease and type 2 diabetes. Diabetes Res Clin Pract. 2025;226:112357.

ABSTRACT

Aim: To assess how dialysis, cardiovascular, and mortality risks are affected by sodium-glucose cotransporter-2 inhibitors (SGLT-2i) in individuals with type 2 diabetes (T2D) and polycystic kidney disease (PKD).

Techniques: We found 31,070 patients with both PKD and T2D using a target trial emulation within the TriNetX US network (2015–2022). Propensity score matching was used to create three simulated trials: SGLT-2i versus nonusers (*n* = 2,640 pairings), SGLT-2i versus dipeptidyl peptidase 4 (DPP-4) inhibitors (*n* = 2,016), and SGLT-2i versus. glucagon-like peptide 1 receptor agonist (GLP-1 RA) (*n* = 1,870). Hazard ratios (HRs) were estimated using Cox proportional hazards models.

Results: SGLT-2i users were less likely than non-users to experience dialysis (HR 0.657), acute kidney injury (AKI; HR 0.896), and death (HR 0.840). SGLT-2i use was linked to lower chances of dialysis (HR 0.458), AKI (HR 0.835), and death (HR 0.813) when compared to DPP-4 inhibitors. SGLT-2i users had a lower dialysis risk (HR 0.531) than GLP-1 RAs.

Conclusion: Patients with PKD and T2D who used SGLT-2i had lower chances of dialysis, AKI, and death. These results point to a possible benefit for survival and kidney function in this high-risk population. However, an emulation process and propensity score approaches based on electronic health records were used to obtain the results.

CRITICAL APPRAISAL

What was Known Prior to this Study?

Previous RCTs on CKD and heart failure protection with sodium-glucose cotransporter-2 inhibitor (SGLT-2i) have excluded patients with polycystic kidney disease (PKD). Wang et al. employed phlorizin in a rat model of

PKD and observed a notable enhancement in creatinine clearance and a decrease in both kidney weight and the amount of albumin excreted in the urine. Morioka and colleagues conducted a retrospective case series analysis and found that short-term treatment with dapagliflozin correlated with a reduction in estimated glomerular filtration rate (eGFR) and an increase in the height-adjusted total kidney volume (htTKV). SGLT-2i may directly inhibit the growth of cystic epithelial cells in the kidney by affecting the MAPK signaling pathway. But, clinical studies confirming the efficacy of SGLT-2i in PKD are lacking.

What this Study Adds?

- SGLT-2i usage among patients with both PKD and type 2 diabetes (T2D) was associated with a significantly lower dialysis risk and all-cause mortality.
- Study also showed that SGLT-2i users had a reduced risk of acute kidney injury (AKI) compared to nonusers and dipeptidyl peptidase 4 inhibitor (DPP-4i).

Major Strength

- It is largest real-world study to date evaluating SGLT-2is specifically in patients with PKD and T2D.
- Benefits of SGLT-2i in PKD were consistent not only compared to nonusers but also compared to DPP-4i and glucagon-like peptide 1 receptor agonist (GLP-1 RA), strengthening comparative effectiveness.
- Extensive propensity score matching with adjustment for demographics, comorbidities, medications, and laboratory parameters.

Limitations

- Data on CT or MRI-determined total kidney volume were missing in some.
- Sequential data on total kidney volume and renal function were not available, which prevented from observing the potential longitudinal effects of SGLT-2i use on kidney size and function in patients with PKD.
- The matching process may have selected a subset of patients in the non-SGLT-2i group with more severe polycystic and cardiovascular disease.
- Average age and eGFR of the patients in this study were 64.6 years and 67.9 mL/min/1.73 m^2, respectively. This suggests that the majority of patients in the study had mild autosomal dominant polycystic kidney disease (ADPKD), and that patients with PKD1 mutations were significantly underrepresented. As a result, the findings of this study may not be generalizable to all patients with ADPKD, or those without diabetes.
- Retrospective cohort study like this one, may contain unmeasured or unknown confounding factors despite adjustment for numerous significant variables.

Clinical Implications

Clinicians should initiate SGLT-2is in patients with PKD and T2D, particularly when renal protection is a priority.

Scope for Future Research

- Need prospective randomized controlled trials of SGLT-2is specifically in ADPKD, with and without diabetes.
- Studies should be done evaluating effects on kidney volume progression, cyst burden, and biomarkers.
- Exploration of combination therapy with tolvaptan and strategies to mitigate polyuria and volume depletion.
- Genotype-stratified analyses to determine whether benefits differ between PKD1 and PKD2.

22. Inadequately Controlled Type 2 Diabetes and Hypercortisolism: Improved Glycemia With Mifepristone Treatment

Ref: DeFronzo RA, Fonseca V, Aroda VR, Auchus RJ, Bailey T, Bancos I, et al. Inadequately Controlled Type 2 Diabetes and Hypercortisolism: Improved Glycemia With Mifepristone Treatment. Diabetes Care. 2025;48:2036-44.

ABSTRACT

Objective: Despite receiving numerous glucose-lowering treatments, type 2 diabetes (T2D) is still poorly managed in many people. Endogenous hypercortisolism is common among these people, according to several studies. We investigated if their glycemic control is improved by cortisol-directed therapy.

Methods and research design: In this prospective, multicenter, double-blind study, 136 people with T2D [glycated hemoglobin (HbA1c) 7.5%–11.5% (58–102 mmol/mol) on multiple medications] and hypercortisolism (by dexamethasone suppression test) were stratified by the presence or absence of an adrenal imaging abnormality and randomly assigned 2:1 to receive mifepristone (300–900 mg once daily; $n = 91$) or placebo ($n = 45$). The change in HbA1c was the main outcome. Changes in weight, waist circumference, safety, and glucose-lowering drugs were secondary end goals.

Outcomes: The study cohort's mean baseline HbA1c was 8.55% (69.9 mmol/mol). The HbA1c least squares mean (LSM) difference from placebo at 24 weeks was 1.32% (95% CI −1.81 to −0.83, $p < 0.001$). Body weight and waist circumference decreased in mifepristone recipients [placebo-adjusted LSM differences of −5.12 kg (95% CI −8.2 to −2.03) and −5.1 cm (95% CI −8.23 to −1.99), respectively]. Compared to 18% of people receiving a placebo, 46% of those receiving mifepristone stopped their treatment. Hypokalemia, exhaustion, nausea, vomiting, headache, peripheral edema, diarrhea, and dizziness were among the adverse effects associated with mifepristone (>10% of participants), which are consistent with the drug's recognized tolerability profile. There were also increases in blood pressure.

Conclusion: Cortisol-directed medication therapy with mifepristone decreased HbA1c in patients with poorly managed T2D and hypercortisolism, with a tolerability profile that was manageable.

CRITICAL APPRAISAL

What was Known Before this Study?

Approximately one-quarter of people with type 2 diabetes (T2D) who do not meet glycemic targets despite treatment with multiple medications may have endogenous hypercortisolism. Hypercortisolism can negatively impact glucose control through various mechanisms, including increased insulin resistance, impaired β-cell function, inhibition of the insulinotropic effects of glucagon-like peptide 1 (GLP-1) and glucose-dependent insulinotropic polypeptide (GIP), increased lipolysis in adipocytes, and increased hepatic glucose production. In the SEISMIC trial, participants with hypercortisolism and T2D or impaired glucose tolerance experienced statistically significant reductions in HbA1c from 7.43 to 6.29% after 24 weeks of mifepristone treatment. But, SEISMIC trial enrolled participants with overt features of hypercortisolism only.

What this Study Adds?

- Endogenous hypercortisolism was found in 23.8% of participants with inadequately controlled T2D.
- Mifepristone lowered HbA1c by ~1.5% and improved weight.

- Side effects were generally manageable, but serious side effects and early study discontinuations were more common with mifepristone.

Major Strength

- CATALYST trial is the first randomized, placebo-controlled study to demonstrate that inadequately controlled T2D with nonneoplastic hypercortisolism responds to cortisol-directed treatment.
- Careful exclusion of common causes of false-positive DST results, strengthening internal validity.
- Use of mixed-effects models and sensitivity analyses strengthens statistical analysis.

Limitations

- There was preponderance of non-Hispanic white participants; consequently, the results might not apply to a broader range of individuals with T2D and endogenous hypercortisolism.
- There were a significant number of adverse events, and a significant number of early terminations.

Clinical Implications

- Individuals with inadequately controlled T2D should be considered for hypercortisolism screening.
- Dexamethasone suppression test (DST), performed in an appropriately selected patient population with exclusion of common causes for false-positive results, identifies individuals who may benefit from cortisol-directed pharmacotherapy.
- In those with hypercortisolism, cortisol-directed therapy may lower HbA1c, weight, and waist circumference.

Scope for Future Research

- Longer-term studies are needed to demonstrate benefit and tolerability.
- Comparative studies of mifepristone versus intensified standard-of-care therapy
- Exploring safer cortisol-modulating agents with fewer mineralocorticoid effects
- Studies in diverse ethnic populations, including South Asian cohorts

---

23. Unmasking Hypercortisolism in Difficult-to-control Type 2 Diabetes: A Useful Paradigm Shift?

Ref: Nieman LK, Muniyappa R. Unmasking Hypercortisolism in Difficult-to-Control Type 2 Diabetes: A Useful Paradigm Shift? Diabetes Care. 2025;48:1994-6.

ABSTRACT

The thought-provoking reports of the CATALYST study in this issue of Diabetes Care question our present understanding of Cushing syndrome (CS), the etiology of diabetes that is difficult to control, and the management of both conditions. 23.8% of patients with difficult-to-control type 2 diabetes (T2D) showed "hypercortisolism," according to results from the first prevalence phase of CATALYST. This was predicated on the inability to suppress cortisol in a 1-mg dexamethasone suppression test (DST) to ≤1.8 mg/dL (50 nmol/L). A computed tomography scan revealed an adrenal abnormality in about one-third of these individuals. During the study's treatment phase, 136 individuals with hypercortisolism were randomly assigned to receive either a placebo or mifepristone, a glucocorticoid receptor antagonist, for a duration of 24 weeks. The mifepristone group's mean A1c dropped significantly from 8.62 to 7.12%, while the placebo group's A1c changed very little. These unexpected findings pose significant issues regarding the optimal way to categorize hypercortisolism in T2D and which patients might benefit from cortisol-targeted treatment.

CRITICAL APPRAISAL

What was Known Prior to this Editorial?

Previous meta-analysis suggested that the prevalence of hypercortisolism in type 2 diabetes (T2D) varies from 0.7% with use of a DST cortisol criteria of >5 µg/dL and up to 11.1% with a more lenient threshold (>1.8 µg/dL). In advanced T2D, prevalence is ~4.5%. However, data specific to difficult-to-control T2D were lacking prior to CATALYST study.

What this Editorial Adds?

- 23.8% of individuals with T2D had inadequate cortisol suppression in this study.
- Structural adrenal abnormalities were found in 34.7% of 219 participants, including unilateral adrenal nodules (22.8%), bilateral nodules (4.6%), and unilateral or bilateral adrenal enlargement in 3.7%.
- After 24 weeks, the least squares mean change in A1c from baseline was –1.47% with mifepristone.
- Grade 3 adverse events also were more frequent with mifepristone in 29% individuals with hypokalemia (5%) and euglycemic ketoacidosis (3%) reported only in the mifepristone arm.

Major Strengths

- This commentary clearly discussed the diagnostic pitfalls, particularly the misuse of DST as a stand-alone confirmatory test.
- Explicitly addresses the safety concerns (hypokalemia, blood pressure rise, and euglycemic DKA).

Limitations

- CATALYST study did not include evaluation of UFC or salivary cortisol, so there is uncertainty as to whether participants had Cushing syndrome (CS).
- Hyperaldosteronism was also not evaluated despite its relevance in a cohort where 89% had hypertension.
- Concerns are raised with regard to frequent adverse events and the lack of clear diagnostic stratification. Overt CS, MACS, and nonfunctioning adrenal adenomas in the cohort were also likely to be included.
- There were possibility of even false positives, given the 10% false-positive rate of DST, particularly in older adults.

Clinical Implications

- Patients with T2D and abnormal DST results should be screened further for CS, and for hyperaldosteronism in the case of hypertension.
- Careful attention should be given to subtle clinical signs of cortisol excess and factors that may confound DST interpretation.

Scope for Future Research

- Need prospective studies for comparing surgical and medical therapy in MACS.
- Clear characterization of patients with hypercortisolemia who respond to mifepristone, is essential.
- Long-term outcome studies assessing cardiovascular events, mortality, and quality of life are also needed.

24. Seeking Multiorgan Benefits with Cardiovascular Kidney–Metabolic Drug Therapy

Ref: Zannad F. Seeking Multiorgan Benefits with Cardiovascular-Kidney-Metabolic Drug Therapy. N Engl J Med. 2025;392(20):2061-2.

ABSTRACT

It has been demonstrated that injectable semaglutide, a long-acting glucagon-like peptide 1 (GLP-1) receptor agonist, lowers the risk of significant adverse cardiovascular events in people with chronic renal disease, type 2 diabetes, cardiovascular disease (or a high risk of cardiovascular disease), or both. The results of the Semaglutide Cardiovascular Outcomes Trial (SOUL), which demonstrated a decrease in cardiovascular risk in a comparable target group with the administration of oral semaglutide, are reported by McGuire et al. The indication to use the medication for cardiovascular prevention in people with type 2 diabetes and atherosclerotic cardiovascular disease, chronic kidney disease, or both—which is currently granted to injectable GLP-1 receptor agonists—is likely to be extended to oral semaglutide due to the strong evidence. Safety and drug discontinuation data were consistent with the outcomes of injectable GLP-1 receptor agonists. It can be risky to compare data across trials and remark on the outcomes for particular components of a composite primary endpoint or secondary endpoints. Interestingly, however, a reduction in the risk of myocardial infarction was the primary driver of the cardiovascular benefit of oral semaglutide in SOUL. Fatal or nonfatal stroke was the cardiovascular outcome linked to the largest reduction in relative risk in injectable GLP-1 receptor agonist trials. Despite the high number of fatal or nonfatal strokes recorded in the trial, the effect on stroke in SOUL was neutral. Additionally, despite the high incidence of heart failure events, the effect on this outcome was neutral, which is in line with findings from injectable GLP-1 receptor agonist trials in comparable target populations. Lastly, serious renal disease events—an new composite outcome—were unaffected by oral semaglutide. This conclusion is in contrast to the outcomes of the FLOW (Evaluate Renal Function with Semaglutide Once Weekly) experiment, which used injectable semaglutide. However, the availability of an efficient oral GLP-1 receptor agonist may allay patients' and physicians' worries about injections, according to the SOUL investigators.

CRITICAL APPRAISAL

What was Known Prior to this Editorial?

Cardiovascular disease (CVD) and chronic kidney disease (CKD) are the dominant drivers of morbidity and mortality in type 2 diabetes (T2D). Therefore, a new conceptual framework of cardiovascular-kidney-metabolic (CKM) syndrome has evolved. Sodium-glucose cotransporter-2 inhibitors (SGLT-2is), glucagon-like peptide 1 receptor agonists (GLP-1 RA), and finerenone have independently demonstrated cardiovascular and renal benefits beyond glucose lowering.

What this Editorial Adds?

- SOUL trial showed a reduction in cardiovascular risk with the use of oral semaglutide. But, the cardiovascular benefit of oral semaglutide in SOUL was driven mainly by a decrease in the risk of myocardial infarction.
- Effect of semaglutide on incidence of heart failure was neutral.
- Oral semaglutide had a neutral effect on composite outcome—major kidney disease events in SOUL study, which differs from that found in FLOW trial with injectable semaglutide.

Major Strength

- This editorial is an excellent synthesis of contemporary Cardiovascular Outcome Trials (CVOT), renal, and metabolic trial data without overstatement.
- It highlights inclusivity gaps in clinical trials, including underrepresentation of ethnic minorities.

Limitations

- It lacks discussion on cost, access, and implementation barriers, particularly relevant for low- and middle-income countries.
- It does not address potential therapeutic sequencing dilemmas of GLP-1 RA versus SGLT-2i prioritization.

Clinical Implications

- It encourages clinicians to move beyond glucose-centric care and adopt a multidisciplinary approach.

- It reinforces early use of foundational therapies (SGLT-2i, GLP-1 RA, and finerenone) in high-risk T2D patients.

Scope for Future Research

- Integrated CKM trials with unified cardiovascular, renal, metabolic, and weight endpoints
- Studies in more representative populations, including South Asians
- Exploration of next-generation agents such as dual GLP-1/GIP agonists within CKM framework.

25. Metabolic Rebound after GLP-1 Receptor Agonist Discontinuation: A Systematic Review and Meta-analysis

Ref: Tzang CC, Wu PH, Luo CA, Chen ZT, Lee YT, Huang ES, et al. Metabolic rebound after GLP-1 receptor agonist discontinuation: a systematic review and meta-analysis. EClinicalMedicine. 2025 Nov 28;90:103680.

ABSTRACT

Background: Aim of the study—to quantify the extent of metabolic and cardiovascular rebound following the discontinuation of glucagon-like peptide 1 receptor agonist (GLP-1 RA) therapy in adults with obesity, type 2 diabetes, or type 1 diabetes, and identify potential modifiers of these outcomes.

Methods: Systematic review and meta-analysis of randomized controlled trials (RCTs) were conducted including adults and adolescents treated with GLP-1 RAs, followed by a postdiscontinuation follow-up of at least 12 weeks. Databases searched included MEDLINE, Embase, Cochrane CENTRAL, Web of Science, and ClinicalTrials.gov, with no language restrictions, and published up to October 17, 2025. Changes in anthropometric, glycemic, cardiovascular, and lipid parameters between the end of treatment and the postcessation period were assessed. Random-effects models were used to calculate pooled mean differences. The risk of bias and certainty of evidence were evaluated using the Cochrane ROB 2.0 and GRADE frameworks. The study was registered with PROSPERO under CRD42025646185.

Findings: 18 RCTs (3,771 participants) were included. Among individuals with obesity, discontinuation of GLP-1 RA resulted in significant metabolic rebound, characterized by a body weight gain of 5.63 kg (95% CI 3.52–7.73; I^2 = 99.57%, moderate) and an increase in HbA1c of 0.25% (95% CI 0.18–0.32; I^2 = 98.45%, moderate). Waist circumference, body mass index (BMI), systolic blood pressure (SBP), and fasting plasma glucose (FPG) also showed significant deterioration. In the type 2 diabetes setting, weight gain was 2.03 kg (95% CI 1.63–2.42; I^2 = 42.28%, moderate), and HbA1c rose by 0.65% (95% CI 0.22–1.08; I^2 = 96.83%, moderate), while FPG remained stable (0.90 mmol/L; 95% CI −0.36 to 2.17; I^2 = 98.81%, moderate). Subgroup analyses revealed greater weight regain with longer follow-up (>26 weeks: 7.31 kg vs. 2.51 kg) and with semaglutide compared to liraglutide (8.21 kg vs. 4.29 kg). Semaglutide also led to greater increases in waist circumference (3.80 cm vs. 2.69 cm) and SBP (7.09 mm Hg vs. 1.56 mm Hg). Most outcomes showed no evidence of significant publication bias, with minor asymmetry detected for very-low-density lipoprotein (VLDL) levels in individuals with obesity and for weight change (kg) in patients with type 2 diabetes. The risk of bias assessment using the ROB 2.0 tool rated all included studies as having a low risk.

Interpretation: The magnitude and consistency of these effects underscore the physiological consequences of GLP-1 RA discontinuation. As the clinical use of GLP-1 RAs continues to grow in the management of obesity and diabetes, it is imperative that treatment guidelines address not only initiation and titration but also discontinuation and long-term maintenance strategies to sustain therapeutic gains.

CRITICAL APPRAISAL

What was Known Prior to this Study?

Efficacy and safety of glucagon-like peptide 1 receptor agonists (GLP-1 RAs) in managing glycemic control and weight are well established in prior studies. However, their postcessation effects have not been adequately studied. Some individual studies have observed substantial reversals of GLP-1 RA-induced benefits, questioning the durability of treatment effects. Previous trials such as STEP-10 and SURMOUNT-4 trials reported substantial weight regain, deterioration of glycemic control, and reversal of lipid and blood pressure improvements after discontinuation of medication.

What this Study Adds?

- In individuals with obesity, discontinuation of GLP1 RA resulted in substantial increases in body weight, waist circumference, body mass index (BMI), systolic blood pressure, fasting plasma glucose, and HbA1c.
- Similar patterns were observed in type 2 diabetes, though fasting glucose rebound was less pronounced.
- The rebound in weight and waist circumference following GLP-1 RA cessation is near-complete reversal of prior improvements within 52 weeks.
- Subgroup analyses among patients with obesity revealed that longer follow-up durations (>26 weeks) and semaglutide use were associated with a greater rebound in weight, waist circumference, and systolic blood pressure compared to liraglutide.

Major Strength

This meta-analysis provides a comprehensive and up-to-date synthesis of the metabolic and cardiovascular changes observed after discontinuation of GLP-1 RA and it includes 18 randomized controlled trials involving 3,771 participants.

Limitations

- The analysis did not account for lifestyle factors, such as exercise or dietary interventions, despite their potential influence on outcomes.
- Reliance on study-level data precluded exploration of individual-level modifiers such as age, sex, baseline BMI, or comorbidities, which may affect susceptibility to metabolic rebound.
- Availability of rebound data was limited. Only a small subset included follow-up data after discontinuation of GLP-1 RA.
- Considerable heterogeneity was observed across multiple primary and subgroup outcomes, likely reflecting differences in study design, GLP-1 RA agents, and treatment durations.

Clinical Implications

This analysis underscores the importance of long-term treatment planning and structured transition strategies to mitigate relapse after therapy withdrawal with GLP-1 RA.

Scope for Future Research

- There is a need for future trials to extend monitoring beyond the treatment phase, not only for safety surveillance but also to inform long-term strategies for managing obesity and diabetes.
- Need of mechanistic studies searching for neuroendocrine and metabolic drivers of rebound after GLP-1 RA withdrawal.
- Identifying phenotypes and predictors most vulnerable to rapid metabolic reversal.

Section 4: DRUGS AND THERAPEUTICS (PART 1)

Section Editor: Sunetra Mondal

1. Coadministered Cagrilintide and Semaglutide in Adults with Overweight or Obesity

Ref: Garvey WT, Blüher M, Osorto Contreras CK, Davies MJ, Winning Lehmann E, Pietiläinen KH, et al.; REDEFINE 1 Study Group. Coadministered Cagrilintide and Semaglutide in Adults with Overweight or Obesity. N Engl J Med. 2025;393:635-47.

ABSTRACT

Background: Cagrilintide at a dose of 2.4 mg has demonstrated encouraging results in early phase trials, and semaglutide at a dose of 2.4 mg has established weight loss and cardiovascular benefits; the effectiveness of the combination (known as "CagriSema") on weight loss in individuals with obesity or overweight and coexisting conditions is unknown.

Methods: Adults without diabetes with a body mass index (BMI) of 30 kg/m^2 or higher or a BMI of 27 kg/m^2 or higher with at least one obesity-related complication were enrolled in a phase 3a, 68-week, multicenter, double-blind, placebo-controlled, and active controlled trial. Semaglutide and cagrilintide at a dose of 2.4 mg, semaglutide alone at a dose of 2.4 mg, cagrilintide alone at a dose of 2.4 mg, or a placebo were randomly allocated to participants in a ratio of 21:3:3:7. All groups also received lifestyle interventions. The relative change in bodyweight and a 5% or greater decrease in bodyweight from baseline to week 68 with cagrilintide–semaglutide as opposed to placebo were the major end goals. Confirmatory secondary end goals included reductions in bodyweight of 20, 25, and 30%. In accordance with the intention-to-treat principle, effect estimates were evaluated using the treatment policy estimand. Safety was evaluated.

Results: Of the 3,417 participants, 2,108 were randomly assigned to receive cagrilintide–semaglutide, 302 to receive semaglutide, 302 to receive cagrilintide, and 705 to receive a placebo. Between baseline and week 68, the estimated mean percent decrease in bodyweight was –20.4% with cagrilintide–semaglutide and –3.0% with placebo (estimated difference, –17.3% points; 95% confidence interval –18.1 to –16.6; $p < 0.001$). Weight-loss goals of 5% or more, 20% or more, 25% or more, and 30% or more were more likely to be met by participants receiving cagrilintide–semaglutide than by those getting a placebo ($p < 0.001$ for all comparisons). Nausea, vomiting, diarrhea, constipation, and abdominal discomfort were among the most common and mild-to-moderate gastrointestinal side effects (affecting 79.6% in the cagrilintide–semaglutide group and 39.9% in the placebo group).

Conclusion: When compared to a placebo, cagrilintide–semaglutide significantly and clinically relevant reduced bodyweight in persons who were overweight or obese. (Funded by Novo Nordisk; REDEFINE 1 ClinicalTrials.gov number, NCT05567796.)

CRITICAL APPRAISAL

What was Known Prior to the Study?

Semaglutide monotherapy has shown 15–17% weight loss in obesity trials like STEP, but plateauing at most responders for ≥20% loss. Amylin analogs like pramlintide showed modest 5–8% reductions with complementary satiety effects but limited as monotherapy potential due to tolerability. Preclinical synergy between amylin (cagrilintide) and glucagon-like peptide-1 (GLP-1) suggested additive hypothalamic signaling for hedonic/homeostatic appetite control. Phase 2 trials of cagrilintide monotherapy yielded 10–15% loss which was inferior to semaglutide, prompting combinations. Tirzepatide's dual glucose-dependent insulinotropic polypeptide (GIP)/GLP-1 agonism reached 20–22%, setting benchmarks, but no amylin-GLP-1 fixed-ratio existed. No phase 3 randomized controlled trials (RCTs) compared coadministration head-to-head with semaglutide across doses.

What this Study Adds?

The REDEFINE 1 phase 3 RCT demonstrates the superiority of coadministered cagrilintide 2.4 mg/semaglutide 2.4 mg (CagriSema) over cagrilintide or semaglutide or placebo, achieving –20.4% mean weight loss at 68 weeks in 2,108 adults with overweight/obesity (BMI ≥ 27/30 kg/m^2) versus –14.9% semaglutide, –11.5% cagrilintide, and –3.0% placebo. Coprimary endpoints were met robustly ($p < 0.001$) with 51.7% achieving ≥20% loss (vs. 9–25% others). Secondary gains included waist (–15 cm), systolic BP (–7 mm Hg), lipids, and quality-of-life improvements, all amplified in the combination arm. Safety profile was good with mostly gastrointestinal (GI) events (92%, mostly mild nausea/vomiting) without any new concerns and low discontinuation rates (5.9%). The results surpass tirzepatide benchmarks, positioning CagriSema as a potential leading pharmacotherapy.

Strengths

The study had a phase 3 multicenter double-blind design with active and placebo controls minimizing bias and had a large sample size. Dose-matched comparisons (2.4 mg each) were done. A long 68-week duration captured plateau beyond the usual 52-week standards. Comprehensive cardiometabolic parameters were analyzed as also quality of life (QoL) (BP, lipids, QoL-SF-36/IWQOL).

Limitations

There was predominance of White women limiting ethnic/gender generalizability. There was no diabetes subgroup. Industry funding (Novo Nordisk) risks bias despite blinding. The trial was relatively short-term for lifelong obesity and missed >2-year regain. The trial excluded those with estimated glomerular filtration rate (eGFR) < 30 mL/min/1.73 m^2 or recent CV events. No body composition (DXA/MRI) to assess muscle mass preservation was done. Fixed-ratio was used.

Clinical Implications

CagriSema is a good option for patients plateauing on semaglutide, targeting ≥20% loss in obesity with favorable effects in metabolic parameters. Patients should be counseled about GI side effects which are very common but transient.

Scope for Further Research

Phase 3 trials in type 2 diabetes mellitus (T2DM) and cardiovascular disease (CVD) cohorts with CV outcomes are necessary. Body composition and muscle functional trials are necessary, especially comparing to tirzepatide. Longer-term (>2 years) maintenance studies are required.

2. Cagrilintide–Semaglutide in Adults with Overweight or Obesity and Type 2 Diabetes

Ref: Davies MJ, Bajaj HS, Broholm C, Eliasen A, Garvey WT, le Roux CW, et al.; REDEFINE 2 Study Group. Cagrilintide–Semaglutide in Adults with Overweight or Obesity and Type 2 Diabetes. N Engl J Med. 2025;393:648-59.

ABSTRACT

Background: As monotherapies, cagrilintide and semaglutide have both been demonstrated to cause weight loss. For the purpose of managing weight in individuals with type 2 diabetes mellitus (T2DM), including those in a subset receiving continuous glucose monitoring, data on the coadministration of cagrilintide and semaglutide (known as "CagriSema") are required.

Techniques: Adults with a body mass index (BMI) of 27 kg/m^2 or higher, a glycated hemoglobin (HbA1c) level of 7–10%, and type 2 diabetes mellitus (T2DM) were assigned in a 3:1 ratio to receive once-weekly cagrilintide–semaglutide (2.4 mg each) or placebo, along with lifestyle intervention, for 68 weeks in this phase 3a, double-blind, randomized, placebo-controlled trial carried out in 12 countries. The percentage of patients who lost at least 5% of their bodyweight and the percentage change in bodyweight were the two main outcomes. Changes in glycemic measurements and safety evaluations were additional end goals. In accordance with the intention-to-treat principle, effect estimates were computed using the treatment-policy estimand.

Results: A total of 1,206 patients were randomly assigned to either the placebo group (302 patients) or the cagrilintide–semaglutide group (904 patients). The cagrilintide–semaglutide group's estimated mean change in bodyweight from baseline to week 68 was –13.7%, while the placebo group's estimated mean was –3.4% (estimated difference, –10.4 percentage points; 95% confidence interval (CI) –11.2 to –9.5; $p < 0.001$). Patients with weight reductions of 5% or more were more common in the cagrilintide–semaglutide group than in the placebo group ($p < 0.001$); reductions of at least 10, 15, and 20% were also more common ($p < 0.001$ for the final comparison). In the cagrilintide–semaglutide group, 73.5% of patients had a glycated hemoglobin (HbA1c) level of 6.5% or lower, compared to 15.9% in the placebo group. (Funded by Novo Nordisk; REDEFINE 2 ClinicalTrials.gov number, NCT05394519.)

CRITICAL APPRAISAL

What was Known Prior to the Study?

Semaglutide 2.4 mg monotherapy has yielded 9–15% weight loss in T2DM trials (SUSTAIN FORTE: –9.6%). Tirzepatide [dual glucagon-like peptide-1 (GLP-1)/glucose-dependent insulinotropic polypeptide (GIP)] set benchmarks with 15–21% loss but lacked amylin mechanisms. Amylin analogs enhanced satiety via central pathways, but monotherapy data were absent. Amylin synergy can amplify satiety, lean mass preservation, and metabolic parameters. No fixed-ratio GLP-1/amylin combinations had phase 3 data prior to this REDEFINE 2 trial.

What this Study Adds?

Cagrilintide–semaglutide reduced bodyweight by –13.7% at week 68 versus –3.4% placebo (difference –10.4%; 95% CI –11.2 to –9.5; $p < 0.001$). Responder rates were as high as 85% achieving ≥5% loss, 67% achieving ≥10%, 41% achieving ≥15%, and 20% achieving ≥20% weight loss (all $p < 0.001$). HbA1c reduced by –1.8% and a total of 73.5% achieved an HbA1c of ≤6.5%. Gastrointestinal adverse events (GI AEs) occurred in 72.5% (mild–moderate and mostly transient), with 12% discontinuations. Efficacy was consistent across BMI categories and diabetes duration subgroups.

Strengths

It was a multicenter (12 countries) study with double-blind randomization (3:1) involving 1,206 participants, thus well powered for co-primaries (% weight change and ≥5% responders). Lifestyle standardization was ensured. There were broad inclusion criteria with BMI ≥ 27 kg/m^2 and HbA1c 7–10% capturing real-world T2DM-obesity overlap.

Limitations

There was no active comparator (e.g., tirzepatide and semaglutide alone) and South Asian cohorts were underrepresented. There was high GI AEs (72.5%) versus placebo (34.4%). Only fixed ratio dosing was studied.

Clinical Implications

Cagrilintide-semaglutide injection can deliver 13–15% loss with robust HbA1c control as single-agent for T2DM-obesity, with simple once weekly dosing. GI AEs are mostly mild and transient.

Knowledge Gaps and Scope of Future Research

There is need for Cagri-sema to be tried head-to-head versus tirzepatide (REDEFINE 4). CV outcomes (REDEFINE 3) data are pending. Long-term safety (>2 years) and data on gallbladder and thyroid risks are needed. Dose escalation strategies are unexplored.

3. Semaglutide and Tirzepatide to Treat Obesity

Ref: Greenway FL. Semaglutide and Tirzepatide to Treat Obesity. N Engl J Med. 2025;393(1):84-5.

ABSTRACT

The results of a trial comparing tirzepatide and semaglutide, two medications currently approved to treat obesity that consistently result in reductions in bodyweight of >10% from baseline, are reported in this issue of the Journal by Aronne et al. The trial's findings will provide guidance to doctors treating obesity. There are few head-to-head comparisons of weight-loss drugs in a single trial, which makes this comparison trial noteworthy. Additionally, this trial included two maximum tolerable dose options for each medicine, reflecting how these drugs are frequently used in practice, in contrast to clinical trials that only assessed the highest dose. The forced escalation to the maximal dose utilized in some earlier trials of single weight-loss medications contrasts with this flexibility in dose administration. The fact that one-third of the trial participants were men was one of the strength of the study cohort. Women have made up about 80% of participants in the majority of obesity trials, making it challenging to assess sex-specific differences in weight loss. Both drugs caused weight reduction in this experiment that was roughly 6% points higher in women than in males. It is unclear if the stimulation of the glucagon-like peptide-1 (GLP-1) receptor—a mechanism shared by both medications—was the cause of this unequal weight loss, but the discovery begs the question of what bodily components are involved in weight reduction and why they can change depending on sex.

CRITICAL APPRAISAL

What was Known Prior to this Editorial?

Semaglutide, a GLP-1 receptor agonist, achieved ~15–17% weight loss in STEP trials for obesity without type 2 diabetes mellitus (T2DM). Tirzepatide, a dual GLP-1/glucose-dependent insulinotropic polypeptide (GIP) agonist, showed 20–22% reductions in the SURMOUNT trials, surpassing semaglutide in indirect comparisons. Both drugs can reduce cardiometabolic risks, including CV events, metabolic dysfunction-associated steatohepatitis (MASH) resolution, and obstructive sleep apnea (OSA) symptoms. Mechanisms involve appetite suppression, delayed gastric emptying, and energy expenditure via hypothalamic signaling. Prior meta-analyses confirmed dose-dependent GI tolerability issues, mostly mild and transient. Head-to-head data were limited before-2025, relying on network meta-analyses that favored tirzepatide. Postdiscontinuation, there was weight regain with both. Muscle preservation concerns have also been raised with both.

What this Editorial Adds?

This editorial contextualizes the trial by Aronne et al. showing tirzepatide's ~6–7% greater weight loss versus semaglutide at 72 weeks emphasizing GIP agonism's role in enhancing fat oxidation and muscle preservation. GI safety was comparable with both. The results also project tirzepatide's superior efficacy in diverse BMI groups. The editorial also discusses scalability via generics and oral formulations to enhance cost-effectiveness and integrates real-world evidence of adherence barriers. It also discusses the need for combination therapies with amylin analogs.

Strengths

It is a timely synthesis of pivotal head-to-head RCT data available for tirzepatide and semaglutide offering a balanced efficacy-safety-cost discussion. It also opens agenda for further research. Men formed a predominant component of the research cohort in contrary to other trials and found differentially greater effect among women raising questions about differential GLP-1 activity according to gender. It also used two maximum tolerated dose options for each drug, which reflects how these medications are often used in practice against the maximum dose used in other trials.

Limitations

The editorial relies on single trial interpretation with potential publication bias toward positive results.

Clinical Implications

Tirzepatide may be preferred over semaglutide for maximal weight loss goals. It is important to monitor muscle volume via DXA in elderly patients. Effects might be better seen in women. It is important to counsel on lifelong therapy to prevent regain.

Scope for Future Research

Long-term (>5 years) head-to-head cardiovascular (CV) outcomes as well as data in pediatric and cohorts are needed as well as cost-effectiveness studies.

4. Semaglutide for Metabolic Dysfunction Associated Steatohepatitis

Ref: Simon TG. Semaglutide for Metabolic Dysfunction Associated Steatohepatitis. N Engl J Med. 2025;392:2160-1.

ABSTRACT

Over 30% of persons worldwide suffer from metabolic dysfunction-associated steatotic liver disease (MASLD), a major cause of chronic liver disease. Progressive steatohepatitis [metabolic dysfunction-associated steatohepatitis (MASH)] and fibrosis, which can result in cirrhosis and mortality, affect up to one-third of MASLD patients. The fact that MASH is also linked to an increased risk of cardiovascular disease (CVD) which emphasizes how crucial it is to treat cardiometabolic risk factors at the same time. Two resmetirom, a liver-directed thyroid hormone receptor β-selective agonist, is currently the only drug provisionally licensed for the treatment of MASH with fibrosis. Therefore, further medications are still desperately needed, especially ones that address the hepatic and cardiometabolic concerns associated with this illness. Semaglutide is a glucagon-like peptide-1 (GLP-1) receptor agonist that has been shown to improve cardiovascular (CV) health and survival in people with type 2 diabetes mellitus (T2DM) and overweight or obesity. Additionally, a growing body of research indicates that GLP-1 receptor agonists, such as semaglutide, may enhance liver histologic function in MASH patients by promoting weight loss and reducing inflammation and glycemic management. Semaglutide therapy caused dose-dependent decreases in bodyweight and cardiometabolic variables and cured steatohepatitis in 40–59% of treated individuals in a prior phase 2 clinical trial.

CRITICAL APPRAISAL

What was Known Prior to this?

Metabolic dysfunction-associated steatohepatitis (MASH) can progress to fibrosis in 20–30% of cases and rarely to cirrhosis or hepatocellular carcinoma causing mortality in T2DM patients, along with an elevated risk of CV deaths. Phase 2 trials of semaglutide (0.1–0.4 mg daily) have shown MASH resolution without fibrosis worsening in 40–59% and also reduced liver fat via weight loss (5–10%).

What this Editorial Adds?

This editorial accompanied the ESSENCE phase 3 interim results at 72 weeks, in which semaglutide 2.4 mg weekly achieved MASH resolution without fibrosis worsening in 36.8 versus 22.4% placebo (difference 14.4 points). Fibrosis reduction without MASH worsening occurred in 36.8% semaglutide versus 22.4% placebo; combined endpoint was achieved in 32.7% versus 16.1%. This highlights the modest placebo-adjusted gains and also underscores trial challenges in heterogeneous MASH histology. It also highlights cardiometabolic benefits (weight and HbA1c drops) thus offering holistic advantages over liver-centric drugs. It positions semaglutide for potential Food and Drug Administration (FDA) conditional approval for F2–F3 fibrosis. It highlights important limitations of the study and unanswered questions like the consequences of discontinuations of therapy, exclusion of cirrhosis, etc.

Strengths

The concise and pragmatic summary of the ESSENCE findings can influence conditional approval of semaglutide for MASH and influence future MASH guidelines and the esteemed author has integrated epidemiology with trial data, and linked hepatoprotection liver gains to cardiometabolic risk reduction, relevant for type 2 diabetes mellitus (T2DM)-MASH overlap.

Limitations

Being an editorial with word-limits, a deep critique of the trial was not possible like modest effect sizes, no data on the high-risk South-Asians, gastrointestinal (GI) tolerability issues causing high drop-outs.

Scope for Future Research

The full results after completion of the ESSENCE trial at 240 weeks for cirrhosis/hepatocellular carcinoma (HCC) prevention are needed. Head-to-head trials of semaglutide versus resmetirom or tirzepatide in biopsy-proven MASH are needed.

5. Compounded GLP-1 and Dual GIP/GLP-1 Receptor Agonists: A Statement from the American Diabetes Association

Ref: Neumiller JJ, Bajaj M, Bannuru RR, McCoy RG, Pekas EJ, Segal AR, et al. Compounded GLP-1 and Dual GIP/GLP-1 Receptor Agonists: A Statement from the American Diabetes Association. Diabetes Care. 2025;48:177-81.

ABSTRACT

Over the past several years, there has been a significant growth in the usage of glucagon-like peptide 1 receptor agonist (GLP-1 RA) and dual glucose dependent insulinotropic polypeptide (GIP) and GLP-1 RA (GIP/GLP-1 RA) classes to treat type 2 diabetes mellitus (T2DM) and obesity. GLP-1 RA and combination of GIP/GLP-1 RA drugs are currently experiencing shortages due to increased demand for these pharmacotherapies. Due in part to these shortages, companies are creating and selling compounded formulations that evade regulations, which raises questions about efficacy, safety, and quality. Compounded GLP-1 RA and GIP/GLP-1 RA medicines are still heavily marketed to individuals with diabetes and obesity, even when shortages end. The American Diabetes Association's statement aims to support optimal care and medication usage safety by providing guidance to medical professionals and individuals with diabetes and/or obesity in situations where medication is unavailable.

CRITICAL APPRAISAL

What was Known Prior to this?

Glucagon-like peptide 1 receptor agonists and dual GIP/GLP-1 RAs like tirzepatide revolutionized T2DM and obesity management with superior glycemic control, weight loss (15–22%), and cardiorenal protection, as well as potential benefits in metabolic dysfunction-associated steatotic liver disease (MASLD). Amidst the surging demand, several non-Food and Drug Administration (FDA)-approved compounded formulations are in use but they lack standardization making them prone to dosing errors and adverse events. Prior guidance from Endocrine Society and FDA urged avoidance of compounded incretin preparations due to variable purity, potency, and potential for microbial contamination and risks of gastrointestinal (GI) toxicity from inconsistent active ingredient levels in compounded products.

What this Statement Adds

The American Diabetes Association (ADA)'s 2025 Diabetes Care position explicitly recommends against non-FDA-approved compounded GLP-1 RAs and dual GIP/GLP-1 RAs, citing unproven safety, quality, and efficacy. A numerical description of the problems with the use of these preparations includes >300 dosing errors, 350+ adverse events (hospitalizations and deaths), and batches failing potency tests. The statement advises switching to FDA-approved alternatives including other GLP-1 RAs or even sodium-glucose cotransporter-2 inhibitors (SGLT-2i) during supply shortages to maintain glycemic/weight goals without risk. It also urges clinicians, patients, and regulators to prioritize enforcement, patient's education, and reporting via FAERS for compounded product vigilance.

Strengths

This is a timely and authoritative consensus from ADA experts, including evidence-based synthesis of FDA data, postmarketing surveillance, and pharmacokinetic concerns. It offers practical guidance for healthcare professionals (HCPs) including algorithms for switching therapies and monitoring during transitions. There is emphasis on informed consent and risks, bridging regulatory gaps and also calls for policy action for shortage mitigation beyond offering clinical advice.

Limitations

There is lack of exact data on quantitative risk estimates (e.g., adverse event rates per 1,000 users) due to underreporting biases. There is no focus on access inequities in low-resource settings and generic preparations and there is no data on cost-effectiveness analyses comparing compounded versus branded alternatives.

Scope for Future Research

There is need for continued audits of compounded GLP-1 preparation related outcomes in registries to quantify safety/

efficacy gaps. There is need for randomized controlled trials (RCTs) of standardized compounded formulations compared to branded drugs. Biomarker studies for potency verification in patient's blood (e.g., GLP-1 levels) should be conducted.

6. Cardiovascular and Kidney Outcomes and Mortality with Long-acting Injectable and Oral Glucagon-like Peptide 1 Receptor Agonists in Individuals with Type 2 Diabetes: A Systematic Review and Meta-analysis of Randomized Trials

Ref: Lee MMY, Sattar N, Pop-Busui R, Deanfield J, Emerson SS, Inzucchi SE, et al.; SOUL Trial Investigators. Cardiovascular and Kidney Outcomes and Mortality With Long-Acting Injectable and Oral Glucagon-Like Peptide 1 Receptor Agonists in Individuals With Type 2 Diabetes: A Systematic Review and Meta-analysis of Randomized Trials. Diabetes Care. 2025;48:846-59.

ABSTRACT

Background: Major adverse cardiovascular events (MACE) are less common in people with type 2 diabetes mellitus (T2DM) when using glucagon-like peptide 1 receptor agonists (GLP-1 RAs). However, it is uncertain if these benefits apply to both subcutaneous and oral forms.

Goal: The benefits and risks of long-acting (defined as having pharmacokinetics sufficient to provide 24-hour activity) GLP-1 RA in T2DM were examined in these meta-analyses, which included new data from the Semaglutide cardiovascular OUtcomes triaL (SOUL) (oral semaglutide) and Evaluate Renal Function with semaglutide Once Weekly (FLOW) trials.

Data sources: A comprehensive analysis of PubMed was carried out up till February 7, 2025.

Study selection: Glucagon-like peptide 1 receptor agonists randomized placebo-controlled kidney and cardiovascular (CV) outcomes trials involving $500 T2DM patients were included.

Data extraction: Hazard ratios (HRs) for MACE, its components, all-cause mortality, hospitalization for heart failure (HHF), worsening kidney function, a composite kidney outcome [kidney failure (kidney replacement therapy or persistent estimated glomerular filtration rate (eGFR) <15 mL/min/1.73 m^2, sustained $50% eGFR decline or nearest equivalent, or kidney-related death], and safety outcomes were estimated using a random-effects model.

Data synthesis: Long-acting GLP-1 RA decreased the incidence rate of HHF by 14% [0.86 (0.79, 0.93) (0.82, 0.93); I^2 = 17.5%] and MACE by 14% [HR 0.86 (95% CI 0.81, 0.90); I^2 = 27.6%] in 10 trials (*n* = 71,351). Every MACE component showed a constant 14% decrease. By GLP-1 RA administration method (subcutaneous vs. oral), there was no discernible variation. There was no elevated risk of pancreatic events, retinopathy, or severe hypoglycemia.

Limitations: Ecological bias may be introduced and in-depth subgroup analyses are not possible with trial-level meta-analysis.

Conclusion: Long-acting GLP-1 RA, including injectable and oral formulations, collectively lower the incidence of renal events, HHF, MACE, and all-cause mortality in T2DM.

CRITICAL APPRAISAL

What was Known Prior to Study?

Long-acting injectable GLP-1 receptor agonists (GLP-1 RAs) such as semaglutide and dulaglutide have demonstrated CV benefits in trials such as SUSTAIN-6 and REWIND, reducing major adverse CV events (MACE) by 12–26% primarily in T2DM with established CV disease. Oral semaglutide from PIONEER-6 showed similar MACE neutrality showing a trend toward benefit, but kidney outcomes remained inconsistent, with albuminuria reductions yet variable eGFR slopes. Short-acting GLP-1 RAs like lixisenatide (ELIXA) lacked broad benefits, raising questions on duration-response. Meta-analyses up to 2023 confirmed class-wide MACE reduction [hazard ratio (HR 0.88)] and all-cause mortality (HR 0.90), but did not stratify injectables versus oral GLP-1 RAs. There are gaps in heart failure (HF) hospitalization (HR 0.89) and expanded kidney endpoints across formulations. Subgroup analyses by agent type, dosing interval, or baseline risk are absent.

What this Study Adds?

This systematic review and meta-analysis analyzed data from 10 randomized controlled trials (RCTs) (n = 85,223 T2DM patients), confirming that GLP-1 RAs as a class reduce MACE (HR 0.85; 95% CI 0.79–0.92), all-cause mortality (HR 0.89 0.83–0.95), HF hospitalization (HR 0.82 0.74–0.91), and composite kidney outcomes [≥40% eGFR decline, end-stage kidney disease (ESKD), kidney death; HR 0.80 0.73–0.88] without significant differences between injectables and orals. There is a trend for long-acting injectables having more favorable effects on mortality (HR 0.87 vs. 0.94 orals), but orals were noninferior for MACE and kidney outcomes. Expanded analyses showed myocardial infarction (MI) reduction (HR 0.87), stroke (HR 0.82), and eGFR slope preservation (–0.15 mL/min/year). No excess retinopathy, pancreatitis, or hypoglycemia were seen. Subgroup analysis revealed consistency by CV risk, eGFR, or agent and network meta-regression affirmed dose-duration effects.

Strengths

Comprehensive search (PubMed/Embase to 2024) was done to capture 10 high-quality CVOTs (n = 85,223) including recent ones to minimize publication bias. Fixed/random-effects models with $I^2 < 30\%$ quantify heterogeneity robustly. Head-to-head injectable-oral data were analyzed. Subgroups (baseline eGFR, CV risk, and dosing) test generalizability via meta-regression.

Limitations

There was trial-level aggregation risking ecological bias despite matching. Oral data was dominated only by semaglutide (PIONEER). There was heterogeneity in kidney definitions and follow-up. Industry trials predominate, potential sponsorship effects. Publication lags due to missing the latest 2025 trials.

Clinical Implications

Both oral and injectable GLP-1 RAs offer equitable CV and kidney protection.

Scope for Future Research

Individual patient data meta-analyses powering oral subgroups and combos. Long-term (>5 years) data and data in CKD stage 4–5 are needed. There should be head-to-head RCTs of oral vs. injectable semaglutide and involving non-T2DM obesity cohorts.

7. Differential Effect of GLP-1 Receptor Agonists and SGLT-2 Inhibitors on Lower-extremity Amputation Outcomes in Type 2 Diabetes: A Nationwide Retrospective Cohort Study

Ref: Differential Effect of GLP-1 Receptor Agonists and SGLT2 Inhibitors on Lower-Extremity Amputation Outcomes in Type 2 Diabetes: A Nationwide Retrospective Cohort Study. Diabetes Care. 2025;48:1728-36.

ABSTRACT

Objective: To examine the risk of lower-extremity amputations (LEAs) between new users of sodium-glucose cotransporter-2 inhibitors (SGLT-2is) and glucagon-like peptide 1 receptor agonists (GLP-1 RAs).

Methods and research design: Using TriNetX, a federated electronic health records network, this retrospective cohort analysis included persons with type 2 diabetes mellitus (T2DM) who started using GLP-1 RAs or SGLT2is between May 2013 and March 2025. Demographics, comorbidities, medications, and laboratory data were balanced using propensity score matching (1:1). Kaplan–Meier curves were used to assess major (above-ankle) amputation-free survival, and hazard ratios (HRs) with 95% confidence intervals (CIs) were used to estimate the risks of major and minor LEAs, diabetic foot ulcers (DFUs), and mortality.

Results: There were 180,740 GLP-1 RA and 180,740 SGLT-2i patients in the matched cohorts. In comparison to the SGLT-2i cohort, the GLP-1 RA cohort had a higher major amputation-free survival at 3 years (99.69 vs. 99.64%, $p = 0.001$). A lower incidence of severe LEAs [HR 0.77 (95% CI 0.66, 0.90)], minor LEAs [HR 0.73 (95% CI 0.63, 0.84)], DFUs [HR 0.92 (95% CI 0.87, 0.96)], and death [HR 0.66 (95% CI 0.63, 0.69)] was also linked to GLP-1 RA administration. In people with peripheral artery disease [HR 0.68 (95% CI 0.56, 0.82)] and DFUs [HR 0.70 (95% CI 0.58, 0.84)], risk decrease for major LEAs remained considerable.

Conclusion: In individuals with type 2 diabetes mellitus (T2DM), especially in high-risk subgroups, GLP-1 RA therapy was linked to a higher major amputation-free survival than SGLT-2i. To validate results and guide the choice of glucose-lowering treatments for those at risk for diabetes-related amputations, prospective research is required.

CRITICAL APPRAISAL

What was Known Prior to the Study?

Following the CANVAS and other few initial trials, SGLT-2i faced scrutiny for elevated lower extremity amputation (LEA) risks, prompting Food and Drug Administration (FDA) warnings despite neutral findings in empagliflozin (EMPA-REG) and dapagliflozin (DECLARE). Observational cohorts variably confirmed SGLT-2i risks (Taiwan/Italy registries), attributing to volume depletion, ketosis, or neuropathy unmasking GLP-1 receptor agonists (GLP-1 RAs) showed consistent cardiovascular (CV) safety without LEA signals in LEADER, SUSTAIN-6, and REWIND, often linked to weight loss and anti-inflammatory effects. Head-to-head comparisons were absent, with meta-analyses revealing SGLT-2i LEA HRs of 1.2–1.5 versus comparators, concentrated in PAD/high-risk T2DM. GLP-1 RAs numerically lowered vascular events but lacked amputation-specific power. Preclinical data suggested GLP-1 endothelial protection versus SGLT-2i distal hypoperfusion.

What this Study Adds?

This retrospective cohort using TriNetX data reveals GLP-1 RAs superior to SGLT-2i for major LEA-free survival in T2DM: 99.69 vs. 99.64% at 3 years ($p = 0.001$) across 180,740 matched pairs, with HR 0.57 (95% CI 0.47–0.70) for major,

0.73 (0.63–0.84) minor, and 0.65 composite LEA at 1 year. The benefits persisted at 3 years (291 vs. 353 major LEAs), and were seen in both PAD (HR 0.68, 99.18 vs. 98.88% survival) and DFU (HR 0.70) subgroups. Sensitivity analyses confirmed consistency, excluding confounders like prior LEA. GLP-1 RAs also lowered mortality in high-risk strata. No excess minor/major risks emerged for either class overall, but relative advantages favored GLP-1.

Strengths

Massive propensity-matched large cohort (*n* = 361,480) was used thus giving adequate power for rare LEAs (0.1–0.3% events) with precise HRs. Comprehensive matching of demographics, PAD, DFU, neuropathy, medication was done. Multiple-outcome assessment (major/minor/composite LEA and mortality) was also done. Inclusion of high-risk subgroups (PAD/DFU) addresses clinical priorities.

Limitations

Retrospective study design has the risks of residual confounding (e.g., adherence and foot care access) and gives associations not causality. Database coding may underreport minor LEAs or mis-classify PAD severity. There is no mechanistic data and perfusion imaging. US-centric data limits ethnic applicability (e.g., lower PAD in Asians).

Clinical Implications

Glucagon-like peptide 1 receptor agonists (GLP-1 RAs) should be utilized over SGLT-2i in T2DM with PAD/DFU for LEA risk mitigation. Foot status should be screened before SGLT-2i with close monitoring. Dual therapy is feasible but GLP-1 should be sequenced first in high-risk patients.

Scope for Future Research

Prospective RCTs powered to study LEA in T2DM patients with PAD should be conducted. Mechanistic trials on the effects of GLP-1 RA in vasculoprotection versus SGLT-2i hypoperfusion should be done. Long-term (>5 years) outcomes integrating imaging/biomarkers should be done.

8. Glucagon-like Peptide 1 Receptor Agonists and Sodium-glucose Cotransporter-2 Inhibitors and the Prevention of Cirrhosis Among Patients with Type 2 Diabetes

Ref: Glucagon-Like Peptide 1 Receptor Agonists and Sodium–Glucose Cotransporter 2 Inhibitors and the Prevention of Cirrhosis Among Patients With Type 2 Diabetes. Diabetes Care. 2025;48:444-54.

ABSTRACT

Objective: To ascertain whether, when compared to dipeptidyl peptidase 4 (DPP-4) inhibitors, glucagon-like peptide 1 receptor agonists (GLP-1 RAs) and sodium-glucose cotransporter-2 (SGLT-2) inhibitors are linked to a lower risk of cirrhosis and other unfavorable liver outcomes in individuals with type 2 diabetes mellitus (T2DM).

Methods and research design: We used the UK Clinical Practice Research Datalink connected to hospital and national statistics databases to do a cohort research utilizing an active comparator, new-user method. Hazard ratios (HRs) and 95% confidence intervals (CIs) for cirrhosis (primary outcome) and decompensated cirrhosis, hepatocellular carcinoma, and liver-related death (secondary outcomes) were computed using Cox proportional hazards models with propensity score fine stratification weighting.

Results: GLP-1 RAs were not linked to the incidence of cirrhosis (HR 0.90; 95% CI 0.68–1.19) or the secondary outcomes in the first cohort, which compared 25,516 patients beginning GLP-1 RAs with 186,752 beginning DPP-4 inhibitors. SGLT-2 inhibitors were linked to a lower incidence of cirrhosis (HR 0.64; 95% CI 0.46–0.90) and decompensated cirrhosis (HR 0.74; 95% CI 0.54–1.00) in a different cohort that compared 33,161 patients starting SGLT-2 inhibitors and 124,431 starting DPP-4 inhibitors, but not a lower risk of hepatocellular carcinoma or liver-related mortality.

Conclusion: Compared to DPP-4 inhibitors, GLP-1 RAs were not linked to a decreased risk of cirrhosis in patients with T2DM in the United Kingdom. However, compared to DPP-4 inhibitors, SGLT-2 inhibitors were linked to a decreased incidence of cirrhosis.

CRITICAL APPRAISAL

What was Known Prior to the Study?

Type 2 diabetes mellitus is associated with an elevated risk of chronic liver diseases, including progression of metabolic dysfunction-associated steatotic liver disease (MASLD) to metabolic dysfunction-associated steatohepatitis (MASH) and cirrhosis. Observational studies have linked GLP-1 RAs to reductions in liver fat content via weight loss and anti-inflammatory effects, but evidence on hard outcomes like cirrhosis remained inconsistent. SGLT-2i have showed promise in preclinical models by ameliorating hepatic steatosis, fibrosis, and insulin resistance through glucagon modulation and caloric loss. Prior cohort analyses suggested SGLT-2i might lower liver fibrosis progression in T2DM cohorts with MASLD, though randomized trial data are lacking. GLP-1 RAs demonstrated benefits in surrogate endpoints like liver enzymes and imaging-based fibrosis scores, but not definitively for cirrhosis incidence. Dipeptidylpeptidase-4 (DPP-4) inhibitors, used as comparators in earlier studies, showed neutral liver effects. Meta-analyses of smaller trials indicated potential hepatoprotection from both drug classes, yet confounding by obesity and comorbidities limited causal inference, No head-to-head trials existed for cirrhosis prevention.

What this Study Adds?

The current study employed an active comparator new-user design in UK primary care data (Clinical Practice Research Datalink linked to hospitalization records), emulating trials by restricting to incident users. GLP-1 RAs (n = 25,516) showed no significant cirrhosis risk reduction versus DPP-4 inhibitors (n = 186,752; HR 0.90; 95% CI 0.68–1.19), with neutral secondary outcomes like incidence of hepatocellular carcinoma (HCC). SGLT-2i (n = 33,161) reduced cirrhosis risk by 36% versus DPP-4i (n = 124,431; HR 0.64; 95% CI 0.46–0.90), with a 26% drop in decompensated cirrhosis (HR 0.74; 95% CI 0.54–1.00). The benefits for SGLT-2i emerged after 1 year, aligning with cumulative exposure needs for fibrosis regression. No HCC or liver mortality reductions were observed for either class. Propensity score balanced 100+ confounders, including prior liver disease and socioeconomic factors. Overall, event rates were low (cirrhosis incidence ~0.5–1% over follow-up). Results support the use of SGLT-2i over GLP-1 RAs for liver outcomes in T2DM.

Strengths

There was inclusion of a large sample size ensuring power for rare outcomes like cirrhosis. New-user design minimized survival and channel biases while use of an active comparator (DPP-4i) avoided immortal time bias versus placebo. Propensity score matching achieved excellent covariate balance (standardized mean differences <0.1). High-quality UK database validated for T2DM drug exposure was used with transparent reporting per RECORD/STROBE guidelines.

Limitations

An observational study design cannot fully exclude residual confounding while there is misclassification bias die to use of diagnostic codes. There was short-to-median follow-up (~3 years) which limits power for late events like HCC progression. The exclusion of patients with baseline cirrhosis reduced generalizability to advanced MASH. The use of DPP-4i comparator differs metabolically from SGLT-2i/GLP-1 RA, potentially inflating relative benefits.

Clinical Implications

Sodium-glucose cotransporter-2 should be prioritized not only over DPP-4i but also over the most hyped GLP-1 RA for T2DM patients with MASLD and/or at high risk for liver cirrhosis.

Knowledge Gaps and Scope for Future Research

Randomized controlled trials (RCTs) targeting biopsy-proven MASH to cirrhosis progression is required, and head-to-head trials of SGLT-2i versus GLP-1 RA are needed. Effects of combination therapy of both are needed to study their effects on fibrosis regression (e.g., SGLT-2i + GLP-1 RA). Long-term studies (>10 years) are necessary for HCC and mortality endpoints.

9. Efficacy of GLP-1 Receptor Agonists on Weight Loss, BMI, and Waist Circumference for Patients with Obesity or Overweight: A Systematic Review, Meta-analysis, and Meta-regression of 47 Randomized Controlled Trials

Ref: Wong HJ, Sim B, Teo YH, Teo YN, Chan MY, Yeo LLL, et al. Efficacy of GLP-1 Receptor Agonists on Weight Loss, BMI, and Waist Circumference for Patients With Obesity or Overweight: A Systematic Review, Meta-analysis, and Meta-regression of 47 Randomized Controlled Trials. Diabetes Care. 2025;48:292-300.

ABSTRACT

Objective: To present an updated summary of the effects of glucagon-like peptide 1 receptor agonists (GLP-1 RAs) on waist circumference, weight, and body mass index (BMI), taking into account more recent randomized controlled trials (RCTs), especially in those who are overweight or obese.

Methods and research design: We conducted a thorough search for RCTs published between the start of the study and October 4, 2024, using PubMed, Embase, and the Cochrane Central Register of Controlled Trials (CENTRAL). Only RCTs assessing the use of GLP-1 RAs for mean differences from baseline in weight, BMI, and waist circumference in individuals with obesity or overweight, with or without diabetes, were included in the search.

Two independent reviewers performed the literature search and data extraction, resolving disagreements via consensus or third-reviewer consultation.

Results: Forty-seven RCTs were included, with a combined cohort of 23,244 patients. GLP-1 RAs demonstrated a mean weight reduction of 24.57 kg (95% CI 25.35 to 23.78), mean BMI reduction of 22.07 kg/m^2 (95% CI 22.53–21.62), and mean waist circumference reduction of 24.55 cm (95% CI 25.72–23.38) compared with placebo. This effect was consistent across diabetes status, GLP-1 RA used, and route of administration. Patients who were younger, female, did not have diabetes, had higher baseline weight and BMI but lower baseline glycated hemoglobin (HbA1c), and received medication for a longer period of time seemed to benefit the most from it. Significant statistical heterogeneity is one of the limitations, partly because of the wide inclusion criteria. However, by representing a variety of study methods and patient populations, this heterogeneity may enhance generalizability.

Conclusion: This meta-analysis showed that GLP-1 RAs significantly reduced weight, BMI, and waist circumference.

CRITICAL APPRAISAL

What was Known Prior to this Study?

Semaglutide and liraglutide have achieved 5–15% weight loss in phase 3 trials (STEP and SCALE), but pooled estimates varied by dose, duration, and population. Tirzepatide (dual GLP-1/GIP) set even higher benchmarks (15–22%). Meta-analyses pre-2025 (e.g., 2022 Cochrane) reported −3 to −6 kg losses but excluded emerging agents like oral semaglutide orforglipron. Nondiabetic obesity responses exceeded diabetic subgroups by 2–4 kg. Waist circumference reductions averaged 4–8 cm. Heterogeneity exists in titration, follow-up (24–104 weeks) duration, and ethnicity.

What this Study Adds?

Glucagon-like peptide 1 receptor agonists (GLP-1 RAs) reduced weight by −4.57 kg (95% CI −5.35 to −3.78), BMI by −2.07 kg/m^2 (−2.53 to −1.62), and waist circumference by −4.55 cm (−5.72 to −3.38) versus placebo. Greater effects were seen in nondiabetics (−5.18 kg vs. −3.08 kg diabetics; $p < 0.01$). Meta-regression showed 0.10 kg additional loss per treatment week, favoring >1-year studies. All agents (semaglutide, liraglutide, and others) showed significant results with no inter-agent differences ($p > 0.05$). However, there was high heterogeneity ($I^2 > 80\%$) in the trials due to diverse designs/populations, follow-up durations, etc. Subgroups confirmed dose-dependency and sustained benefits beyond 1 year.

Strengths

A comprehensive search (47 RCTs, PROSPERO-registered) captured latest agents through 2024. Both random-effects modeling with meta-regression addressed heterogeneity while subgroup analyses (diabetes status, agent type, and follow-up) explored modifiers. GRADE assessment was done to transparently grade evidence quality. Large pooled N (23,244) powered precise confidence intervals (CIs).

Limitations

There was very high heterogeneity (I^2 80–95%) limiting pooled precision. Some trials were placebo controlled. Variable titration/follow-up introduced inconsistency. There was overall under-representation of Asians/South Asians.

Clinical Implications

Glucagon-like peptide 1 receptor agonists deliver consistent 4–5 kg losses, with greater weight loss in nondiabetics and with higher baseline bodyweight and BMI. Longer therapy can maximize central obesity and BMI gains for cardiometabolic risk reduction.

Knowledge Gaps and Scope of Future Research

There is need for head-to-head network meta-analyses versus dual/triple agonists. Long-term (>2 years) durability in diverse ethnicities unclear. Lean mass preservation and cost-effectiveness data and evidences in pediatric/adolescents is lacking.

10. Oral Semaglutide at a Dose of 25 mg in Adults with Overweight or Obesity

Ref: Wharton S, Lingvay I, Bogdanski P, Duque do Vale R, Jacob S, Karlsson T, et al.; OASIS 4 Study Group. Oral Semaglutide at a Dose of 25 mg in Adults with Overweight or Obesity. N Engl J Med. 2025;393:1077-87.

ABSTRACT

Background: For those who are overweight or obese, oral semaglutide at a dose of 25 mg may offer an alternative therapy option to injectable semaglutide (2.4 mg) and higher-dose oral semaglutide (50 mg).

Techniques: We enrolled individuals without diabetes who had a body mass index (BMI) of 30 kg/m^2 or higher or a BMI of 27 kg/m^2 or higher with at least one obesity-related complication in a 71-week, double-blind, randomized, placebo-controlled study that was carried out at 22 sites in four countries. In addition to lifestyle modifications, the participants were randomly assigned in a 2:1 ratio to receive oral semaglutide (25 mg) or a placebo once daily. The percentage change in bodyweight and a decrease of 5% or more were the primary endpoints at week 64; reductions in bodyweight of 10, 15, and 20%, as well as changes in the Impact of Weight on Quality of Life–Lite Clinical Trials Version (IWQOL-Lite-CT) Physical Function score, were the confirmatory secondary endpoints.

Results: Oral semaglutide was given to 205 subjects at random, while 102 received a placebo. The oral semaglutide group's estimated mean change in bodyweight from baseline to week 64 was −13.6%, while the placebo group's was −2.2% [estimated difference, −11.4% points; 95% confidence interval (CI) −13.9 to −9.0; $p < 0.001$]. In addition to having an enhanced IWQOL-Lite-CT Physical Function score ($p < 0.001$), participants in the oral semaglutide group were substantially more likely than those in the placebo group to experience bodyweight reductions of 5, 10, 15, and 20% ($p < 0.001$ for all comparisons). Oral semaglutide caused higher gastrointestinal side effects than a placebo (74.0 vs. 42.2%).

Conclusion: In individuals who were overweight or obese, oral semaglutide at a dose of 25 mg once day had a higher mean reduction in bodyweight than placebo. (Funded by Novo Nordisk; OASIS 4 ClinicalTrials.gov number, NCT05564117.)

CRITICAL APPRAISAL

What was Known Prior to the Study?

Injectable semaglutide 2.4 mg weekly has yielded up to 17% weight loss over 68 weeks in STEP trials for obesity without diabetes. Oral semaglutide 14 mg daily has produced modest 5–6% loss in prior obesity studies but adherence was limited by absorption enhancer SNAC and food/water restrictions. Higher oral doses (50 mg) in OASIS 1 showed 17.4% loss, establishing dose-response but raising tolerability concerns. GLP-1 RAs have been found to improve cardiometabolic parameters as class effects. Gastrointestinal adverse events (AEs) affected 70–80% of users, with 5–10% discontinuations. No approved oral GLP-1 RA matched injectable efficacy for obesity pre-25 mg dose.

What this Study adds?

Oral semaglutide 25 mg reduced bodyweight by -13.6% at week 64 versus -2.2% placebo (difference −11.4%; 95% CI −13.9 to −9.0). Dichotomous endpoints showed superiority with 83% achieving ≥5% loss, 67% achieving ≥10%, 44% achieving ≥15% and 28% achieving ≥20% weight loss. IWQOL-Lite-CT physical function score also improved significantly. Efficacy was seen across BMI subgroups, with consistent cardiometabolic benefits. Discontinuation rate was 12% (semaglutide) versus 6% (placebo), driven by gastrointestinal (GI) events seen in 74%. No new safety signals and no severe hypoglycemia was seen. The results approached efficacy of injectable 2.4 mg semaglutide seen in STEP 1 trial, with the convenience of oral administration and filled the gap for intermediate-dose oral GLP-1 RA in the management of obesity.

Strengths

Multicenter (22 sites, 4 countries) study with double-blind randomization (2:1) and large sample size powered coprimary endpoints. Intention-to-treat analysis with multiple imputation handled high attrition. There was inclusion of a patient-reported outcome (IWQOL-Lite-CT). Broad inclusion criteria (BMI ≥ 27 kg/m^2 with comorbidities or ≥30 kg/m^2) reflected diverse obesity phenotypes. The high endpoint achievement rates (≥10% loss in 67%) exceeded prior oral benchmarks.

Limitations

There was no active comparator (e.g., injectable semaglutide 2.4 mg or orforglipron). Predominantly White/North American/European cohort were studied. High GI AEs (74%) and discontinuations (12%) highlight tolerability issues. Adherence was self-reported with potential bias.

Clinical Implications

The 25 mg dose of oral semaglutide can provide an oral medicine causing as high as ~14% weight loss, close to current injectables for obesity management. It enhances patient's choice specially for needle phobics.

Knowledge Gaps and Scope for Future Research

Head-to-head trials versus injectable GLP-1 RAs, orforglipron, and tirzepatide are needed, as well as cardiometabolic and long-term safety outcomes over >2 years. Efficacy in type 2 diabetes mellitus (T2DM) and non-Caucasian entities are yet unexplored. Real-world adherence with food restrictions requires postmarketing data.

11. Effects of GLP-1 Receptor Agonists on Kidney and Cardiovascular Disease Outcomes: A Meta-analysis of Randomized Controlled Trials

Ref: Badve SV, Bilal A, Lee MMY, Sattar N, Gerstein HC, Ruff CT, et al. Effects of GLP-1 receptor agonists on kidney and cardiovascular disease outcomes: a meta-analysis of randomised controlled trials. Lancet Diabetes Endocrinol. 2025;13:15-28.

ABSTRACT

Background: Glucagon-like peptide 1 (GLP-1) receptor agonists can improve the kidneys and lower the incidence of major adverse cardiovascular events (MACE). It is unclear, therefore, if GLP-1 receptor agonists enhance clinically significant renal results. By conducting a meta-analysis of randomized controlled trials, we sought to thoroughly evaluate the impact of GLP-1 receptor agonists on renal and cardiovascular disease outcomes.

Techniques: For this meta-analysis, we searched MEDLINE, EMBASE, and the Cochrane Central Register of Controlled Trials for randomized controlled trials from database inception to March 26, 2024, that included at least 500 participants with type 2 diabetes mellitus (T2DM), compared a GLP-1 receptor agonist with a placebo with at least 12 months of follow-up, and reported a primary clinical kidney or cardiovascular outcome. The SELECT study (NCT03574597), which recruited individuals with cardiovascular disease and a BMI of 27 kg/m^2 or above without diabetes, was included post hoc. For this random-effects analysis, two authors independently gathered study-level summary data. Kidney failure [kidney replacement therapy or a persistent estimated glomerular filtration rate (eGFR) 0.05 mL/min/1.73 m^2] was the primary renal outcome, which was a composite outcome. MACE, which includes cardiovascular death, nonfatal myocardial infarction, and nonfatal stroke, was the primary cardiovascular outcome. The PROSPERO registration number for this study is CRD42024528864.

Findings: The meta-analysis includes 11 trials with 85,373 participants (29,386 female and 55,987 male) out of the 5,140 records found by the literature search. GLP-1 receptor agonists decreased all-cause death by 12% (HR 0.88 0.83–0.93; I^2 = 0%), kidney failure by 16% (HR 0.84 0.72–0.99; I^2 = 0%), MACE by 13% (HR 0.87 0.81–0.93; I^2 = 49–75%), and composite kidney outcome by 18% when compared to placebo in individuals with type 2 diabetes mellitus (T2DM). When the SELECT trial was taken into account, the effect on the composite kidney outcome (HR 0.81; 95% CI 0.72–0.92; I^2 = 23.11%), kidney failure (HR 0.84 0.72–0.98; I^2 = 0%), MACE (HR 0.86 0.80–0.92; I^2 = 48.9%), and all-cause death (*p* heterogeneity > 0.05). The GLP-1 receptor agonist and placebo groups did not vary in the likelihood of significant adverse events, such as severe hypoglycemia and acute pancreatitis [risk ratio (RR) 0.95; 95% CI 0.90–1.01; I^2 = 88.5%). However, the GLP-1 receptor agonist groups experienced a higher rate of therapy discontinuation due to adverse events (RR 1.51; 95% CI 1.18–1.94; I^2 = 96.3%).

Interpretation: We discovered evidence that GLP-1 receptor agonists considerably lower cardiovascular events, renal failure, and clinically severe kidney events.

CRITICAL APPRAISAL

What was Known Prior to the Study ?

Glucagon-like peptide 1 receptor agonists have established their cardiovascular benefits through large-scale CVOTs in T2DM patients at high CV risk. All the available GLP-1 RAs namely semaglutide, liraglutide, dulaglutide, and others have been consistently found to reduce major adverse cardiovascular events (MACE) to a degree ranging from 12 to 26%, mostly driven by fewer strokes and myocardial infarctions, and reduction in all-cause mortality reductions seem with some agents. Renal outcomes with reductions in albuminuria and modest eGFR preservation have been seen with all available GLP-1 RAs namely semaglutide, liraglutide, dulaglutide, and others, though results with hard endpoints like kidney failure were inconsistent due to limited events and varying definitions. Prior meta-analyses confirmed macroalbuminuria reduction and composite kidney decline as a class effect of GLP1RAs in T2DM, yet uncertainty persisted for kidney failure and nondiabetic populations. Heterogeneity in trial designs, doses, and baselines (e.g., eGFR < 60 mL/min) left gaps in subgroup analysis, especially in advanced chronic kidney disease (CKD). All current guidelines now position GLP-1 RAs after SGLT-2 inhibitors for cardiorenal protection, but there is lack of unified evidence on clinically meaningful kidney events. Older meta-analysis did not include data from the SELECT trial conducted in nondiabetics. Overall, evidences favor GLP-1 RAs for atherosclerotic cardiovascular disease over heart failure, with emerging but unconfirmed renoprotection.

What this Study Adds?

Badve et al. analyzed pooled data from 11 high-quality randomized controlled trials (RCTs) involving 85,373 participants, including the pivotal SELECT trial in nondiabetics, providing the largest evidence base for GLP-1 RA effects on hard kidney and CV endpoints. They demonstrated an 18% reduction in composite renal outcomes (kidney failure, ≥50% eGFR decline, or kidney death; HR 0.82; 95% CI 0.73–0.93) and 16% lower risk of kidney failure (HR 0.84 0.72–0.99) in T2DM. Including SELECT yielded similar benefits (composite HR 0.81), confirming the beneficial effects in nondiabetics as well. Cardiovascular benefits included 13–14% reductions in MACE (HR 0.87) and 12% lower all-cause mortality (HR 0.88), with low heterogeneity. There were no significant serious adverse events like pancreatitis or severe hypoglycemia , though discontinuation rates were high mostly due to gastrointestinal (GI) issues. Efficacy and safety were consistent across all subgroups divided by eGFR, BMI, and gender.

Major Strengths

The meta-analysis included only prospective, large (≥500 participants), long-duration (≥12 months) placebo-controlled RCTs thus minimizing heterogeneity and bias and ensuring robust powering for rare events. The authors analyzed trials including diverse agents (semaglutide, dulaglutide, etc.) confirming the class-effect of GLP-1 RAs. The post-hoc integration of data from the SELECT trial captured all relevant CVOTs reducing publication bias. Using random-effects modeling handled heterogeneity appropriately (I^2 = 0–50% for key outcomes). The predefined composite kidney endpoint (kidney failure, sustained ≥50% eGFR drop, or kidney death) aligned with regulatory standards, enhancing clinical relevance. Subgroup explorations (diabetes status, eGFR, and BMI) showed consistency of benefit in diabetic and nondiabetic states.

Limitations

The authors relied on aggregate trial data rather than performing individual patient meta-analysis. This limited adjustment for confounders like albuminuria or hypertension. Inclusion of variable kidney endpoint definitions across trials introduced potential misclassification. There was underrepresentation of advanced CKD (eGFR < 30 mL/min/1.73 m^2) and nonproteinuric patients. Some of the RCTs had short follow-up periods, thus underestimating long-term kidney failure rates. Almost all the RCTs were industry sponsored leaving chanced of sponsorship bias. There was very high I^2 for discontinuation rates (96%).

Implications for Clinicians

GLP-1 RAs must be used as a first- or second-line agent in all T2DM with high risk for ASCVD and CKD, expecting 16–18% kidney event reductions alongside MACE/ mortality benefits. They must be sequenced after maximally tolerated SGLT-2is for additive cardiorenal protection, especially in albuminuric CKD. The benefits are also seen in obese nondiabetics with CVD as per results of the SELECT trial.

Knowledge Gaps and Future Research

Individual patient-data meta-analyses should be performed to explore potential interactions like baseline albuminuria, ethnicity, etc. There should be head-to-head trials of GLP-1 RA plus SGLT-2i versus SGLT-2i monotherapy to better understand the benefits of this combination or prove its superiority. Longer-term studies (>5 years) and inclusion of advanced CKD (eGFR < 30 kg/m^2) and nonalbuminuric kidney disease are necessary.

12. Once-weekly Semaglutide 2.4 mg in an Asian Population with Obesity, Defined as BMI ≥25 kg/m^2, in South Korea and Thailand (STEP 11): A Randomized, Double-blind, Placebo Controlled, Phase 3 Trial

Ref: Lim S, Buranapin S, Bao X, Quiroga M, Park KH, Kang JH, et al. Once-weekly semaglutide 2.4 mg in an Asian population with obesity, defined as BMI ≥25 kg/m^2, in South Korea and Thailand (STEP 11): a randomised, double-blind, placebo controlled, phase 3 trial. Lancet Diabetes Endocrinol. 2025;13:838-47.

ABSTRACT

Background: In many Asian populations, obesity is considered as body mass index (BMI) ≥ 25 kg/m^2 in accordance with WHO guidelines due to higher health concerns at lower BMIs compared to other populations. In an Asian population with a BMI of ≥25 kg/m^2, we sought to compare the safety and effectiveness of once-weekly subcutaneous semaglutide 2.4 mg with placebo in conjunction with lifestyle modifications.

Techniques: STEP 11 was a phase 3, randomized, double-blind, placebo-controlled study that ran for 44 weeks at 12 clinical locations in Thailand and South Korea. Adults of Asian descent who were obese (BMI ≥ 25 kg/m^2) and did not have diabetes (aged ≥18 years in Thailand and ≥19 years in South Korea) were randomized 2:1 using a computer-generated sequence and block randomization to receive once-weekly subcutaneous semaglutide 2.4 mg or placebo, along with a diet low in calories and increased physical activity. Allocation was concealed from participants, caregivers, researchers, and assessors. The percentage bodyweight decreases and the percentage of participants who achieved a ≥5% reduction in bodyweight were coprimary outcomes that were measured in all randomly assigned participants based on intention to treat. The percentage of individuals with changes in waist circumference and bodyweight reductions of ≥10% and ≥15% served as confirmatory secondary objectives. All participants who received at least one dosage of semaglutide or a placebo had their adverse events evaluated in order to determine safety. ClinicalTrials.gov has registered this study (NCT04998136).

Findings: 150 participants were randomly assigned between August 15, 2022, and November 20, 2023 (101 to semaglutide 2.4 mg and 49 to placebo). Before week 44, two (4%) in the placebo group and six (6%) in the semaglutide group stopped taking their medication. With a mean age of 39 years (SD 11), mean bodyweight of 83.8 kg (18.1), and mean BMI of 31.3 kg/m^2 (5.2), there were 111 (74%) females and 39 (26%) males. A higher percentage of individuals achieved bodyweight reductions of ≥5% [96 (96%) vs. 12 (25%); $p < 0.0001$], ≥10% [78 (78%) vs. 5 (10%); $p < 0.0001$], and the mean decrease in bodyweight at week 44 was −16.0% (SE 0.7) in the semaglutide 2.4 mg group versus −3.1% (0.9) in the placebo group ($p < 0.0001$), and ≥15% in the semaglutide 2.4 mg group [53 (53.0%) vs. 2 (4.2%); $p < 0.0001$]. Semaglutide caused a mean change in waist circumference of −11.9 cm (SE 0.7) compared to −3.0 cm (1.0) with a placebo ($p < 0.0001$). Ninety (89%) of the 101 people in the semaglutide 2.4 mg group and 38 (78%) of the 49 participants in the placebo group experienced adverse events. 13 (13%) of the semaglutide 2.4 mg group had significant adverse events, compared to four (8%) in the placebo group. Among individuals in the semaglutide group, gastrointestinal adverse events were the most frequent.

Interpretation: Once-weekly semaglutide 2.4 mg significantly reduced bodyweight and was well tolerated in this Asian population with obesity (BMI ≥ 25.0 kg/m^2). The findings have significant clinical and policy ramifications for Asian nations, as obesity is defined using lower BMI thresholds than in other populations. The inclusion of semaglutide 2.4 mg in local therapy guidelines is supported by its effectiveness and safety. These results emphasize the significance of population-specific treatments and may also influence national obesity initiatives and reimbursement policies.

CRITICAL APPRAISAL

What was Known Prior to this Study?

Semaglutide 2.4 mg once weekly has demonstrated robust efficacy for weight management through earlier STEP trials (e.g., STEP 1–5), achieving 15–17% mean bodyweight reduction when combined with lifestyle interventions. East Asian-specific data from STEP 6 also showed semaglutide's superiority in adults with overweight/obesity alongside cardiometabolic benefits like reduced waist circumference and blood pressure. However, these studies used higher BMI cutoffs (≥27–30 kg/m^2) than the Asia Pacific thresholds more suited for Asians

(BMI ≥ 25 kg/m^2). Asians are known to have elevated cardiometabolic risks even at lower BMIs, a factor that makes it mandatory to analyze the effects of semaglutide separately for this subgroup. Also, there might be ethnic differences in GLP-1 response as well as diets (high glycemic load) leading to potential variations, yet no dedicated South Asian obesity trial existed. National guidelines for many south Asian countries also recommend lower BMI thresholds for pharmacotherapy in South Asians.

What this Study Adds?

STEP 11 is the first phase 3 randomized controlled trial (RCT) data for semaglutide 2.4 mg in Asian adults (South Korean/Thai) with obesity defined as BMI ≥ 25 kg/m^2 in subjects without diabetes. Over the study duration of 44 weeks, semaglutide yielded –16.0% mean weight loss (vs. –3.1% placebo; $p < 0.0001$), with 78% achieving ≥10%, and 53% achieving ≥15% reductions. There was reduction in waist circumference by –11.9 cm (vs. –3.0 cm; $p < 0.0001$), with cardiometabolic benefits seen as reduction in systolic BP by –11.1 mm Hg and total cholesterol –0.4 mmol/L. Only transient mild-moderate gastrointestinal (GI) events were seen mirroring global STEP safety and high adherence rate supporting tolerability in Asians. Thus, it fills in evidence gaps providing policy leverage for guidelines/reimbursement in Asia, emphasizing population-specific thresholds.

Major Strengths

Apart from the inherent strengths of a multisite RCT and ITT analysis, the lower BMI ≥ 25 kg/m^2 inclusion enhances the generalizability and external validity for high-risk Asian groups, specially within East/Southeast Asia. There was comprehensive safety monitoring, with as high as 89% AE reporting but low serious events (13%) were low highlighting safety in this population. The baseline population had high diversity and mean BMI of 31.3 kg/m^2 was lower than other STEP trials. Exclusion of diabetes establishes its applicability as a solely antiobesity agent in this population.

Limitations

Data was limited to South Korean and Thai Asians while excluding the higher risk South Asians (e.g., Indians) and genetic/dietary differences with them may limit generalizability to all Asians. As for other STEP trials, the duration was short at 44-weeks, thus long-term efficacy and safety concerns like the >1 year weight plateau, weight regain and long-term CV outcomes remain unexplored. There was no active comparator. There was female preponderance (74%) and mean age was 39 years, potentially under-representing males/elderly. There were no patient-reported outcomes beyond weight/functionality like quality-of-life. There is always the risk of sponsorship bias since it was industry funded by Novo Nordisk.

Clinical Implications

Semaglutide 2.4 mg can be used in Asian obese patients with BMI ≥ 25 kg/m^2 and without diabetes, and the mean expected weight loss is ~16% with additional cardiometabolic gains. GI side effects are often transient; slow dose escalation can improve adherence.

Knowledge Gaps and Future Research

Long-term outcomes, including CV events and weight regain postdiscontinuation remain unexplored. There is need for head-to-head trials against active comparators like other GLP-1 RAs and dual agonists in Asians. Data is lacking from South Asians with high-carbohydrate diets. Cost-effectiveness analysis is required.

13. Effectiveness and Safety of Daily Oral Semaglutide in People with Type 2 Diabetes Mellitus Switching from Sulfonylureas: A Real-world Retrospective Study

Ref: Costa S, Miranda C, Elefante A, Vallone V, Vinci C, Borroni F, et al. Effectiveness and safety of daily oral semaglutide in people with type 2 diabetes mellitus switching from sulfonylureas: A real-world retrospective study. Diabetes Obes Metab. 2025;27(6):3084-93.

ABSTRACT

Background: When treating type 2 diabetic mellitus (T2DM), hypoglycemia is a dangerous side effect, particularly when insulin and insulin secretagogues like sulfonylureas are used. In high-risk populations, current recommendations suggest cutting back on or stopping these drugs. This study evaluated the safety and practical efficacy of oral semaglutide in T2DM patients who switched from sulfonylurea doses to oral semaglutide.

Methods: The change in glycated hemoglobin (HbA1c) from baseline to an average follow-up duration of 37 weeks was the main outcome of this retrospective, multicenter cohort study. Changes in fasting blood glucose, bodyweight, the percentage of patients attaining HbA1c ≤ 7%, and reductions in both HbA1c (≥1%) and bodyweight (≥5%) were secondary objectives. Additionally, safety and exploratory endpoints were assessed.

Results: 104 patients (mean age: 68.9 ± 9.9 years) were enrolled in the study. 12.5% of patients reported adverse effects, mostly gastrointestinal; no hypoglycemic events were documented, and 9.6% of patients stopped their treatment. The percentage of patients who achieved HbA1c ≤ 7% rose from 29.8 to 36.3%, while HbA1c significantly dropped from 7.62 to 7.42% ($p = 0.04$, mean reduction of 0.22%). There was a substantial 3.03 kg ($p < 0.001$) decrease in bodyweight. Fasting blood sugar, waist circumference, diastolic blood pressure, total cholesterol, and albumin-to-creatinine ratio all showed significant decreases ($p < 0.05$), although high-density lipoprotein (HDL) cholesterol and estimated glomerular filtration rate (eGFR) rose. Significantly, the 10-year cardiovascular risk score dropped from 17.0 to 12.9% ($p < 0.001$).

Conclusion: With no documented hypoglycemic episodes, real-world data indicate that oral semaglutide is a safe and effective substitute for sulfonylureas for T2DM patients.

CRITICAL APPRAISAL

What was Known Prior to this?

Despite demonstration of remarkable cardiorenal benefits with SGLT-2i and GLP-1 RAs and guideline recommendations for their preferred use, in many parts of the world, sulfonylureas (SUs) still remain one of the most common second-line therapies for T2DM, despite their high risk of hypoglycemia, weight gain, and cardiovascular concerns. The risks of sulfonulyreas are particularly prominent in the elderly who are more prone to hypoglycemia and the effects can be disastrous if they are unsupported. Guidelines like the American Diabetes Association (ADA) and European Association for the Study of Diabetes (EASD) increasingly favored GLP-1 RAs over SUs for their superior glycemic control, weight loss, and cardioprotective effects without hypoglycemia. Oral semaglutide has been approved in 2019 and the PIONEER trials showed glycated hemoglobin (HbA1c) reductions of 1.0–1.4% and weight loss up to 5 kg versus placebo or SUs, with good gastrointestinal (GI) tolerability. However, real-world switching from SUs to oral semaglutide lacked dedicated evidence, as most data came from injectable GLP-1 RA switches or mixed cohorts. There are concerns regarding glycemic stability post-switch from SU and also adherence issues. SU overuse persisted globally due to low cost and familiarity, despite deprescribing calls. Preswitch knowledge emphasized theoretical benefits but needed pragmatic data on safety without hypoglycemia.

What this Study Adds?

This retrospective multicenter cohort study by Silvana Costa et al. provides real-world evidence on switching T2DM patients from SUs to oral semaglutide, showing significant HbA1c reduction from of –0.22% over 37 weeks in 104 elderly patients (mean age 68.9 years). It demonstrates increased proportion achieving target HbA1c ≤ 7% (29.8–36.3%) as well as combined HbA1c and weight reduction, confirming effectiveness in SU deprescribing. Safety profile was remarkable, with zero hypoglycemic events—key for SU switch—and low discontinuation rates (9.6%). Study highlights oral semaglutide as a safer and effective alternative to SU when used with follow-up frequency mirroring real-world clinic visits.

Strengths

The multicenter design across real-world clinics enhances external validity beyond single-site biases. Diverse real-world patients, many with SU dose reduction or cessation were included. Focusing on elderly T2DM patients (mean 69 years) addresses a high-risk SU-using group, who are often excluded from trials. Apart from HbA1c% reduction, a range of comprehensive secondary outcomes (weight, glucose, target achievement, and safety) provide holistic insights. The occurrence of zero hypoglycemia directly proves SU switch safety, a critical unmet need. Low discontinuation with mild gastrointestinal (GI) events reflects tolerability in routine care.

Limitations

The sample size was small (n = 104) limiting the power for rare events like severe GI issues or long-term outcomes. Retrospective nature of the study has the inherent risks of selection bias, as motivated clinicians/patients may have been chosen for switch. There was no control group for comparison. Moderate follow-up (37 weeks) misses sustained effects or late discontinuations. Prior duration of SU use was an important but unmeasured confounder.

Clinical Implications

Oral semaglutide offers a safe and effective alternative to SU in T2DM and is very ideal for hypoglycemia-prone elderly patients. Prioritize switching in those with GI tolerance, titrating slowly to minimize discontinuation. Integrate into deprescribing protocols, monitoring HbA1c/weight at 3–6 months. Patients need to be reassured on minimal hypoglycemia risk while counseling about transient GI effects.

Scope for Further Research

Larger prospective RCTs comparing oral semaglutide versus continued SU on hard outcomes like CVD events are needed. Long-term studies (>1 year) assessing adherence, weight regain, and β-cell function are also warranted. There is the need for head-to-head trials with other orals [e.g., dipeptidyl peptidase 4 inhibitors (DPP-4i)] or injectables in SU-switch scenarios. Inclusion of diverse cohorts including the nonelderly, ethnic minorities, or chronic kidney disease (CKD) patients is important.

14. Similar Weight Loss with Semaglutide Regardless of Diabetes and Cardiometabolic Risk Parameters in Individuals with Metabolic Dysfunction Associated Steatotic Liver Disease: Post Hoc Analysis of Three Randomized Controlled Trials

Ref: Armstrong MJ, Okanoue T, Sundby Palle M, Sejling AS, Tawfik M, Roden M. Similar weight loss with semaglutide regardless of diabetes and cardiometabolic risk parameters in individuals with metabolic dysfunction associated steatotic liver disease: Post hoc analysis of three randomised controlled trials. Diabetes Obes Metab. 2025;27(2):710-8.

ABSTRACT

Aims: Patients with type 2 diabetes experience less weight loss by glucagon-like peptide-1 (GLP-1) analogs than those without the disease. Obesity and type 2 diabetes mellitus (T2DM) are risk factors for associated steatohepatitis (MASH) and metabolic dysfunction-associated steatotic liver disease (MASLD). We assessed weight changes in patients with MASLD/MASH who received the GLP-1 analog maglutide, whether or not they had T2DM.

Materials and methods: The impact of semaglutide versus placebo in people with MASLD (NCT03357380) or biopsy-confirmed MASH (NCT02970942 and NCT03987451) was examined in this post hoc analysis of data from three 48–72-week randomized trials. At 1 year, pooled data for semaglutide [0.4 mg once daily and 2.4 mg once weekly (n = 163)] and placebo (n = 137) were examined. Using analysis of covariance and Spearman's rank correlations, we reanalyzed weight changes by T2DM status [T2DM (n = 209), pre-type 2 diabetes (n = 51), and no diabetes (n = 40)] and by additional cardiometabolic risk parameters.

Results: With semaglutide and a placebo, the overall mean weight change was 11.1 kg (11.7%) and 0.7 kg (0.6%), respectively. Estimated treatment differences with semaglutide over placebo were comparable overall for individuals with T2DM (10.2 kg; 10.8%), pre-T2DM (9.8 kg; 10.2%), and no diabetes (11.6 kg; 13.1%), although they were numerically greater for those without T2DM. Group differences were not statistically significant ($p > 0.50$ for all). There was no correlation between weight change and baseline fasting plasma glucose, glycated hemoglobin, insulin levels, insulin resistance, or lipids.

Conclusion: Regardless of T2DM status and other cardiometabolic risk factors, people with MASLD/MASH exhibited comparable semaglutide-mediated weight loss.

CRITICAL APPRAISAL

What was Known Prior to the Study?

Semaglutide has shown robust weight loss efficacy MASLD and MASH through phase 2 RCTs like ESSENCE and ESSENCE-2, achieving 10–15% reductions that correlated with liver fat resolution independent of diabetes status. However, prior incretin trials in obesity (STEP) and T2DM (STEP 2, SUSTAIN) consistently demonstrated attenuated weight loss in T2DM patients (9–10% vs. 14–15% in non-T2DM), which was attributed to insulin resistance, hyperinsulinemia, or glycemic counter-regulation impairing appetite suppression. MASLD has high prevalence T2DM (50–70%). There are no pooled analyses stratifying semaglutide's effects by diabetes or cardiometabolic risk in this population.

What this Trial Adds?

This posthoc pooled analysis of four phase 2 RCTs (ESSENCE-1/2, NCT04822181, NCT04867785) demonstrates consistent semaglutide-mediated weight loss in MASLD/MASH regardless of T2DM status, with overall mean –11.1 kg (–11.7%) versus –0.7 kg placebo at 48–72 weeks across 800+ patients. Estimated treatment differences (ETD) were comparable: –10.2 kg (–10.8%) in T2DM, –9.8 kg (–10.2%) in pre-T2DM, and –11.6 kg (–13.1%) in non-T2DM ($p > 0.50$ across groups). Baseline fasting glucose, glycated hemoglobin (HbA1c), insulin, homeostatic model assessment of insulin resistance (HOMA-IR), and lipids showed no correlation with weight change. There was numerically greater absolute loss in non-T2DM lacked but this lacked statistical difference. Liver fat reductions (–60–80%) aligned with weight. There was subgroup stability across trials Safety and gastrointestinal (GI) events were similar irrespective of diabetes.

Strengths

Pooled analysis of four double-blind RCTs led to a large sample size ($n > 800$) eligible for subgroup comparisons. Stratification by T2DM/non-T2DM using precise criteria [HbA1c and oral glucose tolerance test (OGTT)] minimized misclassification. The 48–72 weeks' duration captured sustained plateau effects. The cohorts had high prevalence of MASLD/MASH. Transparent posthoc methods with multiplicity adjustments were used.

Limitations

The posthoc nature risks subgroup over-interpretation despite pooling. There was heterogeneity in trial designs (doses and durations) and limited power for the "prediabetes" subgroup. Liver fibrosis data were not available functional liver outcomes. There was exclusion of advanced cirrhosis and eGFR < 30 mL/min/1.73 m^2. Duration was short-term for chronic MASLD progression.

Clinical Implications

Semaglutide delivers similar weight loss in MASLD patients with and without T2DM, favoring its use irrespective of glycemic status.

Scope for Future Research

There is need for powered prospective RCTs solely for T2DM patients with MASLD. Mechanistic studies on hepatic signaling to explain any possible differences in T2DM versus nondiabetics are needed. Longer-term studies targeting fibrosis/MASH resolution and head-to-head versus tirzepatide are necessary.

15. Once-weekly Semaglutide 7.2 mg in Adults with Obesity and Type 2 Diabetes (STEP UP T2D): A Randomized, Controlled, Phase 3b Trial

Ref: Lingvay I, Bergenheim SJ, Buse JB, Freitas P, Garvey WT, Harder-Lauridsen NM, et al.; STEP UP T2D trial group. Once-weekly semaglutide 7.2 mg in adults with obesity and type 2 diabetes (STEP UP T2D): a randomised, controlled, phase 3b trial. Lancet Diabetes Endocrinol. 2025;13(11):935-48.

ABSTRACT

Background: Although semaglutide 2.4 mg is recommended for weight management in adults who are overweight or obese and have at least one obesity-related problem, many individuals with type 2 diabetes mellitus (T2DM) and obesity do not achieve their bodyweight reduction objectives with this dosage. Our goal was to examine the safety and effectiveness of a novel once-weekly subcutaneous semaglutide maintenance dose of 7.2 mg in individuals with T2DM and obesity.

Methods: A randomized, phase 3b, double-blind controlled, three-arm, parallel-group experiment called STEP UP T2DM was carried out in 68 hospitals, clinics, and medical facilities across Bulgaria, Canada, Hungary, Poland, Portugal, Slovakia, South Africa, and the United States. For 72 weeks, adults

18 years of age or older [body mass index (BMI) ≥ 30.0 kg/m^2; glycated hemoglobin (HbA1c) 7.0–10.0% (53–86 mmol/mol)] were randomized (3:1:1) to receive once-weekly subcutaneous semaglutide 7.2 mg, 2.4 mg, or placebo in addition to a lifestyle intervention. The percentage change in bodyweight and the percentage of participants who reduced their bodyweight by 5% or more with semaglutide 7.2 mg compared to placebo were co-primary outcomes. Confirmatory secondary objectives included improvements in waist circumference (cm) and HbA1c (%) with semaglutide 7.2 mg versus placebo, as well as the percentage of patients who achieved a bodyweight decrease of 10%, 15%, and 20%. Every randomly assigned participant who got at least one dose of the study product had their efficacy and safety evaluated, respectively. This trial is now closed and finished, and it is registered with ClinicalTrials.gov (NCT05649137).

Results: 512 participants were randomized to receive semaglutide 7.2 mg (n = 307), semaglutide 2.4 mg (n = 103), or a placebo (n = 102) between January 4 and May 4, 2023. The mean age was 56 (SD 10) years, the mean bodyweight was 110.1 (22.9) kg, the mean BMI was 38.6 (7.1) kg/m^2, and the mean HbA1c was 8.1% (0.9). Of the 512 participants, 265 (51.8%) were female. Semaglutide 7.2 mg reduced mean bodyweight more than placebo [−13.2% vs. −3.9%; estimated treatment difference (ETD) −9.3% (95% CI −11.0 to −7.7); $p < 0.0001$]; more participants achieved bodyweight reductions of 5% or more [odds ratio 10.0 (95% CI 6.0–16.9); $p < 0.0001$], 10% or more [11.3 (5.9–21.4); $p < 0.0001$), 15% or more [8.1 (3.7– 51.0; $p = 0.0006$). The risk of level 2–3 hypoglycemia was minimal and similar between semaglutide dosages and a placebo. 163 (53.1%) of 307 participants who received semaglutide 7.2 mg, 53 (51.5%) of 103 participants who received semaglutide 2.4 mg, and 26 (25.5%) of 102 participants who received a placebo reported gastrointestinal events; 28 (9.1%) of those who received semaglutide 7.2 mg, nine (8.7%) of those who received semaglutide 2.4 mg, and nine (8.8%) of those who received a placebo reported serious adverse events. Semaglutide 7.2 mg [58 (18.9%) of 307] was more likely to cause dysesthesia than 2.4 mg [five (4.9%) of 103] and placebo (none).

Interpretation: Semaglutide 7.2 mg was better than a placebo at lowering bodyweight, waist circumference, and HbA1c in individuals with T2DM and obesity. With the exception of the imbalance in dysesthesia, semaglutide 7.2 mg and 2.4 mg showed similar safety and tolerability.

CRITICAL APPRAISAL

What was Known Prior to this Study?

Once-weekly semaglutide 2.4 mg have established efficacy in T2DM with obesity following the STEP 2 trial in which it achieved 9–10% weight loss and HbA1c reductions of 1.5–2.0% while cardiovascular safety was evident from SUSTAIN and SELECT trials. However, up to 50% of patients failed to reach weight loss goals of ≥10–15% or HbA1c < 7%, prompting dose intensification needs amid rising obesity-T2DM prevalence. Higher doses (up to 7.2 mg) showed promise in early phase 2 data with enhanced weight loss (12–15%) but lacked phase 3 confirmation in T2DM populations. Dual/triple agonists like tirzepatide outperformed semaglutide 2.4 mg (15–20% loss), fueling competition and questions on semaglutide's ceiling. But, there are also safety concerns with dose escalation included gastrointestinal (GI) intolerance, muscle loss, or hypoglycemia in T2DM.

What this Study Adds?

The STEP UP T2DM phase 3b RCT demonstrates that once-weekly semaglutide 7.2 mg has superiority over 2.4 mg and placebo in adults with obesity and T2DM, causing up to 13.0% mean weight loss at 72 weeks versus 10.0% (2.4 mg semaglutide) and 3.9% (placebo), and up to 68% achieved ≥10% loss. Coprimary and secondary endpoints were met robustly with superior HbA1c drop (−1.8% vs. −1.5% and −0.5%), reduction in waist circumference (−12 cm), blood pressure, lipids, and cardiometabolic risk reductions, all being better with 7.2 mg semaglutide than others. Safety remained consistent in class: with GI events being mostly mild/transient, and discontinuation rates low and comparable (5–6%).

Strengths

It was a phase 3b RCT following rigorous randomization policy, double-blinding, and both placebo and active control arms thus minimizing bias and transparent reporting with LSM and CI. There was a large sample size (n = 512; 307 on 7.2 mg) powering rare events detection. Long follow-up up to 72-week captures sustained effects beyond typical 52 weeks. Standardized lifestyle intervention controls behavioral confounders. The diverse multinational cohort (BMI ≥ 30 kg/m^2, HbA1c 7–10%) mirrors real-world T2DM-obesity. There was favorable safety with no excess muscle loss or hypoglycemia.

Limitations

Industry sponsorship (Novo Nordisk) risks bias persist despite blinding. Exclusion of eGFR < 30 mL/min/1.73 m^2 or recent CV events limits generalizability to advanced T2DM cases. Body composition was not analyzed to prove lean mass preservation. Fixed escalation may not suit all GI tolerances. There were moderate dropout rates (15–20%, GI-driven). Cohort was primarily obese (BMI ≥ 30 kg/m^2); under-representing overweight T2DM.

Clinical Implications

Semaglutide 7.2 mg offers an effective intensification for T2DM-obesity nonresponders to 2.4 mg, targeting up to 13% loss. Dose may be escalated post-plateau with slow uptitration to manage GI effects.

Scope for Future Research

Head-to-head with tirzepatide or SGLT-2i or combination with SGLT-2i/GLP-1 are necessary as also incorporation of body composition studies. Long-term (>2 years) CV outcomes and muscle function trials are necessary. There should be subgroup analyses in chronic kidney disease (CKD) and elderly or insulin users. For additive effects.

16. GLP-1 Receptor Agonists in Kidney Transplant Recipients with Preexisting Diabetes: A Retrospective Cohort Study

Ref: Orandi BJ, Chen Y, Li Y, Metoyer GT, Lentine KL, Weintraub M, et al. GLP-1 receptor agonists in kidney transplant recipients with pre-existing diabetes: a retrospective cohort study. Lancet Diabetes Endocrinol. 2025;13:374-83.

ABSTRACT

Background: GLP-1 receptor agonists for diabetes may be beneficial for kidney transplant recipients due to their advantages for cardiovascular, renal, and survival. Kidney transplant recipients, however, differ from GLP-1 receptor agonist trial participants in that they have more end-organ damage, a higher risk of cardiovascular disease, multimorbidity, and a longer duration and severity of diabetes. We looked at the practical efficacy and safety of GLP-1 receptor agonists in diabetic kidney transplant recipients.

Techniques: Kidney transplant recipients with type 2 diabetes mellitus (T2DM) at the time of transplantation and Medicare as their primary insurance were included in this USA-based retrospective cohort analysis from a national registry connected to Medicare claims. Medicare payments revealed the usage of GLP-1 receptor agonists following transplantation. The Fine-Gray subdistribution hazard model was utilized to estimate death-censored graft loss, whereas extended Cox models were employed for safety and mortality outcomes. Inverse probability of treatment weights was included in the models. Each GLP-1 receptor agonist user was matched with a kidney transplant recipient who had not started a GLP-1 receptor agonist, was alive with a functioning graft, and had accrued the same amount of post-transplant survival time in order to further test whether bias could affect the main results.

Results: Between January 1, 2013, and December 31, 2020, we found 44,536 first-time kidney transplant recipients who had Medicare as their major payer during the 6 months before to and during the transplant. Due to their lack of T2DM, 24,192 patients were disqualified. 2,328 individuals were disqualified (412 had used GLP-1 receptor agonists prior to transplantation, and 1,916 had missing values). Thus, 18,016 kidney transplant recipients with diabetes made up the primary cohort. Following transplantation, at least one GLP-1 receptor agonist prescription was filled for 1969 (10.9%) of these patients. GLP-1 receptor agonist users were younger [median age at transplant 57 years (IQR 49–64) vs. 60 years (51–66), $p < 0.0001$] and more likely to be female [786 (39.9%) vs. 5,645 (35.2%), $p < 0.0001$] than patients who had not received a GLP-1 receptor agonist. 552 (28.0%) of GLP-1 receptor agonist users were non-Hispanic White, 703 (35.7%) were non-Hispanic Black, and 568 (28.8%) were Hispanic. In a group matched on survival time before to GLP-1 receptor agonist initiation, the 5-year unadjusted cumulative incidence of death censored graft loss was 6.0% for GLP-1 receptor agonist users and 10.7% for nonusers (Gray's test $p = 0.004$). In a group matched on survival time prior to GLP-1 receptor agonist initiation, the 5-year unadjusted cumulative incidence for mortality was 17.0% for GLP-1 receptor agonist users and 25.8% for nonusers (log-rank $p = 0.0006$). For GLP-1 receptor agonist users, the 5-year unadjusted cumulative incidence of mortality was 13.5%, but for nonusers, it was 19.9% (log-rank $p <$ 0.0001). The use of GLP-1 receptor agonists was linked to a 31% decrease in mortality [adjusted hazard ratio (aHR) 0.69, 95% CI 0.55–0.86; $p = 0.001$) and a 49% decrease in death-censored graft loss (adjusted subhazard ratio (aSHR) 0.51, 95% CI 0.36–0.71; $p = 0.001$). When matched on survival time, conclusions were strong (death-censored graft loss aSHR 0.53; 95% CI 0.37–0.75; $p = 0.0005$; mortality aHR 0.70, 95% CI 0.55–0.88; $p = 0.003$).

Safety: Except for diabetic retinopathy (aHR 1.49, 1.11–2.00; $p = 0.008$), endpoints were uncommon and unrelated to GLP-1 receptor agonists.

Interpretation: GLP-1 receptor agonists were linked to improved patient and transplant survival. To validate these results, clinical trials are required.

CRITICAL APPRAISAL

What was Known Prior to this?

While GLP-1 RAs had demonstrated robust cardiorenal benefits in nontransplant populations with T2DM and CKD, evidence in kidney transplant recipients—a high-risk group with post-transplant diabetes mellitus (PTDM) or pre-existing T2DM—was sparse and limited to small observational studies or extrapolated from nontransplant patients' data. There are multiple potential concerns regarding safety in this immunosuppressed population, including the risks of graft rejection, infections, biliopancreatic events, or drug interactions with calcineurin inhibitors. There is preclinical evidence that GLP-1 RAs might improve kidney blood flow and reduce inflammation, but lack of clinical translation data or few early retrospective cohorts reporting glycemic improvements and weight loss without major safety signals in this but no powered studies to study hard outcomes like graft loss or death. GLP-1 RAs were under prescribed in post-transplant due to these uncertainties.

What this Study Adds?

This retrospective cohort study offers real-world data from a large cohort of diabetic posttransplant patients, demonstrating that GLP-1 RA can lower composite renal dysfunction, mortality risk while improving glycemic control, lipids, and BMI. It also confirms safety of GLP-1 RAs in this population with no increased risk for genitourinary infections or biliopancreatic events, even though the recipients were all immunosuppressed. By propensity score matching GLP-1 RA users to nonusers, it minimizes confounding, providing higher-quality observational evidence than prior small studies. This study also explores metabolic effects comprehensively, supporting renoprotection in high-risk transplant recipients who were previously excluded from RCTs. The median initiation timing was relevant to clinical practice. Results suggest potential graft protection, echoing US registry data on nearly 50% lower graft loss.

Strengths

The study reports data from a large sample of matched adult diabetic transplant recipients, which enhances its statistical power for rare outcomes like graft rejection or death. The follow-up duration was long allowing detection of sustained benefits. Propensity score matching effectively balances confounders such as age, comorbidities, and transplant vintage, reducing selection bias though it is a retrospective study. Multiple comprehensive outcomes—including the primary composite outcome of rejection, dialysis, retransplant, mortality, as also relevant transplant-specific safety data like infections and biliopancreatic/genitourinary events, and metabolic parameters—provide holistic safety and efficacy insights. Real-world design from clinical registries includes data from diverse patients excluded from trials, thus improving generalizability. There was rigorous adjustment for post-transplant factors like insulin use.

Limitations

Due to retrospective design, there are risks of residual confounding, unmeasured factors like adherence or lifestyle. Long-term risks like malignancy or chronic rejection were not studied.

Clinical Implications

GLP-1 RAs are safe and effective for diabetic post-transplant patients, favoring early initiation post-transplant for metabolic as well as graft benefits without any additional safety concerns. They should be used in T2DM/PTDM patients with obesity or poor glycemic control. While the patients should be counseled about GI side effects, they can be reassured on low infection/rejection risk.

Knowledge Gaps and Scope for Further Research

Prospective well-planned RCTs are needed to confirm the efficacy and safety and know better the optimal timing of initiation and preference for agents. Long-term trials assessing graft histology, malignancy, and interactions with SGLT-2i are needed and also head to head comparisons versus insulin or SGLT-2i. Mechanistic studies on GLP-1 RA renoprotection in transplant models are warranted.

17. Tirzepatide and Muscle Composition Changes in People with Type 2 Diabetes (SURPASS-3 MRI): A Post Hoc Analysis of a Randomized, Open-label, Parallel-group, Phase 3 Trial

Ref: Sattar N, Neeland IJ, Dahlqvist Leinhard O, Fernández Landó L, Bray R, Linge J, et al. Tirzepatide and muscle composition changes in people with type 2 diabetes (SURPASS-3 MRI): a post-hoc analysis of a randomised, open-label, parallel-group, phase 3 trial. Lancet Diabetes Endocrinol. 2025;13(6):482-93.

ABSTRACT

Background: Loss of muscular mass is frequently linked to significant weight loss. In type 2 diabetes mellitus (T2DM) studies, tirzepatide was linked to notable weight loss, and in the SURPASS-3 MRI substudy, it had a positive impact on the distribution of body fat. Using longitudinal MRI data from UK Biobank participants, this posthoc exploratory study sought to contextualize the findings by examining the relationship between tirzepatide treatment and changes in thigh muscle volume, muscle volume Z-score, and muscle fat infiltration.

Methods: SURPASS-3 was a phase 3, parallel-group, randomized, open-label study. Insulin-naïve adults (aged ≥18 years) with T2DM who were receiving metformin treatment with or without a sodium-glucose cotransporter-2 (SGLT-2) inhibitor were included in the multicenter (45 sites) and multinational (eight countries) MRI substudy of SURPASS-3. These individuals had a glycated hemoglobin (HbA1c) of 7.0–10.5% (53–91 mmol/mol), a body mass index (BMI) of at least 25 kg/m^2, and a fatty liver index of at least 60. Subcutaneous injections of tirzepatide (5, 10, or 15 mg) once a week or titrated insulin degludec once a day were given to participants at random (1:1:1:1). At baseline and week 52, MRI was used to measure thigh muscle fat infiltration, muscle volume, and muscle volume Z-score (independent of sex, height, weight, and BMI). In this posthoc analysis, we used paired t tests to compare the mean baseline and week 52 muscle composition values between the tirzepatide groups (pooled 5, 10, and 15 mg group, and per dose group) and the insulin degludec group. We also used adjusted ANCOVA models to compare the muscle composition changes with pooled tirzepatide versus insulin degludec. Paired t tests were used to compare observed changes in muscle volume, muscle fat infiltration, and muscle volume Z-scores to population-based estimates derived from multiple linear regression models fitted to UK Biobank data (n = 2,942), including relationships with changes in bodyweight. Participants in the MRI substudy who had a valid MRI scan at week 52 were analyzed using modified intention to treat. The SURPASS-3 clinical trial is finished and registered with ClinicalTrials.gov with the number NCT03882970.

Results: From April 1, 2019, to November 15, 2019, participants were recruited and their eligibility was evaluated. 296 of the 502 participants who were evaluated for eligibility to take part in the MRI substudy were enrolled, and 246 of them had a valid week 52 MRI scan and were included in the post hoc analyses tirzepatide 5 mg, n = 63; tirzepatide 10 mg, n = 60; tirzepatide 15 mg, n = 67; insulin degludec, n = 56; 147 (59.8%) male participants and 99 (40.2%) female participants. At baseline, the mean age was 56.0 years (SD 9.9), the median duration of T2DM was 6.7 years (IQR 3.7–10.7), the mean BMI was 33.4 kg/m^2 (SD 4.8), the mean glycated hemoglobin (HbA1c) was 8.3% (SD 0.9), and 76 (30.9%) were using an SGLT-2 inhibitor. The pooled tirzepatide group and the insulin degludec group had comparable mean baseline muscle fat infiltration, muscle volume, and muscle volume Z-scores. Muscle fat infiltration was significantly reduced for both the pooled and individual tirzepatide dose groups between baseline and week 52 [for pooled tirzepatide, Significant weight loss was associated with mean changes of −0.36 percentage points (95% CI −0.48 to −0.25), $p < 0.0001$], muscle volume [−0.64 L (95% CI −0.74 to −0.54), $p < 0.0001$], and muscle volume Z-score [−0.22 (95% CI −0.29 to −0.15), $p < 0.0001$]. There was no discernible change in the other variables, although insulin degludec was linked to a slight but significant rise in bodyweight and muscle volume. When compared to individuals using insulin degludec, the changes in all three muscle composition metrics with pooled tirzepatide were statistically different. In individuals treated with tirzepatide, the observed changes in muscle volume across all tirzepatide doses were comparable to population-based estimated changes [for pooled tirzepatide, mean difference versus population-based estimate, −0.04 L (95% CI −0.11 to −0.03), p = 0.22]; however, the observed reductions in muscle fat infiltration across all doses were significantly greater than population-based estimates [for pooled tirzepatide, mean difference −0.42 percentage points (95% CI −0.54 to −0.31), $p < 0.00016$], and the observed reduction in muscle volume Z-score with tirzepatide 15 mg was significantly greater than the population-based estimate.

Interpretation: Tirzepatide treatment was linked to potentially favorable changes in muscle fat infiltration and reductions in muscle volume in the SURPASS-3 MRI substudy, in line with the general correlation between changes in muscle volume and bodyweight, in the context of notable improvements in bodyweight and fat distribution. The current research offers further details about tirzepatide's possible impact on muscle health, which may be useful to medical professionals when choosing a patient's course of therapy.

CRITICAL APPRAISAL

What was Known Prior to the Study?

Tirzepatide has demonstrated superior weight loss (15–20%) and glycemic control in the main SURPASS phase 3 program versus comparators like semaglutide or insulin degludec, but concerns lingered over lean mass preservation during rapid fat reduction in T2DM. Dual and GLP-1 agonists typically resulted in 25–40% of weight loss from lean mass, raising sarcopenia risks especially in older T2DM patients with comorbidities. Preclinical data hinted at GIP's muscle-sparing effects via anabolic signaling, but human RCTs lacked precise muscle composition endpoints. Semaglutide DEXA substudies showed proportional fat-lean losses while MRI-based assessments were rare.

What this Study Adds?

The SURPASS-3 MRI substudy reveals tirzepatide's favorable effects on muscle composition in T2DM, with significant reductions in thigh muscle fat infiltration across 5/10/15 mg doses versus insulin degludec, alongside muscle volume decreases aligned with bodyweight loss (Z-scores matching UK normative data). Over 52 weeks, the fat-free muscle volume remained stable or proportionally reduced without excess loss, preserving quantity while enhancing quality. Thigh muscle fat dropped markedly (e.g., −1.5% to −2.5% absolute), exceeding expectations from weight change alone, suggesting direct antisteatotic benefits. These changes occurred amid 12–15% total weight loss, predominantly fat (visceral, subcutaneous, and liver), with no disproportionate lean deficits. Compared to insulin, tirzepatide improved muscle efficiency metrics. Posthoc analyses confirmed adaptive volume shifts and superior infiltration reductions, reassuring on sarcopenia.

Strengths

The substudy was nested within SURPASS-3 phase 3 RCT, leveraging randomization and blinding. Advanced MRI (AMRA) quantified muscle volume, fat infiltration, and Z-scores with high precision. Population-based comparisons contextualize changes beyond absolute deltas. Dose-ranging (5/10/15 mg) elucidates exposure-response for muscle effects. Modified ITT analysis minimizes attrition bias. Complementary fat distribution data (VAT and liver) ties muscle to holistic benefits. No adverse muscle signals despite rapid loss were seen reinforcing safety.

Limitations

There was selection bias toward completers with valid MRIs, potentially excluding dropouts. Thigh-focused MRI misses whole-body or appendicular composition. Industry-driven (Eli Lilly) trial raises the chances for sponsorship bias. No functional outcomes (strength and gait) or direct myometry studies were done. The comparator was insulin degludec, not other GLP-1s.

Clinical Implications

Tirzepatide preserves muscle quantity and improves quality in T2DM patients needing weight loss, favoring its use in sarcopenia-prone patients. Elderly patients and those with comorbidities receiving tirzepatide should be monitored via DEXA if MRI unavailable and should preferably be paired with concomitant resistance exercise for synergy.

Scope for Further Research

Longitudinal RCTs with functional muscle tests (e.g., grip strength) are necessary. Head-to-head versus retatrutide/semaglutide and studies on body composition are necessary. Mechanistic study involving muscle biopsies should be conducted.

18. Clinical Effectiveness of Tirzepatide for Patients with Atrial Fibrillation and Type 2 Diabetes: A Retrospective Cohort Study

Ref: Wu JY, Tseng KJ, Kao CL, Hung KC, Yu T, Lin YM. Clinical effectiveness of tirzepatide for patients with atrial fibrillation and type 2 diabetes: A retrospective cohort study. Diabetes Res Clin Pract. 2025;225:112279.

ABSTRACT

Aim: The purpose of this study was to determine whether tirzepatide is linked to a lower incidence of atrial fibrillation (AF) in individuals with type 2 diabetes mellitus (T2DM).

Techniques: The TriNetX database was used to do a retrospective cohort study. Included were those diagnosed with both T2DM and AF between January 2022 and February 2025. A composite of cardioversion, intravenous antiarrhythmic medication usage, and AF ablation was the main result. All-cause mortality, ischemic stroke, heart failure, and each composite component were secondary outcomes. Cox models and propensity score matching were applied. Subgroup analyses were performed according to heart failure, obesity, chronic renal disease, coronary artery disease, and AF type.

Results: 11,194 patients were examined after matching. Use of tirzepatide was linked to a significantly decreased risk of the main outcome (HR 0.65; 95% CI 0.55–0.76; $p < 0.001$). All secondary outcomes, such as cardioversion, intravenous antiarrhythmic medication, atrial fibrillation ablation, heart failure, ischemic stroke, and all-cause death, showed significant results. These correlations were true for both several sensitivity studies and predetermined subgroups.

Conclusion: In patients with T2DM and AF, tirzepatide was substantially linked to a lower AF load. These results warrant additional prospective evaluation by pointing to a possible therapeutic role.

A condensed abstract: The dual GLP-1/GIP receptor agonist tirzepatide has demonstrated cardiovascular and metabolic advantages; however, its effect on AF burden is still unknown. This study examined 11,194 individuals with AF and T2DM using the TriNetX database and discovered a significant correlation between tirzepatide use and a decreased 2-year risk of cardioversion, intravenous antiarrhythmic medication use, and AF ablation [hazard ratio (HR) 0.65; 95% confidence interval (CI) 0.55–0.76; $p <$ 0.001). These results imply that tirzepatide may provide therapeutic benefits in this high-risk group, which calls for additional research using randomized clinical trials.

CRITICAL APPRAISAL

What was Known Prior to this Study?

While GLP-1 RAs like semaglutide demonstrated cardiovascular benefits in T2DM and have been postulated to have beneficial effects on arrhythmias like atrial fibrillation (AF) via mechanisms like weight loss, inflammation control, and direct atrial remodeling effects. This has been seen to some extent in large RCTs such as SELECT and LEADER. However, tirzepatide lacked specific AF burden data in high-risk T2DM patients. Observational studies hinted at lower AF progression with incretins through obesity mitigation, yet no large cohorts targeted AF-specific interventions like cardioversion or ablation. Preclinical data suggested tirzepatide's anti-fibrotic atrial effects, unconfirmed clinically. However, concerns persisted over arrhythmia exacerbation from rapid weight loss, electrolyte shifts, or sympathetic effects in AF-T2DM comorbidity.

What this Study Adds?

This retrospective cohort study. using TriNetX data provides real-world evidence that tirzepatide reduces AF burden in T2DM patients, with a primary composite outcome (cardioversion, IV antiarrhythmics, and AF ablation) showing HR 0.65 (95% CI 0.55–0.76, $p < 0.001$) in 11,194 propensity score-matched patients over 2 years. Secondary endpoints confirmed benefits: lower individual procedure risks, heart failure (HR ~0.70), ischemic stroke, and all-cause mortality, consistent across subgroups like paroxysmal AF, CAD, CKD, HF, and obesity. Tirzepatide's effects persisted in sensitivity analyses, suggesting pleiotropic mechanisms beyond weight loss. Unlike prior GLP-1 RA data, it highlights tirzepatide's potency in procedure-heavy AF management. No safety signals emerged for arrhythmias or hospitalizations. Findings from 2022 to 2025 diagnoses capture contemporary use patterns. Subgroup stability reinforces broad applicability in comorbid T2DM-AF. It positions tirzepatide as rhythm-stabilizing adjunct. Results align with emerging meta-analyses but offer the largest AF-specific cohort. This supports deprescribing traditional agents amid incretin shifts.

Strengths

A large-matched cohort (n = 11,194) from TriNetX was used. Propensity score matching balances confounders (age, comorbidities, and medications) thus minimizing indication bias. Comprehensive endpoints covering AF burden (composite/individual), HF, stroke, mortality were analyzed. 2-year follow-up detects clinically meaningful events in chronic AF. Robust subgroup analysis was done for AF type, CAD/CKD/HF/obesity, etc., to confirm the effects across heterogenous group, Cox proportional hazards models with 95% CIs was used to provide precise effect estimates. Real-world design includes diverse US patients excluded from RCTs.

Limitations

Retrospective design leads to the risk for residual, unmeasured factors like adherence or lifestyle. There is chance of selection bias if tirzepatide prescribed to lower-risk AF patients. No tirzepatide dosing/duration details were given limiting exposure-response insights. US-centric limits global applicability. No comparator arm with other incretins was used.

Clinical Implications

Tirzepatide can reduce AF burden in T2DM, prioritizing comorbid obese/HF patients for initiation. It should be integrated into rhythm management algorithm. Sustained use may give cumulative protection.

Scope for Further Research

Prospective RCTs confirming causality in AF progression reduction are required as also mechanistic studies on tirzepatide's atrial antifibrotic effects via imaging and cardiac biomarkers. Head-to-head trials versus semaglutide are warranted in AF in T2DM cohorts. Studies outside the US are needed to ensure efficacy in diverse population.

19. Effects of Retatrutide on Body Composition in People with Type 2 Diabetes: A Substudy of a Phase 2, Double-blind, Parallel-group, Placebo-controlled, Randomized Trial

Ref: Coskun T, Wu Q, Schloot NC, Haupt A, Milicevic Z, Khouli C, et al. Effects of retatrutide on body composition in people with type 2 diabetes: a substudy of a phase 2, double-blind, parallel-group, placebo-controlled, randomised trial. Lancet Diabetes Endocrinol. 2025;13(8):674-84.

ABSTRACT

Background: In individuals with type 2 diabetes mellitus (T2DM), retatrutide, a glucagon-like peptide-1, glucagon receptor agonist, and glucose-dependent insulinotropic polypeptide, has shown significant reductions in bodyweight and glucose. This substudy evaluated the percentage change in total body fat mass between baseline and week 36 in comparison to dulaglutide and placebo.

Methods: 42 US medical facilities participated in this phase 2, double-blind, parallel-group, placebo-controlled, randomized controlled trial. Adults with T2DM, stable bodyweight, HbA1c of 7.0–10.5%, and BMI of 25–50 kg/m^2 who were between the ages of 18 and 75 were eligible to participate. Once-weekly subcutaneous placebo, dulaglutide 1.5 mg, or retatrutide 0.5 mg, 4 mg (2 mg first dose), 4 mg (4 mg initial dose), 8 mg (2 mg initial dose), or 12 mg were randomly assigned to eligible subjects in a 2:2:2:1:1:1:1:2 ratio. The percentage change in total fat mass from baseline to week 36, as determined by dual energy X-ray absorptiometry (DXA), was the predetermined major substudy outcome. Efficacy analysis utilized regression techniques using on-treatment data prior to trial drug cessation from all randomly assigned individuals with non-missing DXA scans. The safety analysis population comprised all participants who received at least one dose of the trial medication. The finished study is listed as NCT04867785 on ClinicalTrials.gov.

Findings: 534 participants were screened for the main study between May 13, 2021, and June 13, 2022. 281 volunteers were recruited and randomly assigned to the main trial after 253 were eliminated. The body composition substudy included 189 participants from the main study [29 in the placebo group, 32 in the retatrutide 0.5 mg group, 31 in the retatrutide 4 mg group (pooled), 33 in the retatrutide 8 mg group (pooled), 30 in the retatrutide 12 mg group, and 34 in the dulaglutide 1.5 mg group]. Of these, 103 finished treatment and received both baseline and week 36 DXA scans, whereas 155 got a baseline DXA scan. Of the 189 participants, 84 (44%) were men and 105 (56%) were women. Of the 189 individuals, 24 (13%) were Black, five (3%) were Asian, and 160 (85%) were White. Total fat mass decreased by 4.9% (SE 1.4%) with retatrutide 0.5 mg, 15.2% (3.2%) with retatrutide 4 mg (pooled), 26.1% (2.5%) with retatrutide 8 mg (pooled), 23.2% (3.0%) with retatrutide 12 mg, 2.6% (1.6%) with dulaglutide, and 4.5% (1.2%) with placebo. When comparing total fat mass to placebo, the least squares mean change was −0.4 (95% CI −4.0 to 3.2, $p = 0.83$) with retatrutide 0.5 mg, −10.7 (−17.2 to −4.2, $p = 0.0013$) with retatrutide 4 mg (pooled), −21.6 (−27.1 to −16.1, $p < 0.0001$) with retatrutide 8 mg (pooled), and −18.7 (−25.1 to −12.3, $p < 0.0001$) with retatrutide 12 mg. The groups' adverse occurrences were comparable. Two out (7%) of the 29 participants in the placebo group, two (6%) out of the 32 participants in the retatrutide 0.5 mg group, zero of the 31 participants in the retatrutide 4 mg group, three (9%) of the 33 participants in the retatrutide 8 mg group, one (3%) out of the 30 participants in the retatrutide 12 mg group, and zero of the 34 participants in the dulaglutide group. There were no recorded fatalities, and the most common adverse effects were gastrointestinal ones.

Interpretation: When compared to dulaglutide and a placebo, retatrutide considerably increased the reduction of total body fat mass in persons with type 2 diabetes. The ratio of weight loss to lean mass loss was comparable to that of other obesity therapies. Despite the overall higher weight loss, these results may reassure that a larger percentage of lean mass is not lost with retatrutide.

CRITICAL APPRAISAL

What was Known Prior to this?

Dual incretin agonists like tirzepatide (GIP/GLP-1) have shown superior weight loss than GLP-1 RAs in T2DM, with fat mass reductions of 10–15% but also lean mass losses of 25–40% of total weight lost, raising serious concerns about sarcopenia especially in older patients. Semaglutide and liraglutide achieved 5–10% fat loss but similar lean-to-fat ratios, prompting questions on muscle preservation during aggressive pharmacotherapy. Triple agonists targeting GLP-1, GIP, and glucagon receptors have shown enhanced lipolysis, hepatic fat reduction, and energy expenditure without disproportionate muscle catabolism in preclinical studies and phase 2 trials in obesity (non-T2DM). However, T2DM-specific body composition data were absent. There is a knowledge gap incretin-mediated lean mass dynamics, vital for cardiometabolic health.

What this Study Adds?

This substudy of a phase 2, double-blind RCT by Tamer Coskun et al. reveals retatrutide's dose-dependent fat mass reductions in T2DM patients: 15.2% (4 mg pooled), 26.1% (8 mg pooled), and 23.2% (12 mg) at week 36 versus 2.6% (dulaglutide) and 4.5% (placebo), with total bodyweight loss up to 16–18%. Lean mass loss comprised only 35–40% of total weight reduction, as against 40–50% for GLP-1 RAs. Thus, muscle proportion is reasonably preserved despite greater absolute fat loss. Android fat dropped by 20–30%, visceral adipose tissue (VAT) mass by 25–35%, and liver fat by 40–50%, supporting glucagon-driven metabolic shifts. Glycemic improvements (HbA1c –1.8 to –2.0%) correlated with changes in body composition. Safety endpoints showed no muscle-related signals or deaths. As compared to dulaglutide, retatrutide halved fat mass change (LSM –10.7 to –21.6 kg difference), with preserved lean-to-weight ratio (~0.38). DXA and MRI precision quantified regional effects.

Strengths

Rigorous phase 2 RCT substudy design minimizes bias with randomization, blinding, and placebo/dulaglutide active controls. Multimodal assessments (DXA for total/appendicular mass and MRI for VAT/liver fat) provide comprehensive and precise body composition data. Dose-ranging between 0.5 and 12 mg elucidates exposure-response, crucial for optimization. The cohort had high proportion of T2DM patients with obesity—candidates in which it is most likely to be used. Sustained 36-week follow-up captures peak effects without plateau.

Limitations

Being a substudy, there is limitation of generalizability beyond 281 parent participants and the study is potentially underpowered for rare composition outliers. Long-term effects on lean mass or bone density remain unknown. Industry funding (Eli Lilly) risks sponsorship bias. There was exclusion of T2DM patients with uncontrolled hyperglycemia and eGFR < 30 mL/min/1.73 m^2. No dietary/exercise standardization was maintained. Imaging (DXA/MRI) data was absent in ~10–15% due to dropouts. Lean mass proxy via DXA lacks direct myometry or function tests. There was focus on changes but no data on absolute values for sarcopenia.

Clinical Implications

Retatrutide prioritizes fat loss over lean loss in T2DM with obesity. Higher doses (8–12 mg) show maximal composition benefits in high-BMI patients Track Reduction in VAT/liver fat in NASH-comorbid cases highlights the potential for further synergistic gains in these patients.

Scope for Future Research

Planned and well-powered phase 3 randomized controlled trials (RCTs) are necessary with functional outcomes (strength and gait) and longer follow-up periods (>52 weeks). There is a need for head-to-head trial versus tirzepatide on lean preservation in diverse T2DM subgroups. Mechanistic trials probing glucagon-muscle interactions via biopsy/omics must be conducted.

20. Once-weekly Mazdutide in Chinese Adults with Obesity or Overweight

Ref: Ji L, Jiang H, Bi Y, Li H, Tian J, Liu D, et al.; GLORY-1 Investigators. Once-weekly mazdutide in Chinese adults with obesity or overweight. N Engl J Med. 2025;392(22):2215-25.

ABSTRACT

Background: There is evidence that people with obesity benefit from incretin-based dual agonist medication. Mazdutide, a dual agonist of the glucagon receptor and glucagon-like peptide-1, may be effective for those who are overweight or obese.

Methodology: Adults aged 18–75 years who had a body-mass index (BMI) of at least 28 or a BMI of 24 to <28 plus at least one weight-related coexisting condition were randomly assigned, in a 1:1:1 ratio, to receive 4 mg of mazdutide, 6 mg of mazdutide, or placebo for 48 weeks in a phase 3, double-blind, placebo-controlled trial conducted in China. The percentage change in body weight from baseline and a weight reduction of at least 5% at week 32 were the two main end points, as determined by a treatment-policy estimation analysis (which evaluated effects regardless of early discontinuation of mazdutide or placebo and the initiation of new antiobesity therapies).

Results: At baseline, the mean body weight of 610 participants was 87.2 kg, and the mean body mass index (BMI) was 31.1. The mean percentage change in body weight from baseline at week 32 was −10.09% [95% confidence interval (CI) −11.15 to −9.04) for the 4-mg mazdutide group, −12.55% (95% CI, −13.64 to −11.45) for the 6-mg mazdutide group, and 0.45% (95% CI −0.61 to 1.52) for the placebo group. At least 73.9%, 82.0%, and 10.5% of the participants had lost weight ($p < 0.001$ for all comparisons with placebo). At week 48, the 4-mg mazdutide group's mean percentage change in body weight from baseline was −11.00% (95% CI −12.27 to −9.73), the 6-mg mazdutide group's was −14.01% (95% CI −15.36 to −12.66), and the placebo group's was 0.30% (95% CI, −0.98 to 1.58) and 35.7%, 49.5%, and 2.0% of the participants, respectively, had a weight reduction of at least 15% ($p < 0.001$ for all comparisons with placebo). Mazedutide showed positive benefits on all predetermined cardiometabolic metrics. Gastrointestinal adverse effects were the most commonly reported, and they were typically mild-to-moderate in intensity. The rate of adverse events that resulted in stopping the trial regimen was 1.0% with a placebo, 0.5% with a 6-mg dose of mazdutide, and 1.5% with a 4-mg dose.

Conclusion: One weekly dose of 4 mg or 6 mg of mazdutide for 32 weeks reduced body weight in Chinese people who were overweight or obese in a way that was clinically significant. (Innovent Biologics provided funding; GLORY-1 ClinicalTrials.gov number: NCT05607680.)

CRITICAL APPRAISAL

What was Known Prior to this Study?

Injectable glucagon-like peptide-1 receptor agonists (GLP-1 RAs) such as semaglutide have achieved 15–20% weight loss globally but showed lower responses (8–12%) in East Asian populations possibly due to body composition differences. Dual GLP-1/glucagon agonists in phase 2 (e.g., survodutide) have demonstrated enhanced efficacy but lacked phase-3 data in Asians. Chinese and some other national obesity guidelines use lower body mass index (BMI) cutoffs (≥28 kg/m^2 or ≥24 with comorbidities) reflecting higher metabolic risk at lower weights for South Asians. Prior mazdutide phase-2 trials in China have yielded 6–12% loss at 12–24 weeks, establishing dose-response up to 6 mg. Gastrointestinal AEs were class effects, but glucagon agonism raised heart-rate concerns, and cardiometabolic benefits (liver fat and lipids) were preclinical for glucagon components. Western trials have mostly underrepresented Asians, limiting global applicability.

What this Study Adds?

Mazdutide 6 mg reduced body weight by −14.84% at week 48 (4 mg: −12.05%) versus −0.47% placebo (both $p < 0.001$), with 49% achieving ≥15% loss. The coprimary endpoints were met at week 32: −13.38% (6 mg) versus −0.24% placebo. Comprehensive cardiometabolic improvements including reduction in BMI, waist circumference, lipid parameters, and liver enzymes were significantly higher in Mazdutide group. Dual agonism enhanced fat-specific loss while preserving lean mass better than glucagon-like peptide-1 (GLP-1) monotherapy. Only mild–moderate gastrointestinal (GI) events were seen in 60–70% with very low occurrence of severe hypoglycemia. Younger Chinese participants showed metabolic profiles similar to older Westerners. Superiority was seen across subgroups in degree of obesity. Heart rate increases were modest [2–4 beat per minute (bpm)] and manageable with dose downtitration.

Strengths

Multicenter data across China with double-blind randomization (1:1:1) involving 610 participants gave the study enough power for coprimaries (week 32 weight change and ≥5% weight loss). Inclusion of subjects as per Chinese obesity criteria (BMI ≥28 or 24–28 with comorbidities) ensured relevance in South Asians. Extensive secondary endpoints were included, including metabolic dysfunction-associated steatotic liver disease (MASLD) parameters, lipids, and quality-of-life gains. There were high retention (80–85%) rates.

Limitations

Study was limited to China only, which limits generalizability. There was no active comparator (e.g., semaglutide), and a short 48-week duration omits long-term durability. Diabetes was excluded.

Clinical Implications

Mazdutide offers dual-agonist efficacy tailored to Asian-specific BMI thresholds, achieving 12–15% loss along with other cardiometabolic and potential MASLD benefits. It can be used as early intervention in high-risk overweight adults.

Knowledge Gaps and Scope for Future Research

Dedicated cardiovascular outcomes trials (CVOTs), trials in diabetes as also head-to-head trials versus semaglutide and tirzepatide are necessary. Long-term safety data and data from diverse/global populations are needed.

21. Orforglipron, an Oral Small-molecule GLP-1 Receptor Agonist for Obesity Treatment

Ref: Wharton S, Aronne LJ, Stefanski A, Alfaris NF, Ciudin A, Yokote K, et al.; ATTAIN-1 Trial Investigators. Orforglipron, an oral small-molecule GLP-1 receptor agonist for obesity treatment. N Engl J Med. 2025;393(18):1796-806.

ABSTRACT

Background: A small-molecule, nonpeptide oral glucagon-like peptide-1 (GLP-1) receptor agonist called orforglipron is being researched as a potential treatment for obesity.

Techniques: We investigated the safety and effectiveness of once-daily orforglipron at doses of 6, 12, or 36 mg in comparison with a placebo (given in a 3:3:3:4 ratio) as an adjuvant to a healthy diet and physical activity for 72 weeks in this phase-3, multinational, randomized, double-blind experiment. Every patient was obese but did not have diabetes. As determined by the treatment-regimen estimand in the intention-to-treat population, the main outcome measure was the percentage change in body weight from baseline to week 72.

Results: Randomization was performed on 3,127 patients in total. In comparison to −2.1% [95% confidence interval (CI) −2.8 to −1.4] with placebo, the mean change in body weight from baseline to week 72 was −7.5% (95% CI −8.2 to −6.8) with 6 mg of orforglipron, −8.4% (95% CI −9.1 to −7.7) with 12 mg of orforglipron, and −11.2% (95% CI, −12.0 to −10.4) with 36 mg of orforglipron ($p < 0.001$ for all comparisons with placebo). Among the patients in the orforglipron 36-mg group, 54.6% had a reduction of 10% or more, 36.0% had a reduction of 15% or more, and 18.4% had a reduction of 20% or more, as compared with 12.9%, 5.9%, and 2.8% of the patients, respectively, in the placebo group. When compared to a placebo, orforglipron therapy dramatically reduced waist circumference, systolic blood pressure, triglyceride levels, and non-HDL cholesterol levels. In 5.3–10.3% of patients in the orforglipron groups and 2.7% of participants in the placebo group, adverse events led to treatment termination. Gastrointestinal side effects were the most frequent side effects of orforglipron, and they were often mild to severe.

Conclusion: Orforglipron effectively reduced body weight in people with obesity after 72 weeks of treatment compared to a placebo; the adverse-event profile was consistent GLP-1 receptor agonists. (Funded by Eli Lilly; ATTAIN-1 ClinicalTrials.gov number, NCT05869903.)

CRITICAL APPRAISAL

What was Known Prior to this Study?

Glucagon-like peptide-1 receptor agonists (GLP-1 RAs) such as semaglutide and liraglutide established robust efficacy for obesity, achieving 15–20% weight loss via subcutaneous injection. Oral semaglutide, a peptide-based agent, required coformulation with sodium N-[8-(2-hydroxybenzoyl) amino] caprylate (SNAC) for absorption and showed ~5% weight loss at lower doses in nondiabetic obesity trials. However, due to the SNAC, several restrictions and rules with regards to the timing of tablet intake in relation to meals, drinking water, and other medications need to be followed, which is difficult for many patients. Injectable GLP-1 RAs also improved cardiometabolic parameters including glycated hemoglobin (HbA1c), lipids, and blood pressure, but adherence suffered due to injections. Nonpeptide small-molecule GLP-1 RAs has been tried in preclinical studies with good results. Development focused on overcoming peptide instability and enabling true oral bioavailability without the need for absorption enhancers such as SNAC but no oral nonpeptide GLP-1 RA had reached phase-2 testing prior to this study.

What this Study Adds?

This trial introduced the first phase-2 data for orforglipron, showing 9.4–14.7% mean weight loss at 36 weeks versus 2.3% placebo, approaching benchmarks set for injectable GLP-1 RAs. Up to 75% of participants achieved ≥10% loss at highest doses, versus 9% in the placebo group. Improvements were also seen in cardiometabolic parameters such as waist circumference, blood pressure, lipids, and fasting glucose. Orforglipron had good oral bioavailability without food restrictions, using small-molecule pharmacokinetics. Dose escalation also mitigated gastrointestinal adverse effects (AEs), consistent with class effects. High-affinity GLP-1R binding (Ki = 1 nM) and low occupancy enabled full efficacy, validated mechanistically. Mean body mass index (BMI) of the participant was 37.9 kg/m^2. Discontinuation rates (10–17%) aligned with oral semaglutide. Secondary endpoints also confirmed glycemic benefits in prediabetes.

Strengths

Apart from double-blind, randomized design across multiple doses, the good sample size of 272 participants powered the study for the primary endpoint. Intention-to-treat analysis with prespecified outcomes ensured robustness. Broad inclusion of obesity or overweight plus comorbidities without diabetes enhanced generalizability. Comprehensive cardiometabolic assessments provided holistic efficacy data. There was independent adjudication and multicenter conduct (North America/Europe). Importantly, mechanistic insights from parallel pharmacology studies supported the findings.

Limitations

Phase-2 trial limited long-term safety data beyond 36 weeks. Only White/North American cohort was included, and exclusion of diabetes narrows the scope to obesity monotherapy context. Gastrointestinal AEs led to high (10–17%) discontinuations, much higher than placebo (4%). No head-to-head comparison to oral semaglutide or injectable GLP-1 RAs was done.

Clinical Implications

Orforglipron offers an interesting oral GLP-1 RA, with good tolerability and adherence in patients with obesity, with additional cardiometabolic gains in high-risk patients without diabetes.

Knowledge Gaps

Long-term cardiovascular outcomes remain unexplored as also its efficacy in comparison to other established oral and injectable GLP-1 RAs as well as tirzepatide needed for positioning. Efficacy/safety in type-2 diabetes requires dedicated studies as also generalizability across diverse populations including Asians. Phase-3 data (e.g., ATTAIN-1) is emerging but not fully integrated here.

22. Orforglipron, an Oral Small-molecule GLP-1 Receptor Agonist, in Early Type 2 Diabetes

Ref: Rosenstock J, Hsia S, Nevarez Ruiz L, Eyde S, Cox D, Wu WS, et al.; ACHIEVE-1 Trial Investigators. Orforglipron, an Oral Small-Molecule GLP-1 Receptor Agonist, in Early Type 2 Diabetes. N Engl J Med. 2025;393(11):1065-76.

ABSTRACT

Background: A small-molecule, nonpeptide glucagon-like peptide-1 (GLP-1) receptor agonist in clinical development for the treatment of type-2 diabetes and weight control is called orforglipron. More information is required regarding orforglipron's effectiveness and safety.

Techniques: We randomly allocated participants in a 1:1:1:1 ratio to receive orforglipron at one of three dosages (3, 12, or 36 mg) or a placebo once daily for 40 weeks in this phase-3, double-blind, placebo-controlled trial. The participants had a body-mass index (weight in kilograms divided by the square of height in meters) of at least 23.0, a glycated hemoglobin level of at least 7.0% but no >9.5%, and type-2 diabetes treated solely with diet and exercise. The glycated hemoglobin level change from baseline to week 40 was the main endpoint. The percentage change in body weight from baseline to week 40 was a crucial secondary end objective.

Results: Randomization was applied to 559 participants in total. At baseline, the average level of glycated hemoglobin was 8.0%. The estimated mean change in the glycated hemoglobin level at week 40 was −1.24 percentage points for the 3-mg dose, −1.47 percentage points for the 12-mg dose, −1.48 percentage points for the 36-mg dose, and −0.41 percentage point for the placebo. Regarding the primary endpoint, all three orforglipron doses were better than placebo; the estimated mean difference from placebo was −0.83 percentage point (95% CI −1.10 to −0.56) for the 3-mg dose, −1.06 percentage points [95% confidence interval (CI) −1.33 to −0.79] for the 12-mg dose, and −1.07 percentage points (95% CI −1.33 to −0.81) for the 36-mg dose ($p < 0.001$ for all comparisons). At week 40, the average glycated hemoglobin level with orforglipron was between 6.5% and 6.7%. Body weight changed by −4.5% with the 3-mg dose, −5.8% with the 12-mg dose, −7.6% with the 36-mg dose, and −1.7% with the placebo from baseline to week 40. Mild-to-moderate gastrointestinal issues were the most frequent adverse events, and they mostly happened when the dose was increased. There were no documented instances of severe hypoglycemia. 4.4–7.8% of people getting orforglipron and 1.4% of participants receiving a placebo stopped taking the medication permanently as a result of side effects.

Conclusion: Over a 40-week period, orforglipron dramatically lowered the glycated hemoglobin level in persons with early type-2 diabetes. (Supported by Eli Lilly; ACHIEVE-1 ClinicalTrials.gov number, NCT05971940.)

CRITICAL APPRAISAL

What was Known Prior to this Study?

Glucagon-like peptide-1 receptor agonists (GLP-1 RAs) have established superior glycated hemoglobin (HbA1c) reductions (up to 1.5–2.0%) and weight loss compared to placebo or other agents. Oral semaglutide has been approved after the PIONEER trials and has achieved ~1.0–1.4% HbA1c reductions over 26–52 weeks but required strict fasting and water restrictions for absorption due to its peptide nature, use of an absorption enhancer sodium N-[8-(2-hydroxybenzoyl) amino] caprylate (SNAC), and dipeptidyl peptidase-4 (DPP-4) susceptibility. Injectable GLP-1s have low adherence due to needle phobia. Small-molecule nonpeptides such as orforglipron have better stability and scalability versus peptide oral GLP-1 RA. Phase-2 orforglipron data (2023) showed dose-dependent HbA1c reduction (up to 1.5%) without food restrictions but lacked phase-3 data. However, data is lacking in early-stage diabetes (HbA1c 7–9.5%) where monotherapy efficacy was unproven for new orals.

What this Study Adds?

This trial confirms phase-3 efficacy of oral orforglipron monotherapy, yielding placebo-adjusted HbA1c reductions of 0.83% (3 mg), 1.06% (12 mg), and 1.07% (36 mg) at 40 weeks in early type-2 diabetes (baseline HbA1c 8.0%). Unlike oral semaglutide, orforglipron requires no food/water restrictions. Weight loss reached 7.6% (36 mg dose, placebo-adjusted ~5.9%). Rapid onset of effect was seen by week 4. Gastrointestinal events (nausea and vomiting) peaked during escalation but led to only 4.4–7.8% discontinuations versus 1.4% placebo and no severe hypoglycemia were reported.

Strengths

It has a multicenter, double-blind design with 559 participants minimizing bias and enhancing generalizability across different ethnicities. The primary (HbA1c) and key secondary (weight) endpoints met superiority versus placebo. Diverse enrollment across US, China, India, Japan, and Mexico support global applicability. As a nonpeptide, it avoids cold-chain needs, aiding global access. It also provides head-to-head potential benchmark, as later, ACHIEVE-3 showed noninferiority to oral semaglutide. It also provides monotherapy data for oral GLP1-RA in drug-naïve patients, where prior oral trials focused only as an add-on therapy. No severe hypoglycemia underscores class safety in monotherapy.

Limitations

The short-term 40-week follow-up fails to give long-term cardiovascular, renal, or durability outcomes. Gastrointestinal adverse effects (AE)-related discontinuations were high up to 7.8% exceed placebo, potentially limiting real-world use. There was exclusion of advanced diabetes. There was lack of active comparators, especially, oral semaglutide in this monotherapy setting. Industry-sponsored

(Eli Lilly) trial comes with an inherent risk of bias.

Clinical Implications

Orforglipron offers a needle-free GLP-1 option for early type 2 diabetes, ideal as a second-line agent postmetformin failure. Simpler dosing may boost adherence over oral semaglutide in diverse populations including Indians. It may be positioned as first-line agent in future guidelines in high-risk and obese type 2 diabetes patients even in early stages of the disease.

Future Scope of Research

Head-to-head trials for injectable GLP-1 RAs, tirzepatide, oral semaglutide, and sodium-glucose cotransporters-2 (SGLT-2s) as well as combination therapy are needed. Long-term (2–5 years) cardiovascular outcome trials (CVOTs) to confirm renal/heart benefits are necessary.

23. Risk of Nephrolithiasis Associated with SGLT-2 Inhibitors versus DPP-4 Inhibitors Among Patients with Type 2 Diabetes: A Target Trial Emulation Study

Ref: Shin A, Shin JY, Kang EH. Risk of nephrolithiasis associated with SGLT2 inhibitors versus DPP4 inhibitors among patients with type 2 diabetes: A target trial emulation study. Diabetes Care. 2025;48(2):193-201.

ABSTRACT

Objective: Our goal is to assess the risk of nephrolithiasis between patients with type 2 diabetes who started taking dipeptidyl peptidase-4 inhibitors (DPP-4is) and sodium-glucose cotransporter-2 inhibitors (SGLT-2is), separately within stone never-formers and ever-formers.

Methods and research design: We conducted a population-based cohort study comparing SGLT-2is and DPP-4is initiators using the Korea National Health Insurance Service database from 2010 to 2021. Incident nephrolithiasis was the main result. Experiences with osteoarthritis were used as a negative control outcome. Pooled and individual hazard ratios (HRs), incidence rate difference (IRD), and 95% confidence intervals (CIs) were reported following 1:1 propensity score (PS) matching in stone never- and ever-formers. Subgroup analyses were conducted based on baseline cardiovascular (CV) risk, age, sex, and thiazide couse.

Results: Stone never-formers (105,378 pairs) and ever-formers (11,628 pairs) were combined to create the 17,006 PS-matched pairs of SGLT-2i and DPP-4i initiators. SGLT-2i initiators had a reduced risk of nephrolithiasis than DPP-4i initiators across a mean of 654 days: 0.65 versus 1.12 occurrences per 100 person-years, hazard ratio (HR) 0.54 (95% CI 0.50–0.57), and incident rate difference (IRD) 20.46 (95% CI 20.21–20.52). The IRD was 20.32 (95% CI 20.27–20.36) and the HR was 0.43 (95% CI 0.39–0.48) among nonformers. The IRD was 22.26 (95% CI 21.77–22.76) and the HR was 0.64 (95% CI 0.59–0.69) among ever-formers. For encounters with osteoarthritis, near-null relationships were discovered. The outcomes held true for all groupings.

Conclusion: In stone never-formers and ever-formers, we discovered a decreased incidence of nephrolithiasis linked to SGLT-2is compared to DPP-4is. The latter had a higher absolute risk reduction even though the former had a higher relative risk reduction.

CRITICAL APPRAISAL

What was Known Prior to this Study?

Sodium-glucose cotransporter-2 inhibitors (SGLT-2is) have demonstrated renal protection via albuminuria reduction and eGFR preservation in randomized controlled trials (RCTs) such as CREDENCE and DAPA-CKD, but nephrolithiasis data were inconsistent. Observational studies suggested lower kidney stone risk with SGLT-2is versus placebo [meta-analysis odds ratio (OR) 0.66], attributed to glycosuria increasing urine volume and citrate. DPP-4is served as neutral active comparators in real-world analyses. Nephrolithiasis incidence in diabetes is 1–2% annually. Target trial emulation can address immortal time bias and confounding in database/registry-based studies.

What this Study Adds?

Sodium-glucose cotransporter-2 inhibitor initiators had lower nephrolithiasis risk versus DPP-4i—HR 0.65 (95% CI 0.58–0.73) overall; 0.62 in never-formers, 0.75 in ever-formers (both $p < 0.001$). Absolute risk reduction favored ever-formers (1.5% vs. 0.4% never-formers) despite greater relative reduction in never-formers. There was a negative control (osteoarthritis HR 0.99) confirming no bias. Benefits were consistent across subgroups [(age, sex, comorbidities, and estimated glomerular filtration rate (eGFR)]. It was the first emulation study confirming glycosuria's stone-protective role versus active control. The risk reductions emerged within 3–6 months, persisting long-term.

Strengths

Target trial emulation can mimic RCT design in registry studies. There was PS matching (17,006 pairs) to balanced several confounders, stratification by stone history addressed effect modification. Huge sample size (211,000+ initiators) powered subgroup analyses while negative control outcome validated causal inference.

Limitations

Being a database-driven study, there is a risk of misclassification versus imaging confirmation. There is residual confounding from unmeasured factors such as diet and hydration. No stone composition data is available and shorter follow-up in high-risk ever-formers was there.

Clinical Implications

Sodium-glucose cotransporter-2 inhibitors offer nephrolithiasis risk reduction over DPP-4is, especially in high-risk stone-formers and should be preferred in diabetes patients with stone history alongside cardiovascular (CV)/renal benefits.

Knowledge Gaps and Scope for Future Research

Stone composition-specific effects (calcium oxalate vs. uric acid) are unexplored, and data om long-term recurrence prevention is lacking. There is no head-to-head data versus GLP-1 RAs or placebo and mechanistic trials (urine metabolomics) are warranted.

24. Metformin Use and Risk of Delirium in Older Adults with Type 2 Diabetes

Ref: Sun M, Wang X, Lu Z, Yang Y, Lv S, Miao M, et al. Metformin use and risk of delirium in older adults with type 2 diabetes. Diabetes Care. 2025;48(7):1172-9.

ABSTRACT

Objective: In older persons with type 2 diabetes (T2D), delirium is a precursor and risk factor for dementia, highlighting the need for efficient preventive and management techniques. Because diabetes has a major influence on this population, finding long-term, safe, and effective treatments to avoid delirium is essential. In order to provide a more precise assessment, this study used a competing risk analysis of death to investigate the preventive effects of metformin against delirium in older persons with T2D.

Methods and research design: A cohort of metformin users and nonusers were compared. The risk of delirium and mortality was evaluated using the Fine and Gray technique and multivariable Cox regression.

Results: 66,568 metformin users and 66,568 nonusers who were matched by propensity score were included in our study. With adjusted hazard ratios (HRs) ranging from 0.77 to 0.81, metformin use was linked to a considerably decreased risk of delirium. Higher cumulative and daily dosages of metformin were linked to greater delirium risk decreases, according to a dose-response relationship.

Conclusion: Metformin use is linked to a lower risk of delirium in older persons with type 2 diabetes, with higher dosages providing more protection.

CRITICAL APPRAISAL

What was Known Prior to this Study?

Delirium can affect 20–30% of hospitalized older adults with diabetes, often serving as a precursor for dementia. Metformin's neuroprotective effects have been suggested by preclinical data [adenosine monophosphate-activated protein kinase (AMPK) activation, anti-inflammation, and gut microbiome modulation], and observational studies have showed cognitive benefits. Prior cohorts linked metformin to lower dementia incidence [hazard ratio (HR) 0.7–0.9] but lacked delirium-specific endpoints. Dipeptidyl peptidase-4 (DPP-4) inhibitors and sulfonylureas showed neutral or adverse neuropsychiatric profiles in diabetes.

What this Study Adds?

Metformin use can reduce the risk of delirium [adjusted subdistribution HR (sdHR) 0.77, 95% confidence interval (CI) 0.74–0.81], with dose-response, i.e., high cumulative dose (>360 DDD/year) sdHR 0.71 and daily dose ≥1 g having sdHR 0.74. The benefits emerged within 1 year and persisted long-term and were consistent across sub-groups including age ≥80 years and comorbidities. Competing mortality risk was lower (sdHR 0.85) supporting causality. This trial provided first evidence of metformin as delirium prophylactic in community-dwelling elderly diabetics.

Strengths

Propensity score matching (1:1, 66,568 pairs) enabled balancing 30+ confounders (demographics, comorbidities, medications, and frailty). Competing risk analysis (Fine-Gray model) accurately estimated delirium hazards accounting for death. Large sample powered dose-response and subgroups (n > 133,000) while 20-year span captured long-term effects (median 4.2 years). Taiwan database offered universal coverage with validated delirium codes [International Classification of Diseases (ICD)-9/10].

Limitations

Observational design has the risk of residual confounding (lifestyle and cognition proxies) factors. There was no data on delirium severity or subtype. Taiwan population base study limits its generalizability to multiethnic groups. No neuroimaging or biomarkers for underlying neurodegeneration were studied.

Clinical Implications

Metformin reduces delirium risk in older diabetics, favoring its continuation at high-dose in suitable patients and supporting its first-line status despite age-related concerns. The dose-response guides titration for neuroprotection.

Knowledge Gaps and Scope for Future Research

Mechanistic randomized controlled trials (RCTs) (neuroimaging and biomarkers) are needed as also head-to-head versus GLP-1 RAs/SGLT-2i. Delirium subtypes (hypoactive/hyperactive) were unexamined. Multiethnic/global cohorts are underrepresented. Importantly, long-term dementia conversion postdelirium is yet unclear.

25. Efruxifermin in Compensated Liver Cirrhosis Caused by MASH

Ref: Noureddin M, Rinella ME, Chalasani NP, Neff GW, Lucas KJ, Rodriguez ME, et al. Efruxifermin in compensated liver cirrhosis caused by MASH. N Engl J Med. 2025;392(24):2413-24.

ABSTRACT

Background: Efruxifermin, a bivalent fibroblast growth factor-21 (FGF21) analog, decreased fibrosis and cured metabolic dysfunction-associated steatohepatitis (MASH) in phase-2 trials including patients with stage 2 or 3 fibrosis. Information is required about the safety and effectiveness of efruxifermin in patients with MASH-induced compensated cirrhosis (stage-4 fibrosis).

Techniques: Patients with MASH who had biopsy-confirmed compensated cirrhosis (stage-4 fibrosis) were randomly assigned to receive subcutaneous efruxifermin (at a dose of 28 mg or 50 mg once weekly) or a placebo in this phase 2b, randomized, placebo-controlled, double-blind trial. At week 36, the main result was a decrease in at least one stage of fibrosis without a worsening of MASH. At week 96, secondary outcomes included the same criterion.

Outcomes: 181 patients in all were randomly assigned to receive either a placebo or efruxifermin at least once. A liver biopsy was done on 154 of these patients at 36 weeks and 134 of these patients at 96 weeks. At 36 weeks, a reduction in fibrosis without worsening of MASH occurred in 8 out of 61 patients (13%) in the placebo group, 10 out of 57 patients (18%) in the 28-mg efruxifermin group [difference from placebo, 3 percentage points; 95% confidence interval (CI) –11 to 17; $p = 0.62$], and 12 out of 63 patients (19%) in the 50-mg efruxifermin group (difference from placebo, 4 percentage points; 95% CI –10 to 18; $p = 0.52$). At week 96, a reduction in fibrosis without worsening of MASH occurred in 7 out of 61 patients (11%) in the placebo group, 12 out of 57 patients (21%) in the 28-mg efruxifermin group (difference from placebo, 10 percentage points; 95% CI –4 to 24), and 18 out of 63 patients (29%) in the 50-mg efruxifermin group (difference from placebo, 16 percentage points; 95% CI 2–30). Efruxifermin increased the frequency of gastrointestinal adverse effects, the majority of which were mild or severe.

Conclusion: Efruxifermin did not significantly lessen fibrosis at 36 weeks in patients with compensated cirrhosis brought on by MASH. (Funded by Akero Therapeutics; SYMMETRY ClinicalTrials.gov number, NCT05039450.)

CRITICAL APPRAISAL

What is Known Prior to this Study?

There was no approved pharmacotherapy for metabolic dysfunction-associated steatohepatitis (MASH) cirrhosis reversal prior to this trial; and management relied on lifestyle management. fibroblast growth factor-21 (FGF21) analogs have showed preclinical antifibrotic effects via metabolic regulation, lipid reduction, and stellate cell inhibition, but human data were limited to phase 2a in noncirrhotic MASH (HARMONY trial ~40% MASH resolution). Resmetirom (thyroid agonist) has gained approval for noncirrhotic MASH but not in cirrhosis due to safety concerns. Biopsy-proven cirrhosis carries 10–20% decompensation risk over 5 years. Prior trials in cirrhosis failed primary fibrosis endpoints. Glucagon-like peptide-1 receptor agonists (GLP-1 RAs) improved early MASH but lacked cirrhosis data. Dual endpoints (≥1-stage fibrosis improvement without MASH worsening) have become standard post Food and Drugs Administration (FDA) guidance.

What this Study Adds?

At 96 weeks, 50 mg efruxifermin achieved 29% fibrosis reduction without MASH worsening (ITT: completers 39% vs. 15% placebo; difference 16–24%; p = 0.009–0.031). MASH resolution reached 24–30% (50 mg) versus 11% placebo at 96 weeks. Noninvasive improvements included enhanced liver fibrosis (ELF) score reduction in -0.5, Pro-C3 reductions, and liver stiffness stabilization. Metabolic benefits encompassed low-density lipoprotein cholesterol (LDL-C) lowering (15–20%), triglycerides (20%), and glycated hemoglobin (HbA1c) stabilization. Cirrhosis reversal (F4–F3) was seen in 39% (completers, 50 mg) versus 15% placebo. Response was consistent across subgroups by diabetes status and body mass index (BMI) category. Gastrointestinal (GI) adverse effects (AEs) were mostly mild (50–60%), with low discontinuations (10–15%). It provided the first evidence of histologic cirrhosis regression in a MASH trial.

Strengths

Randomized, double-blind design across 40+ United States (US)/European sites involving 181 F4 patients powered hierarchical endpoints (fibrosis at 36/96 weeks and MASH resolution). Serial biopsies (baseline, 36, and 96 weeks) were done by expert pathologists minimizing assessment bias, and high biopsy compliance (73% at 96 weeks) was seen. Comprehensive noninvasive correlates (ELF, Fib-4, and vibration-controlled elastography) validated histologic findings. Metabolic/lipid-related secondary endpoints were analyzed. The trial results were mentioned in a dedicated editorial in the journal.

Limitations

Primary endpoints were not noted at 36 weeks, raising concerns regarding early efficacy. There was as high as 25% dropout rate. There was no active comparator like resmetirom. Short-term clinical outcomes (decompensation and mortality) were not analyzed.

Clinical Implications

Efruxifermin might be a potential disease-modifying therapy for MASH cirrhosis, targeting fibrosis regression over 96 weeks of use but needs further studies.

Knowledge Gaps

The results of its phase-3 clinical outcomes (SYNCHRONY outcomes) are pending. There is a need for head-to-head versus resmetirom or GLP-1 RAs. Long-term safety beyond >2 years is needed and the dose optimization is unclear, as also safety and efficacy in decompensated cirrhosis.

26. Weekly Insulins and Therapeutic Burden in Type 2 Diabetes

Ref: Ingelfinger JR, Rosen CJ. Weekly insulins and therapeutic burden in type 2 diabetes. N Engl J Med. 2025;393(4):401-2.

ABSTRACT

When to add or switch to daily insulin therapy is one of the more challenging choices for patients with poorly controlled type 2 diabetes, as well as for their doctors. Glycated hemoglobin levels can be effectively lowered by starting longer-acting insulins, such as glargine or degludec, before bedtime. However, daily dosing also necessitates a significant change in lifestyle for many patients. An alternative regimen for the treatment of type 2 diabetes has been made available by the recent licensing of novel glucagon-like peptide-1 (GLP-1) receptor agonists administered weekly; however, the expense of these medications may limit their use. One strategy that is receiving increased attention is the creation of novel, longer-acting insulin analogs. Insulin therapy is currently administered to 7–15% of people with type 2 diabetes, though this percentage is probably going to rise. Since 2024, patients with blood glucose levels of 300 mg/dL or higher (≥16.7 mmol/L), glycated hemoglobin levels greater than 10%, symptoms of hyperglycemia, evidence of generalized catabolism, or those who have received three or more oral noninsulin glucose lowering therapies have been advised to start insulin therapy. However, glycated hemoglobin levels of 8.5% or higher (or >7% in patients with complications) at diagnosis, the emergence of intolerable side effects from different hypoglycemic medications, and the existence of coexisting conditions would be additional indications for a switch to insulin in this new era of stricter glycemic control.

CRITICAL APPRAISAL

What was Known Prior to this Editorial?

Daily basal insulins such as glargine and degludec can achieve glycemic control in type-2 diabetes mellitus (T2DM) but daily pricks can contribute to nonadherence in 20–50% of patients. Phase-2 trials of once-weekly insulins (e.g., insulin icodec and insulin Fc) have shown noninferior glycated hemoglobin (HbA1c) reductions (–1.3 to –1.6%) compared to daily analog insulins, with more stable control of fasting glucose. Hypoglycemia rates were comparable for severe events, though level 1 (asymptomatic) hypoglycemia increased slightly. Patient-reported outcomes indicated preference for weekly dosing.

What this Editorial Adds?

This editorial synthesizes phase-3 data from ONWARDS trial, confirming the superiority of icodec in HbA1c reduction (–0.29% vs. glargine U100) and improvement in time-in-range for insulin-naïve T2DM patients. It emphasizes reduced treatment burden: 52 versus 365 injections/year and enhancement of the quality-of-life scores by 10–15 points. The expert author balances benefits against the increased risk for mild hypoglycemia and highlights the need for clinician education on dose adjustments.

Strengths

The author has wonderfully integrated trial data with practical insights on implementation, including patient-centered outcomes such as adherence and burden reduction. There is highlight on the real-world relevance for T2DM escalation, where 25% require basal insulin and is very relevant amid icodec insulin's 2024 approvals, influencing American Diabetes Association (ADA)/European Association for the Study of Diabetes (EASD) guidelines on the choice of basal insulin.

Limitations

Being an editorial, it was not possible to discuss all limitations including subgroup analyses such as in chronic kidney disease (CKD) patients, where icodec showed increased hypoglycemia and lacks cost-effectiveness discussion and issues about global access. The long-term data (>2 years) for immunogenicity or durability remain unexplored. Further studies focusing on type-1 diabetes are required.

Scope for Future Research

Head-to-head trials of icodec insulin and other long-acting basal insulins such as Fc-pegged insulins are required as also long-term randomized clinical trials (RCTs) (>5 years) and combination studies with glucagon-like peptide-1 receptor agonists (GLP-1 RAs) to minimize total injections further.

27. Finerenone and New-onset Diabetes in Heart Failure: A Prespecified Analysis of the FINEARTS-HF Trial

Ref: Butt JH, Jhund PS, Henderson AD, Claggett BL, Desai AS, Viswanathan P, et al; FINEARTS-HF Committees and Investigators. Finerenone and new-onset diabetes in heart failure: a prespecified analysis of the FINEARTS-HF trial. Lancet Diabetes Endocrinol. 2025;13(2):107-18.

ABSTRACT

Background: There is conflicting information regarding how mineralocorticoid receptor antagonist medication affects new-onset diabetes and glycated hemoglobin (HbA1c) levels. In the Finerenone experiment to Investigate Efficacy and Safety Superior to Placebo in Patients with Heart Failure (FINEARTS-HF), we sought to determine the impact of oral finerenone versus placebo on incident diabetes.

Techniques: 6,001 participants with heart failure who had New York Heart Association functional class II–IV, left ventricular ejection fraction 40% or higher, evidence of structural heart disease, and elevated N-terminal pro-B-type natriuretic peptide levels were randomly assigned to receive finerenone or a placebo orally in this double-blind, randomized, placebo-controlled study. Concealed allocation was used for randomization. The composite of cardiovascular death and total (first and recurring) heart failure events (such as hospitalization or urgent heart failure visit) was the trial's main endpoint. Participants having diabetes at baseline (investigator-reported history of diabetes or baseline HbA1c ≥6.5%) were not included in this study. A HbA1c reading of 6.5% or above on two consecutive follow-up visits or the start of new glucose-lowering medication were considered indicators of new-onset diabetes. Regardless of the therapy received (i.e., intention to treat), the full-analysis set included all participants who were randomly assigned to study treatment and analyzed based on their treatment assignment. Participants who took at least one dosage of the investigational product and were randomly allocated to study therapy made up the safety analysis set, which was analyzed based on the actual treatment received. This study is no longer accepting new participants and is registered with ClinicalTrials.gov with the number NCT04435626.

Results: 6,001 participants were recruited between September 14, 2020, and January 10, 2023, and they were randomized to receive either finerenone or a placebo. The study population consisted of 3,222 (53.7%) individuals who did not have diabetes at baseline. 115 (7.2%) individuals in the finerenone group and 147 (9.1%) in the placebo group experienced new-onset diabetes during a median follow-up period of 31.3 months (IQR 21.5–36.3). This translates to a rate of 3.0 events per 100 person-years [95% confidence interval (CI) 2.5–3.6] in the finerenone group and 3.9 events per 100 person-years (3.3–4.6) in the placebo group. Finerenone significantly decreased the risk of new-onset diabetes by 24% when compared to placebo [hazard ratio (HR) 0.76 (95% CI 0.59–0.97), $p = 0.026$]. When the competing risk of mortality was taken into consideration, Fine–Gray competing risk analysis produced a similar result [subdistribution HR 0.75 (0.59–0.96), $p = 0.024$]. Sensitivity analyses yielded similar results when the definition of new-onset diabetes was limited to HbA1c measurements only, restricted to new initiation of glucose-lowering medications only [excluding sodium-glucose cotransporter-2 (SGLT-2)] inhibitor treatment), and expanded to include initiation of SGLT-2 inhibitor treatment with diabetes as indication. When individuals who had received glucose-lowering medication at baseline were eliminated ($n = 15$), the results remained the same. Across important participant subgroups, finerenone had a consistent effect on new-onset diabetes when compared to placebo. Seven patients experienced a novel diabetes adverse event that did not fall under any of the aforementioned categories.

Interpretation: Oral finerenone decreased the risk of new-onset diabetes in heart failure patients with modestly reduced or retained ejection fraction who did not have diabetes. This represents a significant additional clinical advantage of this medication in these patients.

CRITICAL APPRAISAL

What was Known Before this Study?

Steroidal mineralocorticoid receptor antagonist (MRA) spironolactone has consistently been associated with elevations in glycated hemoglobin (HbA1c) in individuals with and without diabetes. In the EMPHASIS-HF trial, the steroidal MRA eplerenone did not reduce the risk of incident diabetes among patients with heart failure and reduced ejection fraction. Nonsteroidal MRA finerenone led to a reduction in kidney and cardiovascular events, including hospitalizations for heart failure in two large RCTs. FINEARTS-HF trial enrolled participants with heart failure with mildly reduced or preserved ejection, with and without diabetes. Finerenone reduced the hazard of the primary composite outcome of total (first and recurrent) worsening heart failure events and cardiovascular death, and improved health-related quality of life.

What this Study Adds?

Nonsteroidal MRA finerenone reduced the hazard of new-onset diabetes by 24% among patients with heart failure with mildly reduced or preserved ejection fraction.

Results were similar in sensitivity analyses, in which the definition of new-onset diabetes was expanded to include initiation of sodium-glucose cotransporter-2 (SGLT-2) inhibitor treatment with diabetes as indication, restricted to HbA1c measurements only.

Major Strengths

- Large, randomized, double-blind, placebo-controlled trial with robust methodology
- Prespecified analysis, reducing the risk of bias
- Long median follow-up (~31 months), allowing adequate assessment of incident diabetes
- Adds clinically relevant insight into cardiometabolic prevention in heart failure

Limitations

Participants enrolled in clinical trials are selected according to specific inclusion and exclusion criteria, and the results might not be generalizable to all individuals with heart failure. Specially, the proportion of non-White participants recruited was not globally representative.

The study did not have measurements of plasma insulin or glucometabolic investigations.

The confidence interval (CI) of the point estimates in these analyses were wide, and the associations should therefore be interpreted with caution.

Clinical Implications

In participants with heart failure with mildly reduced or preserved ejection fraction, without diabetes, finerenone reduced the hazard of new-onset diabetes, representing an additional clinical benefit of this treatment.

Scope for Future Research

- Dedicated trials assessing finerenone for diabetes prevention in high-risk populations without heart failure
- Comparative studies with SGLT-2 inhibitors and GLP-1 receptor agonists
- Mechanistic studies exploring insulin sensitivity, β-cell function, inflammation, and aldosterone-mediated pathways
- Long-term studies assessing whether diabetes prevention translates into outcome benefits (mortality and renal failure)

Section 5: DRUGS AND THERAPEUTICS (PART 2)

Section Editor: Pritam Biswas

1. Phase 3 Trial of Semaglutide in Metabolic Dysfunction-associated Steatohepatitis

Ref: Sanyal AJ, Newsome PN, Kliers I, Østergaard LH, Long MT, Kjær MS, et al. Phase 3 Trial of Semaglutide in Metabolic Dysfunction-Associated Steatohepatitis. N Engl J Med 2025;392:2089-99.

ABSTRACT

Background: One potential treatment for metabolic dysfunction-associated steatohepatitis (MASH) is semaglutide, an agonist of the glucagon-like peptide-1 receptor.

Techniques: We randomly assigned 1,197 patients with biopsy-defined MASH and fibrosis stage 2 or 3 in a 2:1 ratio to receive once-weekly subcutaneous semaglutide at a dose of 2.4 mg or placebo for 240 weeks in this ongoing phase 3, multicenter, randomized, double-blind, placebo-controlled trial. Here (part 1) are the findings of a scheduled interim study including the first 800 patients that was carried out at week 72. The cure of steatohepatitis without worsening hepatic fibrosis and a decrease in liver fibrosis without worsening steatohepatitis were the main goals of part 1.

Results: In 62.9% of the 534 patients in the semaglutide group and 34.3% of the 266 patients in the placebo group, steatohepatitis resolved without the fibrosis getting worse [estimated difference, 28.7 percentage points; 95% confidence interval (CI) 21.1 to 36.2; $p < 0.001$]. 36.8% of patients in the semaglutide group and 22.4% of patients in the placebo group reported a decrease in liver fibrosis without a worsening of steatohepatitis (estimated difference, 14.4 percentage points; 95% CI 7.5–21.3; $p < 0.001$). The following were the findings for the three secondary outcomes that were part of the multiple testing adjustment plan: 32.7% of patients in the semaglutide group and 16.1% of patients in the placebo group experienced both steatohepatitis resolution and a decrease in liver fibrosis (estimated difference, 16.5 percentage points; 95% CI 10.2–22.8; $p < 0.001$). Semaglutide caused a mean change in body weight of −10.5%, while a placebo caused a mean change of −2.0% (estimated difference, −8.5 percentage points; 95% CI −9.6 to −7.4; $p < 0.001$). There was no discernible difference between the two groups' mean changes in body pain scores. The semaglutide group experienced higher gastrointestinal side effects.

Conclusion: Semaglutide at a dose of 2.4 mg once weekly improved liver histology outcomes in patients with MASH with moderate or severe liver fibrosis (Supported by Novo Nordisk; NCT04822181 on ClinicalTrials.gov.).

CRITICAL APPRAISAL

What was Known Prior to this Study?

Noncirrhotic MASH with stage 2–3 fibrosis is strongly associated with progression to cirrhosis and increased liver-related and all-cause mortality, yet until recently no drug had full regulatory approval; resmetirom holds accelerated FDA approval with confirmatory outcome data pending. Phase 2 data with daily semaglutide up to 0.4 mg showed high rates of steatohepatitis resolution but a nonsignificant effect on fibrosis regression, and GLP-1 receptor agonists were already established for weight loss and cardiometabolic risk reduction in obesity and type 2 diabetes.[1-4]

What this Study Adds?

This phase 3 interim analysis demonstrates that a higher-dose, once-weekly semaglutide regimen (2.4 mg) in a larger, global cohort with stage 2–3 fibrosis achieves significant improvements in both steatohepatitis resolution and fibrosis regression versus placebo over 72 weeks. The study also shows concordant improvements in noninvasive fibrosis markers (ELF, liver stiffness, FAST, PRO-C3, transaminases) and cardiometabolic risk factors, suggesting a broad disease-modifying effect in a population enriched for diabetes, obesity, and high cardiovascular risk.

Strengths

Robust design and conduct; Rigorous histologic assessment; Clinically relevant endpoints; Comprehensive phenotyping.

Limitations

- *Interim, histology-focused analysis:* This report covers only part 1 (72-week histologic outcomes) and not the full 240-week clinical outcome data.
- The trial underrepresents Black patients and lean metabolic dysfunction-associated steatotic liver disease (MASLD), and excludes other chronic liver diseases.
- Confounding by weight loss and cointerventions.
- *Short-term and safety nuances:* The 72-week time frame may be insufficient to fully assess rare or long-latency adverse events.

Clinical Implications

In adults with biopsy-proven MASH and stage 2–3 fibrosis, semaglutide 2.4 mg once weekly appears to be a promising disease-modifying option that can achieve regulatory-relevant histologic endpoints while concurrently treating obesity and type 2 diabetes, making it attractive as a single agent addressing multiple cardiometabolic axes. If part-2 outcome data confirm reductions in cirrhosis-related events and maintain acceptable safety, semaglutide could be integrated alongside or in sequence with agents like resmetirom within guideline-directed MASLD pathways, particularly in patients with obesity/diabetes and high cardiovascular risk.

The trial also reinforces the importance of early identification of stage 2–3 disease using noninvasive tests and referral for disease-modifying therapies before cirrhosis develops.

Knowledge Gap and Scope for Future Research

Key unanswered questions include whether semaglutide-induced histologic improvements translate into durable reductions in cirrhosis, decompensation, hepatocellular carcinoma, and mortality over many years, which will be addressed only once the full 240-week ESSENCE data are available. Further work is needed to clarify differential efficacy across racial/ethnic groups, lean versus obese MASLD, and varying genetic risk profiles, as well as to understand the relative contributions of weight loss versus direct hepatic effects, and to explore combination or sequencing strategies with agents targeting other pathways [e.g., Thyroid hormone receptor-β (THR-β) agonists, farnesoid X receptor (FXR) agonists].

2. Tirzepatide as Compared with Semaglutide for the Treatment of Obesity

Ref: Aronne LJ, Horn DB, le Roux CW, Ho W, Falcon BL, Gomez Valderas E, et al.; SURMOUNT-5 Trial Investigators. Tirzepatide as Compared with Semaglutide for the Treatment of Obesity. N Engl J Med. 2025;393(1):26-36.

ABSTRACT

Background: Two very successful drugs for managing obesity are semaglutide and tirzepatide. It is unknown whether tirzepatide is safer and more effective than semaglutide in adults who are obese but do not have type 2 diabetes.

Techniques: Adult participants who were obese but did not have type 2 diabetes were randomly assigned in a 1:1 ratio to receive either the maximum tolerated dose of tirzepatide (10 mg or 15 mg) or the maximum tolerated dose of semaglutide (1.7 mg or 2.4 mg) subcutaneously once weekly for 72 weeks in this phase 3b, open-label, controlled trial. The percentage change in weight from baseline to week 72 was the main outcome measure. A change in waist circumference from baseline to week 72 and weight reductions of at least 10%, 15%, 20%, and 25% were important secondary end goals.

Results: Randomization was performed on 751 participants. At week 72, the least-squares mean percent change in weight was −20.2% (95% CI −21.4 to −19.1) for tirzepatide and −13.7% (95% CI −14.9 to −12.6) for semaglutide ($p < 0.001$). With tirzepatide, the least-squares mean change in waist circumference was −18.4 cm (95% CI −19.6 to −17.2), while with semaglutide, it was −13.0 cm (95% CI −14.3 to −11.7) ($p < 0.001$). Weight reductions of at least 10%, 15%, 20%, and 25% were more common in the tirzepatide group than in the semaglutide group. Gastrointestinal adverse effects were the most frequent in both treatment groups; they were mostly mild-to-moderate in severity and mostly happened during dose escalation.

Conclusion: When it came to the reduction of body weight and waist circumference at week 72, tirzepatide treatment outperformed semaglutide treatment in individuals with obesity but no diabetes (Eli Lilly provided funding; SURMOUNT-5 ClinicalTrials.gov number, NCT05822830).

CRITICAL APPRAISAL

Knowledge Prior to this Study

Glucagon-like peptide-1 (GLP-1) agonists like semaglutide (STEP trials) achieved 15–17% weight loss at 68–104 weeks in obesity without diabetes, with sustained effects but plateaus. Tirzepatide (SURMOUNT-1) showed up to 21% loss via dual glucose-dependent insulinotropic polypeptide (GIP)/GLP-1 action, outperforming semaglutide indirectly in type 2 diabetes (T2D) (SURPASS-2) and real-world data (4–5% more loss). Head-to-head data were lacking in nondiabetics.[5-8]

What this Study Adds?

This first direct randomized controlled trial (RCT) confirms tirzepatide superiority (6.5% more weight loss, 5.4 cm waist reduction) in nondiabetics using maximum tolerated doses, with 2× likelihood of ≥ 25% loss and dose-escalation mitigation. It links higher losses to cardiometabolic gains [e.g., systolic blood pressure (SBP) drop 10.2 vs. 7.7 mm Hg].

Strengths

Multicenter design (32 sites); diverse participants (24% Hispanic, 19% Black); robust study power; multiplicity-controlled analyses, and real-world-relevant flexible dosing enhance generalizability.

Limitations

Open-label risks performance or expectation bias, though aligns with blinded priors; male underrepresentation (35%) and U.S./Puerto Rico sites limit broader applicability. Short-term (72 weeks) safety; no long-term cardiovascular (CV) outcomes or quality-of-life primacy.

Clinical Implications

Tirzepatide offers greater weight/waist loss for obesity management, potentially improving prediabetes/hypertension (HTN) remission thresholds (>15–20% loss). Favor for patients needing aggressive targets, but semaglutide viable if tolerability prioritized; shared decision-making key given gastrointestinal (GI) risks.

Knowledge Gap and Scope for Future Research

Long-term durability, especially of post-72 weeks data; detailed CV event reduction data (awaiting SURMOUNT-MMO trial results); head-to-head trial designs.

3. Relationship between Metabolic and Histological Responses in People with Metabolic Dysfunction Associated Steatohepatitis with and without Type 2 Diabetes: Participant-level Exploratory Analysis of the SYNERGY-NASH Trial with Tirzepatide

Ref: Caussy C, Cusi K, Rosenstock J, Bugianesi E, Thomas MK, Tang Y, et al. Relationship Between Metabolic and Histological Responses in People With Metabolic Dysfunction Associated Steatohepatitis With and Without Type 2 Diabetes: Participant-Level Exploratory Analysis of the SYNERGY-NASH Trial With Tirzepatide. Diabetes Care 2025;48:2074-83.

ABSTRACT

Objective: To investigate the connection between histological and metabolic reactions in a tirzepatide phase 2 trial for metabolic dysfunction-associated steatohepatitis (MASH).

Methods and research design: The 52-week, double-blind, randomized, placebo-controlled SYNERGY-NASH experiment (NCT04166773) is the subject of this participant-level post hoc analysis. Tirzepatide (5, 10, or 15 mg) or a placebo were given once weekly to participants (*n* = 190) with MASH and stage 2/3 fibrosis at random. The main goal was to resolve MASH without making fibrosis worse. Fibrosis improvement of at least one stage without MASH worsening was one of the secondary end objectives. 154 patients who finished the therapy study had their metabolic alterations assessed for histological end goals in both responders and nonresponders.

Results: The mean body mass index (BMI) was 35.7 kg/m^2 at baseline, and 59% of people had type 2 diabetes. Respondents showed higher body weight reductions for fibrosis improvement (–13.6% vs. –9.8%; $p = 0.023$) and MASH resolution (–16.0% vs. –7.0%; $p < 0.001$) than nonresponders. HbA1c decreased more for fibrosis responders (–1.2% vs. –0.7%; $p = 0.004$) and MASH responders (–1.2% vs. –0.6%; $p < 0.001$) than for nonresponders. MASH responders showed higher improvements in liver fat and markers of adipose tissue insulin sensitivity (adiponectin and the adipose tissue insulin resistance index) than nonresponders ($p < 0.001$). Normalization of liver fat was a major mediator of both fibrosis improvement and MASH resolution in causal mediation analyses.

Conclusion: MASH resolution and fibrosis improvement were linked to improved glycemic control, normalization of liver fat, and body weight decrease in this post hoc exploratory research. Treatment with tirzepatide may have helped MASH patients lose weight and improve their metabolism.

CRITICAL APPRAISAL

What was Known Prior to this Study?

Prior to this investigation, several key findings had been established in the MASH treatment landscape. Body weight reduction of at least 10% through lifestyle modification or bariatric surgery was known to be associated with MASH resolution and regression of liver fibrosis. Incretin-based therapies, particularly glucagon-like peptide-1 (GLP-1) receptor agonists like semaglutide, had demonstrated beneficial effects in achieving MASH resolution and fibrosis improvement compared with placebo. The primary SYNERGY-NASH trial had already shown that tirzepatide, a dual glucose-dependent insulinotropic polypeptide (GIP)/GLP-1 receptor agonist, resolved MASH in up to 62% and improved fibrosis in up to 55% of participants. However, the specific mechanistic relationships between metabolic improvements and histological outcomes remained incompletely understood.[9-11]

What this Study Adds?

This exploratory analysis provides novel insights into the mechanistic underpinnings of tirzepatide's efficacy in MASH. A key contribution is the identification through causal mediation analyses that normalization of liver fat [magnetic resonance-proton density fat fraction (MRI-PDFF) < 5%] is a significant mediator of both MASH resolution (68% mediated) and fibrosis improvement (66% mediated). The study reveals that 82.4% of patients achieving liver fat normalization also achieved MASH resolution compared to only 31.9% who did not normalize liver fat. Importantly, the analysis shows differential relationships between metabolic parameters and histological outcomes in patients with versus without type 2 diabetes, suggesting that metabolic dysfunction may be a larger contributor to hepatic fibrosis in individuals with diabetes. The finding that unmediated treatment effects of tirzepatide remained significant even after controlling for weight and metabolic improvements suggests additional mechanisms beyond simple weight loss may contribute to MASH resolution.

Strengths

It employed rigorous histological assessment with central pathologist review of liver biopsies using validated NASH Clinical Research Network scoring criteria; the analysis incorporated comprehensive metabolic assessments; Inclusion of participant-level data allows for detailed examination of individual response patterns through waterfall plots and density curves. The study also benefits from the high quality of the parent SYNERGY-NASH trial, which was a well-designed, multicenter, double-blind, randomized controlled trial.

Limitations

The authors appropriately acknowledge several important limitations. As a post hoc exploratory analysis, the findings are hypothesis-generating rather than confirmatory, and no adjustments were made for multiple comparisons, increasing the risk of Type I error. The relatively small sample size (n = 154 completers) may have limited statistical power, particularly for mediation analyses and subgroup comparisons. The per-protocol analysis approach, including only participants who completed the study with both baseline and postbaseline measures, introduces potential selection bias and limits generalizability. The 52-week duration is insufficient to fully assess effects on fibrosis regression and major adverse liver outcomes such as cirrhosis, hepatic decompensation, or hepatocellular carcinoma. The study pooled all tirzepatide doses (5, 10, 15 mg) with placebo for responder analyses, which may obscure dose-response relationships. Baseline differences between responders and nonresponders for fibrosis improvement—particularly higher baseline fibrosis stage and liver stiffness in nonresponders—suggest that disease severity may confound the relationship between metabolic improvements and histological outcomes. The presence of concomitant glucose-lowering and lipid-lowering medications may have influenced metabolic outcomes independently of tirzepatide.

Clinical Implications

The findings have several important clinical implications for MASH management. The strong association between body weight reduction and MASH resolution suggests that achieving substantial weight loss (> 15%) should be a primary therapeutic target in MASH patients. The observation that normalization of liver fat is a significant mediator of histological improvement supports the potential use of MRI-PDFF as a noninvasive biomarker for monitoring treatment response and predicting histological outcomes. For patients with MASH and type 2 diabetes, the findings emphasize the importance of intensive glycemic control, with data showing that achieving HbA1c < 5.7% (diabetes remission range) was associated with higher odds of MASH resolution. The improvements in adipose tissue insulin sensitivity markers (Adipo-IR, adiponectin) suggest that tirzepatide's dual GIP/GLP-1 receptor agonism may offer advantages over GLP-1-only agonists by targeting adipose tissue dysfunction. However, the observation that unmediated treatment effects persisted after controlling for weight and metabolic factors suggests that tirzepatide may have direct hepatic or anti-inflammatory effects beyond metabolic improvements. These findings support the potential use of tirzepatide as a disease-modifying therapy in MASH, particularly for patients with concurrent obesity and type 2 diabetes.

Knowledge Gap and Scope for Future Research

Future studies should investigate the mechanisms underlying the unmediated treatment effects of tirzepatide, including potential direct anti-inflammatory or antifibrotic effects on hepatocytes and hepatic stellate cells. Comparative effectiveness studies are needed to determine whether tirzepatide's dual GIP/GLP-1 agonism provides superior outcomes compared to GLP-1-only agonists or other emerging MASH therapies. Finally, investigations into predictors of treatment response could enable personalized medicine approaches to identify which patients are most likely to benefit from tirzepatide therapy.

4. Tirzepatide Associated with Reduced Albuminuria in Participants with Type 2 Diabetes: Pooled Post Hoc Analysis from the Randomized Active- and Placebo-controlled SURPASS-1–5 Clinical Trials

Ref: Apperloo EM, Tuttle KR, Pavo I, Haupt A, Taylor R, Wiese RJ, et al. Tirzepatide Associated With Reduced Albuminuria in Participants With Type 2 Diabetes: Pooled Post Hoc Analysis From the Randomized Active- and Placebo-Controlled SURPASS-1–5 Clinical Trials Diabetes Care. 2025;48:430-6.

ABSTRACT

Objective: In the SURPASS-4 trial, tirzepatide, a long-acting, glucose-dependent insulinotropic polypeptide/glucagon like peptide 1 receptor agonist, decreased the decline in the estimated glomerular filtration rate (eGFR) and urine albumin-to-creatinine ratio (UACR) in individuals with type 2 diabetes and high cardiovascular risk. We evaluated change from baseline in UACR for tirzepatide (5, 10, and 15 mg) compared with active and placebo treatment in a large sample from the SURPASS-1–5 trials in order to assess the generalizability of these findings.

Research design and methods: Data from the entire pooled SURPASS-1–5 population and subgroups identified by baseline UACR ≥ 30 mg/g were evaluated in this post hoc analysis. On-treatment data from baseline to the end-of-treatment visit were analyzed using a mixed model for repeated measures. The model incorporated the study identification as a covariate.

Outcomes: In comparison to all pooled comparators, the adjusted mean percent change from baseline in UACR for tirzepatide 5, 10, or 15 mg was −19.3% (95% CI −25.5, −12.5), −22.0% (−28.1, −15.3), and −26.3 (−32.0, −20.0), respectively. Pooled placebo, active, and insulin comparator studies showed comparable outcomes. In subgroups with UACR ≥ 30 mg/g, UACR decrease was more noticeable. According to the results of the mediation analysis, weight loss may be responsible for almost half of the albuminuria reduction linked to tirzepatide. At week 40/42, there was no difference in eGFR between pooled comparators and tirzepatide.

Conclusion: Tirzepatide was linked to a clinically significant lower UACR compared to comparators in individuals with type 2 diabetes, including those with chronic renal disease, in this post hoc study, indicating a possible kidney-protective effect.

CRITICAL APPRAISAL

What was Known Prior to this Study?

- Glucagon-like peptide-1 (GLP-1) receptor agonists, particularly semaglutide, had demonstrated nephroprotective effects (FLOW trial); sodium-glucose cotransporter-2 (SGLT-2) inhibitors and RAS blockers were established as first-line agents for kidney protection in diabetic kidney disease.
- Post hoc analysis from the single SURPASS-4 trial showed tirzepatide reduced albuminuria and eGFR decline versus insulin glargine in high cardiovascular risk patients.
- Changes in UACR of ≥ 25–30% have been validated as surrogate endpoints predictive of long-term kidney outcomes, with each 30% reduction associated with 19% lower hazard for kidney failure.
- The mechanisms of incretin-based kidney protection were incompletely understood, with mediation through glycemic control and weight loss partially explaining benefits.[12-14]

What this Study Adds?

This is the first comprehensive pooled analysis demonstrating consistent UACR reduction (exceeding 40% for all doses) with tirzepatide across a broad diabetes population (n = 5,299) in a dose-dependent fashion. 46% of UACR reduction is mediated through metabolic effects (primarily HbA1c reduction at 21.7%, with additional 15.6% via HbA1c changes from weight loss), while 54% appears to be direct kidney effects. Concurrent SGLT-2i or RAS inhibitor usages support potential combination therapeutic strategies.

Strengths

Large sample size and individual patient data; Comprehensive comparator groups; Prespecified subgroup analyses. Results replicated across multiple trial populations with different baseline characteristics and background therapies, enhancing external validity.

Limitations

Post hoc exploratory analysis; Single spot urine samples; Short follow-up duration; Lack of hard kidney outcomes (clinical endpoints like kidney failure, sustained eGFR decline ≥40%, or renal replacement therapy initiation). Open-label design; Exclusion criteria limited enrollment of patients with eGFR < 30–45 mL/min/1.73 m^2, reducing generalizability to advanced chronic kidney disease (CKD).

Clinical Implications

- *Potential nephroprotective agent*: Tirzepatide demonstrates clinically relevant albuminuria reduction comparable to established kidney-protective therapies, supporting its consideration in diabetic kidney disease management.

- *Triple therapy potential*: Consistent benefits observed with concurrent SGLT-2i and RAS inhibitor use suggest tirzepatide could be added to existing nephroprotective regimens for additive benefit.
- *Early intervention strategy:* Substantial benefits in patients with UACR ≥ 30 mg/g suggest potential for early intervention in microalbuminuria stage to prevent progression.

Knowledge Gaps and Scope for Future Research

- Dedicated kidney outcomes trial, like TREASURE-CKD, is essential.
- Long-term eGFR trajectory, Studies with ≥ 2–3 years follow-up.
- Advanced CKD populations, in patients with eGFR < 30–45 mL/min/1.73 m^2 to establish efficacy and safety across the full spectrum of kidney disease.
- Head-to-head trials and combination studies with SGLT-2 inhibitors.

5. Metabolic Improvements with Tirzepatide in Lipodystrophy: A Novel Option?

Ref: Meral R, Celik Guler M, Kaba D, Prativadi J, Frontera ED, Foss-Freitas MC, et al. Metabolic Improvements With Tirzepatide in Lipodystrophy: A Novel Option? Diabetes Care. 2025;48:756-62.

ABSTRACT

Objective: A collection of uncommon conditions linked to serious metabolic disease is called lipodystrophy. These conditions are characterized by aberrant fat distribution and near-total [generalized lipodystrophy (GL)] or partial [partial lipodystrophy (PL); such as familial partial lipodystrophy (FPLD)] lack of adipocyte bulk, which results in a reduced capacity to safely store lipids. The metabolic symptoms are more likely to result from the storage of excess lipids in nonadipose tissues. Glucagon-like peptide-1 (GLP-1) agonists have been linked to metabolic improvements in FPLD, as we recently shown. Here, we speculate that patients with lipodystrophy may benefit metabolically from tirzepatide, a dual incretin.

Research design and methods: In the framework of ongoing natural history investigations, an observational cohort of lipodystrophy patients who received tirzepatide clinically was monitored.

Outcomes: Tirzepatide was administered to 17 patients, 14 of whom had FPLD (n = 12 female and 2 male; ages 30–74 years). Following a median follow-up of 8.7 months, the following were considerably decreased: Triglycerides [median difference, -65 mg/dL (–0.73 mmol/L, range –3820 to 43 mg/dL [–43.2 to 0.49 mmol/L), $p = 0.003$), BMI (median difference –1.7; range –05.9 to 0.9 kg/m^2, $p = 0.008$) HbA1c (median difference, –1.1%; range, –6.3% to –0.1%; $p < 0.001$),. We also detail three more patients with less common types of lipodystrophy who also responded well to tirzepatide (atypical PL, n = 1; acquired GL, n = 2; all female; aged 35–64 years). Benign stomach discomfort were the only adverse effects.

Conclusion: Patients with lipodystrophy may benefit from tirzepatide.

CRITICAL APPRAISAL

What was Known Prior to this Study

Prior to this investigation, metreleptin (recombinant leptin) was established as the only Food and Drug Administration (FDA)-approved treatment for generalized lipodystrophy, demonstrating dramatic improvements in glycemic control, triglyceride levels, and hepatic steatosis in patients with severe leptin deficiency. Metreleptin showed variable and only modest effects in partial lipodystrophy. Emerging case reports and small series suggested that pure GLP-1 receptor agonists might provide metabolic benefits in familial partial lipodystrophy in a retrospective cohort of 14 patients. However, the efficacy of dual incretin agonism with tirzepatide, the most potent approved anti-obesity medication, remained unexplored in this patient population.[15-18]

What this Study Adds?

This study provides the first systematic evidence that tirzepatide demonstrates robust metabolic efficacy in lipodystrophy syndromes, particularly in familial partial lipodystrophy. The magnitude of HbA1c reduction with tirzepatide (–1.1%) exceeded that previously reported with pure GLP-1 agonists (–0.5%) and approached the efficacy seen with metreleptin in generalized lipodystrophy (–2.0%), despite substantial concurrent insulin reduction. The study extends preliminary observations by including patients with various lipodystrophy subtypes and demonstrates that metabolic improvements with tirzepatide may be independent of baseline body mass index (BMI). Additionally, the research suggesting the therapeutic benefit does not stem from hormone deficiency but rather from enhanced incretin pathway activation.

Strengths

The study's primary strength lies in addressing a rare disease with significant unmet medical need, capturing data from the largest cohort of lipodystrophy patients treated with tirzepatide to date. The collaborative approach between two major academic centers [University of Michigan and National Institutes of Health (NIH)] enhanced data collection from this ultra-rare population. The median follow-up duration of 8.7 months provides meaningful insight into intermediate-term efficacy and tolerability.

Limitations

The retrospective observational design without a randomized control group represents the most significant limitation, precluding definitive causal inferences and leaving open the possibility of Hawthorne effect or regression to the mean. Notably, quantitative dietary intake data were not collected. Body composition analysis via dual-energy X-ray absorptiometry (DEXA) scanning was not consistently performed, preventing determination of whether weight loss came from adipose tissue, ectopic lipid stores, or lean mass. The relatively short follow-up period (median 8.7 months) cannot address long-term tolerability, durability of metabolic benefits, or potential for adverse events that emerge with prolonged exposure. The small sample size limits statistical power and generalizability.

Clinical Implications

Tirzepatide emerges as a potentially valuable therapeutic option for patients with partial lipodystrophy who have limited treatment alternatives, particularly those who do not respond adequately to metreleptin or are not leptin-deficient. The substantial reduction in insulin requirements (median –109 units/day) while maintaining improved glycemic control suggests tirzepatide can reduce treatment burden and potentially improve quality of life. Clinicians should recognize that traditional BMI thresholds for obesity medication use do not apply to lipodystrophy patients, as metabolic health in this population may require achieving BMIs that would typically be considered underweight. Aggressive insulin down-titration protocols should be implemented when initiating tirzepatide to prevent hypoglycemia.

Knowledge Gap and Scope for Future Research

Randomized, placebo-controlled trials are urgently needed to definitively establish efficacy, optimal dosing strategies, and long-term safety profiles of tirzepatide in lipodystrophy syndromes. Future studies should incorporate comprehensive body composition assessments using DEXA or magnetic resonance imaging (MRI) to determine whether metabolic improvements correlate with changes in ectopic fat deposition (hepatic, visceral) versus subcutaneous fat or lean mass. Longer-term studies (≥2–3 years) are essential to assess durability of metabolic benefits, tolerance development, effects on hard clinical endpoints (cardiovascular events, liver cirrhosis progression, renal outcomes), and survival benefits. Investigation of tirzepatide in treatment-naïve patients with congenital generalized lipodystrophy who have not been exposed to metreleptin would help determine whether incretin agonism can substitute for or complement leptin replacement. Comparative effectiveness studies would inform treatment algorithms.

6. Tirzepatide Treatment and Associated Changes in β-cell Function and Insulin Sensitivity in People with Obesity or Overweight with Prediabetes or Normoglycemia: A Post Hoc Analysis from the SURMOUNT-1 Trial

Ref: Mari A, Stefanski A, van Raalte DH, Ma X, LaBell ES, Fan L, et al. Tirzepatide Treatment and Associated Changes in β-Cell Function and Insulin Sensitivity in People With Obesity or Overweight With Prediabetes or Normoglycemia: A Post Hoc Analysis From the SURMOUNT-1 Trial. Diabetes Care. 2025;48:1622-7.

ABSTRACT

Objective: We evaluated β-cell activity and insulin sensitivity in persons without diabetes who were overweight or obese and receiving tirzepatide for 72 weeks.

Methods and research design: This post hoc analysis examined tirzepatide versus placebo in 2,539 patients with body mass index (BMI) ≥ 27 kg/m^2 and either prediabetes or normoglycemia at baseline from the Study of Tirzepatide (LY3298176) in patients With Obesity or Overweight (SURMOUNT-1) study. Oral glucose tolerance tests were used to evaluate model-derived characteristics of insulin sensitivity and β-cell function.

Results: In individuals with prediabetes or normoglycemia, tirzepatide therapy was linked to improvements in insulin sensitivity and β-cell function parameters as well as a decrease in body weight at week 72. Increases in β-cell function were primarily linked to tirzepatide treatment, while increases in insulin sensitivity were primarily linked to weight loss and somewhat to tirzepatide treatment in multivariate regression models.

Conclusion: Treatment with tirzepatide was linked to increased β-cell activity and insulin sensitivity in persons with obesity/overweight who did not have type 2 diabetes, partially independently of weight loss.

CRITICAL APPRAISAL

What was Known Prior to this Study?

Tirzepatide, a dual glucose-dependent insulinotropic polypeptide (GIP) and glucagon-like peptide-1 (GLP-1) receptor agonist, had demonstrated substantial weight reduction effects (>20% at highest dose) in the SURMOUNT-1 trial for obesity management. Previous studies in patients with type 2 diabetes showed that tirzepatide improved β-cell function and insulin sensitivity compared to selective GLP-1 receptor agonists like dulaglutide. Preclinical evidence suggested that GIP receptor activation contributed to insulin sensitivity improvements independent of GLP-1 effects. However, comprehensive mechanistic data on β-cell function and insulin sensitivity changes in individuals with obesity or overweight without diabetes remained limited.[19-21]

What this Study Adds?

This analysis provides novel mechanistic insights by demonstrating that tirzepatide's benefits extend beyond weight loss in non-diabetic individuals with obesity. The study uniquely differentiates the contributions of weight reduction versus direct drug effects using multivariate regression models, revealing that β-cell function improvements (β-cell glucose sensitivity and basal insulin secretion) are predominantly drug-mediated rather than weight-dependent. Conversely, insulin sensitivity improvements were primarily weight-related but with a partial independent tirzepatide effect observed through oral glucose insulin sensitivity (OGIS) measurements. The findings were consistent across both prediabetes and normoglycemia subgroups, demonstrating broad applicability. Notably, participants with normoglycemia and normal baseline β-cell function still experienced significant improvements, suggesting potential preventive benefits even before metabolic dysfunction becomes apparent.

Strengths

- Large sample size (n = 2,539) from a well-conducted randomized controlled trial with 72-week duration providing adequate time to assess metabolic changes.
- *Sophisticated methodology:* Mari model, multiple insulin sensitivity indices (Matsuda index, OGIS).
- *Clinically relevant endpoints:* Assessment of parameters directly related to diabetes pathophysiology (β-cell function and insulin resistance) rather than just glycemic or weight outcomes.
- *Multiple dose evaluation:* Three tirzepatide doses (5, 10, 15 mg) allowed dose-response assessment.

Limitations

- The study was not prospectively designed to assess β-cell function and insulin sensitivity as primary endpoints, introducing potential bias in hypothesis testing.
- 70% White participants and small percentage meeting overweight criteria limits generalizability to diverse ethnic populations and true overweight category.
- *Lack of active comparator:* Absence of selective GLP-1 receptor agonist control group prevents direct assessment of GIP receptor contribution to observed benefits.
- *Confounding factors:* Lifestyle modifications were part of the intervention, making it difficult to isolate pure pharmacological effects.
- No long-term follow-up.

Clinical Implications

These findings support tirzepatide's role as a promising agent for diabetes prevention in high-risk populations with obesity or overweight. The demonstration of β-cell function preservation independent of weight loss suggests therapeutic benefits beyond traditional weight management approaches. Clinicians managing patients with prediabetes should consider that tirzepatide offers dual metabolic benefits—both reducing insulin resistance through weight loss and enhancing β-cell function through direct mechanisms. The consistent effects across normoglycemic individuals suggest potential for early intervention strategies before prediabetes develops. These results align with the recently published 3-year SURMOUNT-1 extension data showing marked reduction in progression to type 2 diabetes with tirzepatide treatment. For endocrinologists, this mechanistic understanding helps inform treatment selection and patient counseling regarding expected metabolic benefits beyond glycemic control and weight reduction.

Knowledge Gap and Scope for Future Research

Several important research questions remain unanswered:

- Comparative effectiveness studies.
- Long-term durability assessment.
- Ethnic and age-group (e.g., pediatrics) diversity evaluation.
- Genetic and biomarker predictors to check heterogeneity.

7. Gradual Titration of Semaglutide Results in Better Treatment Adherence and Fewer Adverse Events: A Randomized Controlled Open-label Pilot Study Examining a 16-week Flexible Titration Regimen versus Label-recommended 8-week Semaglutide Titration Regimen

Ref: Eldor R, Avraham N, Rosenberg O, Shpigelman M, Golan-Cohen A, Cukierman-Yaffe T, et al. Gradual Titration of Semaglutide Results in Better Treatment Adherence and Fewer Adverse Events: A Randomized Controlled Open-Label Pilot Study Examining a 16-Week Flexible Titration Regimen Versus Label-Recommended 8-Week Semaglutide Titration Regimen. Diabetes Care. 2025;48:1607-11.

ABSTRACT

Objective: To ascertain if, in patients with type 2 diabetes (T2D), a slower, more flexible semaglutide titration regimen would improve adherence and lower gastrointestinal adverse events (GI-AEs) in comparison to the label-recommended regimen.

Methods and research design: For 26 weeks, 104 T2D patients were randomized to either flexible titration [beginning at 0.0675 mg (measured by five clicks made by the dose selector dial), with gradual increases by 0.0675 mg/week and delays for GI-AEs] or label-recommended titration (0.25 mg, 0.5 mg, and 1 mg at 4-week intervals).

Results: Only 2% of patients in the flexible arm withdrew because of GI-AEs compared to 19% in the label arm, despite the fact that final doses were comparable between the groups ($p = 0.005$). The flexible arm reported lower rates of asthenia (9.8% vs. 24.5%; $p = 0.047$) and nausea (45.1% vs. 64.2%; $p = 0.051$), as well as fewer days with nausea (2.88 vs. 6.3 days; $p = 0.017$). Changes in body mass index (BMI) and HbA1c were comparable across groups.

Conclusion: Without sacrificing effectiveness, slower, more flexible titration increased adherence and decreased side effects.

CRITICAL APPRAISAL

What was Known Prior to this Study?

Semaglutide is a highly effective glucagon-like peptide-1 (GLP-1) receptor agonist for glycemic control and weight reduction in type 2 diabetes, but gastrointestinal adverse events during dose escalation represent a major barrier to treatment persistence. Real-world data showed discontinuation rates of 10–20% due to gastrointestinal (GI) side effects in diabetic populations, with overall adherence rates as low as 42.7% at 6 months for semaglutide. Evidence from insulin/GLP-1 fixed-ratio combination studies suggested that GI-AEs might stem from titration speed rather than the final dose achieved, with slower titration strategies associated with improved tolerability. Gastrointestinal adverse events were known to be dose-dependent and typically decline over time, with most events occurring within the first week or month of treatment.[22-24]

What this Study Adds?

This is the first randomized controlled trial specifically testing a gradual, patient-driven flexible titration protocol for semaglutide using the injection pen's click-counting system for precise micro-dosing. The study demonstrates that extending titration from 8 weeks to approximately 16 weeks with symptom-guided dose adjustments reduced treatment discontinuation nearly 10-fold (2% vs. 19%) while maintaining equivalent therapeutic efficacy. Importantly, the study showed that 6 of 10 patients who initially discontinued under standard titration successfully restarted and continued with the flexible approach, providing evidence for rescue strategies in patients who fail initial titration. The finding that mean days with nausea were reduced by more than half (2.88 vs. 6.3 days) demonstrates clinically meaningful symptom burden reduction.

Strengths

The study employed a pragmatic design using readily available technology (pen click-counting) that can be easily implemented in routine clinical practice without additional costs or specialized equipment. Randomization ensured a balanced approach.

Limitations

The open-label design represents a significant methodological limitation. The sample size was relatively small for a pilot study, and power calculations were based on assumptions rather than prior data. The COVID-19 pandemic necessitated mostly telephone-based biweekly follow-up rather than in-person visits. Participants were from two centers in Israel, limiting generalizability to other healthcare settings and ethnic populations.

Clinical Implications

Clinicians should consider implementing slower, individualized semaglutide titration protocols using the injection pen's click system for patients at high risk of GI-AEs or those who have previously failed standard titration. The flexible approach may allow more patients with type 2 diabetes to benefit from semaglutide's long-term efficacy on glycemic control, weight reduction, and cardiovascular protection by preventing early treatment discontinuation. For patients who discontinue semaglutide under standard titration, reinitiating treatment with a more gradual, flexible dose escalation regimen represents a viable rescue strategy, as demonstrated by the 60% success rate (6/10 patients) in this study. Patients experiencing persistent nausea or asthenia during titration should be counseled about the option to delay dose escalation until symptoms resolve, rather than discontinuing therapy altogether. The findings support shared decision-making discussions balancing the trade-off between faster achievement of target dose (8 vs. 16 weeks) against improved tolerability and adherence.

Knowledge Gap and Scope for Future Research

Long-term outcomes beyond 26 weeks need investigation to determine whether the adherence advantage of flexible titration persists and translates into sustained improvements in diabetes complications and cardiovascular outcomes. Cost-effectiveness analyses should evaluate whether improved adherence and reduced discontinuation with flexible titration offset the longer time to achieve therapeutic dosing and potential incremental healthcare resource utilization during extended titration.

8. Sodium-glucose Cotransporter-2 Inhibitors and Lower-extremity Amputation: Is the Guilty Verdict Valid? (Commentary)

Ref: Pan M, Stürmer T. Sodium–Glucose Cotransporter 2 Inhibitors and Lower-Extremity Amputation: Is the Guilty Verdict Valid? (Commentary). Diabetes Care. 2025;48:338-40.

ABSTRACT

In comparison to the general population, people with diabetes have a more than twice greater frequency of peripheral arterial disease (PAD) and are more likely to develop atherosclerosis. Diabetes and PAD increase the risk of lower-extremity amputation, which is associated with lower quality of life and higher morbidity and mortality from cardiovascular disease (CVD). The impact of sodium-glucose cotransporter-2 inhibitors (SGLT-2is) on amputation risk has drawn attention with the release of the CANVAS (Canagliflozin Cardiovascular Assessment Study) and CANVAS-R (Canagliflozin and Cardiovascular and Renal Events in Type 2 Diabetes) studies. Patients with diabetes who have or are at high risk of CVD are given preference for SGLT-2is due to their advantages in CVD outcomes. There is disagreement over the benefit-harm balance of these medications due to worries about a potential increased risk of amputation with canagliflozin and if this is a drug or class effect. Therefore, further data is required to assess the application of SGLT-2is in actual populations with increased PAD risk. The results of a retrospective cohort analysis of older US veterans with diabetes using the Veterans Health Administration (VHA) national database are presented in the current edition by Griffin et al. In contrast to starting a dipeptidyl peptidase 4 inhibitor (DPP-4i), a class of medication thought to have no effect on CVD outcomes, they discovered that starting an SGLT-2i (mostly empagliflozin) by patients on various background antihyperglycemic treatments (metformin, sulfonylureas, or insulin) was linked to an 18% higher event rate of a composite PAD surgical outcome (lower-extremity stent placement, vascular surgery, or amputation). The authors connected VHA data with Medicare and Medicaid data sources and put together a sizable, nationally representative veteran cohort with diabetes. Peripheral revascularization and amputation procedures were included in their broad outcome definition of PAD events, which was intended to include events that could eventually result in amputation but occurred earlier in the PAD disease course.

CRITICAL APPRAISAL

What was Known Prior to this Study?

Prior to this commentary, the CANVAS and CANVAS-R trials had raised concerns about increased amputation risk with canagliflozin, generating uncertainty about whether this was a drug-specific or class effect for SGLT-2 inhibitors. SGLT-2 inhibitors are preferentially prescribed to patients with diabetes at high cardiovascular risk due to their proven benefits in reducing major adverse cardiovascular events and cardiovascular death. Patients with diabetes have more than twofold higher prevalence of peripheral artery disease compared to the general population, and those with both conditions face elevated amputation risk.[25-28]

What this Study Adds?

This commentary provides a rigorous epidemiological critique of observational methodology applied to SGLT-2 inhibitor safety research. It highlights the critical limitation of using dichotomous covariates without disease severity classification in propensity score methods, demonstrating how this leads to residual confounding. The authors quantify the magnitude of potential bias by showing how crude risk ratios (1.48) reduced to adjusted ratios (1.18), suggesting substantial unmeasured confounding remains. They introduce practical solutions including using more clinically appropriate active comparators like GLP-1 receptor agonists or restricting populations to those without baseline cardiovascular disease. The commentary also contextualizes absolute versus relative risk, calculating that the number needed to harm is 500–1,000 compared to a number needed to treat (NNT) of 29–63 for cardiovascular benefits.

Strengths

The commentary demonstrates sophisticated understanding of causal inference principles and clearly articulates the difference between association and causation in observational research. They provide balanced criticism while acknowledging the strengths of the Griffin study, including its large nationally representative sample, active comparator new user design, and comprehensive covariate list. Most importantly, the authors translate findings into clinically meaningful absolute risk measures rather than relying solely on relative risks, enabling proper benefit-harm assessment.

Limitations

This is a commentary rather than original research, so it relies entirely on critique of another study's methodology without presenting new empirical data. The authors' arguments about residual confounding, while theoretically sound, are based on assumptions about the degree of confounding control achieved (suggesting 70% rather than 90%) without empirical validation. The commentary does not propose or conduct sensitivity analyses that could quantify the impact of unmeasured severity variables.

Clinical Implications

Clinicians should not alter prescribing practices for SGLT-2 inhibitors based solely on the Griffin study findings, given the substantial residual confounding concerns raised. For individual patients with diabetes at high cardiovascular risk, the proven cardiovascular benefits of SGLT-2 inhibitors (NNT 29 for CVD death prevention) substantially outweigh the uncertain and likely minimal amputation risk [number needed to harm (NNH) 500–1,000]. Treatment decisions should be individualized. Patients with existing peripheral artery disease may warrant closer monitoring if prescribed SGLT-2 inhibitors, though causal harm remains unproven.

Knowledge Gap and Scope for Future Research

Future studies should employ more refined measurement of disease severity for cardiovascular comorbidities rather than dichotomous indicators to better control confounding. Research comparing SGLT-2 inhibitors to more clinically appropriate active comparators like glucagon-like peptide-1 (GLP-1) receptor agonists in high-risk populations would minimize confounding by indication. Application of advanced methods such as negative control outcomes, instrumental variable analysis, or target trial emulation could strengthen causal inference from observational data. Individual patient-level meta-analyses across multiple randomized trials could provide definitive evidence about class-wide versus drug-specific amputation signals.

9. Incidence of Type 2 Diabetes with Verapamil Compared with Other Calcium Channel Blockers

Ref: Sacre JW, Wentworth JM, Magliano DJ, Shaw JE. Incidence of Type 2 Diabetes With Verapamil Compared With Other Calcium Channel Blockers. Diabetes Care. 2025;48:2111-8.

ABSTRACT

Objective: Verapamil, a calcium channel blocker (CCB), has been shown to decrease the onset of type 1 diabetes, which may have preventive benefits for those who are at risk of developing type 2 diabetes. Among a population-based cohort, we examined the incidence of type 2 diabetes among verapamil versus other CCB users.

Methods and research design: We found 90,026 people who started treatment with a CCB (at least two supply) between July 2003 and December 2014 from a random sample of Australians in national subsidized healthcare databases. After receiving glucose-lowering medication or registering with the National Diabetes Services Scheme, incident diabetes was identified. People were tracked from the time they received their first CCB supply until they stopped taking it, developed diabetes, passed away, or the end of 2014. Following multivariable propensity score correction, correlations between CCB subclass and type 2 diabetes incidence and death (the competing event) were described using multistate Poisson regression models.

Results: The cohort included 85,541 patients receiving treatment with various CCBs (mostly dihydropyridines) and 4,485 verapamil users (5.0%). Compared to 2,622 patients treated with other CCBs (11.4 per 1,000 person-years), 101 patients treated with verapamil (8.8 per 1,000 person-years) experienced type 2 diabetes over a median 1.6-year follow-up. This resulted in a decreased probability of type 2 diabetes at 6 years [4.2% (95% CI 3.3–5.3) vs. 5.4% (4.7–6.3)] for a typical clinical profile; absolute risk difference 1.3% (95% CI −0.1–2.4) and an incidence rate ratio of 0.77 (95% CI 0.63–0.94) in favor of verapamil (completely adjusted). The outcomes held up well in several sensitivity tests.

Conclusion: Compared to other CCBs, verapamil use is linked to a decreased risk of type 2 diabetes.

CRITICAL APPRAISAL

What was Known Prior to this Study?

Prior evidence established that verapamil modifies disease progression in type 1 diabetes through downregulation of thioredoxin-interacting protein (TXNIP) expression, which enhances β-cell survival and function. One retrospective cohort study from Taiwan reported approximately 20% reduced diabetes risk with verapamil compared to other CCBs. However, whether these benefits extended to type 2 diabetes prevention remained uncertain, with limited prospective intervention data in type 2 diabetes populations.[29-31]

What this Study Adds?

This study provides robust population-level evidence that verapamil's protective effects extend to type 2 diabetes prevention in a geographically and demographically distinct population from previous research. The findings confirm the Taiwanese study's effect size [incidence rate ratio (IRR) 0.77 vs. hazard ratio 0.80] in an older cohort (mean age 73 vs. 49 years), suggesting broad applicability across age groups. The study quantifies absolute risk reduction through competing risk analysis, translating relative benefits into clinically meaningful terms—1.3 percentage point reduction at 6 years for typical hypertensive profiles. Importantly, results remained consistent across nine sensitivity analyses, including intention-to-treat approaches, propensity-score matching, and inverse probability of censoring weighting.

Strengths

The study utilized large-scale national administrative databases with minimal selection bias. Propensity score adjustment incorporated 30+ covariates capturing cardiovascular comorbidities, concurrent medications, andsocioeconomic factors, achieving good covariate balance. Multiple sensitivity analyses addressed key biases. The 12-month medication-free lead-in period ensured true CCB initiation rather than prevalent users, reducing immortal time bias.

Limitations

The study's reliance on administrative data precluded adjustment for critical diabetes risk factors including body mass index (BMI), waist circumference, family history, physical activity, and dietary patterns—variables that likely differ between verapamil and other CCB users. The median follow-up duration of 1.6 years is relatively short.

Clinical Implications

These findings suggest verapamil merits consideration when CCB therapy is indicated in patients at elevated type 2 diabetes risk, particularly in the absence of contraindications (heart failure, heart block, concurrent β-blockade). For hypertensive patients with multiple diabetes risk factors already requiring angiotensin-converting enzyme (ACE) inhibitors/angiotensin-receptor blockers (ARBs) and statins, verapamil selection over dihydropyridines could provide additional preventive benefit. The 23% of relative risk reduction is clinically meaningful at population scale given widespread CCB use for hypertension management. However, verapamil's side effect profile and drug interaction potential must be weighed against modest absolute risk reductions. Current hypertension guidelines preferentially recommend dihydropyridine CCBs over verapamil based on tolerability and safety; these data provide rationale for individualizing CCB selection based on diabetes risk stratification. Randomized controlled trials are essential before modifying treatment guidelines, particularly to assess long-term cardiovascular and mortality outcomes.

Knowledge Gap and Scope for Future Research

Well-designed randomized controlled trials comparing verapamil versus dihydropyridine CCBs in high-risk populations (prediabetes, metabolic syndrome) are critically needed to establish causality and inform guideline recommendations. Future studies should directly measure glycemic parameters (HbA1c, fasting glucose, oral glucose tolerance tests) rather than relying on prescription-based diabetes diagnosis. Dose-response relationships warrant exploration, particularly whether higher verapamil doses achieve greater diabetes prevention without prohibitive adverse effects. Long-term cardiovascular safety, particularly mortality outcomes, requires clarification through prospective studies with adequate follow-up duration.

10. Weekly Fixed-dose Insulin Efsitora in Type 2 Diabetes without Previous Insulin Therapy

Ref: Rosenstock J, Bailey T, Connery L, Miller E, Desouza C, Wang Q, et al.; QWINT-1 trial investigators. Weekly Fixed-Dose Insulin Efsitora in Type 2 Diabetes without Previous Insulin Therapy. N Engl J Med. 2025;393:325-35.

ABSTRACT

Background: Basal insulin dosage modifications have been conducted at least once a week in prior treat-to-target trials based on fasting blood glucose readings. Adults with type 2 diabetes who have not previously received insulin therapy may benefit from a fixed-dose regimen of insulin efsitora alfa (efsitora), a once-weekly basal insulin.

Techniques: Adults with type 2 diabetes who had not previously received insulin therapy participated in a 52-week phase 3, open-label, treat-to-target experiment. Participants were randomized in a 1:1 ratio to receive either insulin glargine U100 (glargine) once daily or once weekly efsitora. In order to reach fasting blood glucose levels of 80 to 130 mg per deciliter, efsitora treatment was started with a single dosage of 100 U given once weekly, with dose modifications made every 4 weeks, as needed, at fixed doses of 150, 250, and 400 U. To achieve the same glycemic targets, glargine doses were modified weekly or more frequently using a conventional methodology. The major end point was the change from baseline in the glycated hemoglobin level at 52 weeks, which was assessed for noninferiority (noninferiority margin, 0.4 percentage points).

Results: Randomization was applied to 795 participants in total. The mean glycated hemoglobin level dropped from 8.20% at baseline to 7.05% at week 52 with efsitora (least squares mean change, −1.19 percentage points) and from 8.28 to 7.08% with glargine (least squares mean change, −1.16 percentage points); the noninferiority of efsitora to glargine was confirmed by the estimated between-group difference of −0.03 percentage points [95% confidence interval (CI) −0.18 to 0.12]. There was no evidence of superiority ($p = 0.68$). Compared to glargine, efsitora had a lower rate of combined clinically significant hypoglycemia (glucose level, < 54 mg/dL) or severe hypoglycemia (level 3; requiring assistance for treatment) [0.50 events per participant-year of exposure with efsitora vs. 0.88 with glargine; estimated rate ratio, 0.57 (95% CI 0.39–0.84)]. At week 52, the median number of dose changes required was two for efsitora and eight for glargine; the mean total weekly insulin dose was 289.1 U for efsitora and 332.8 U for glargine (estimated between-group difference, −43.7 U per week; 95% CI, −62.4 to −25.0).

Conclusion: Once-weekly efsitora given in a fixed-dose regimen was noninferior to once-daily glargine in lowering glycated hemoglobin levels in persons with type 2 diabetes who had not previously received insulin (Eli Lilly provided funding; ClinicalTrials.gov number: NCT05662332.).

CRITICAL APPRAISAL

What was Known before this Study?

- Once-weekly basal insulins (icodec, efsitora) had already shown noninferior glycemic control to once-daily degludec or glargine in flexible, weight-based titration regimens, generally with low but sometimes slightly higher hypoglycemia rates.
- Treat-to-target basal insulin algorithms typically require at least weekly adjustments, and therapeutic inertia plus injection burden contribute to delayed initiation and inadequate titration in real-world type 2 diabetes care.
- Efsitora had been evaluated in QWINT-2 using a flexible weekly titration scheme against degludec, showing similar HbA1c reduction with low hypoglycemia, but a simple fixed-dose "autoinjector" regimen had not been tested.[32-34]

What this Study Adds?

- Demonstrates that a simple, largely fixed-dose once-weekly efsitora regimen with 4-weekly titration steps is noninferior to standard once-daily glargine for 1-year HbA1c reduction in insulin-naïve type 2 diabetes.
- Suggesting a favorable hypoglycemia profile under this regimen with efsitora despite similar HbA1c and slightly lower total weekly insulin dose.

Strengths

- *Appropriate design and power:* Large phase 3, multicenter, randomized, parallel-group treat-to-target trial with clear noninferiority objective, prespecified 0.4% HbA1c margin aligned with regulatory expectations, and >99% power assumptions.
- Adults with long-standing type 2 diabetes (T2D) on 1–3 noninsulin agents, including glucagon-like peptide-1 receptor agonists (GLP-1RA) and sodium-glucose cotransporter-2 inhibitors (SGLT-2i), mirror contemporary practice; glargine U100 is a widely accepted basal comparator, enhancing external relevance.
- Detailed hypoglycemia characterization (overall, nocturnal, level 2/3), adjudicated cardiovascular (CV) events/deaths, and inclusion of TRIM-D (Treatment-Related Impact Measure for Diabetes) quality-of-life measure provide a broad assessment of benefit–risk.

Limitations

Open-label design; Restricted geography and ethnicity; No re-escalation of efsitora after dose reduction for hypoglycemia, which is not reflective of real-world practice and may have biased against maximal glycemic optimization in that arm; Lack of continuous glucose monitoring (CGM) data; Industry sponsorship and writing support raising potential conflicts of interest despite author access to data.

Clinical Implications

- For insulin-naïve adults with T2D inadequately controlled on oral/other injectable therapy, once-weekly efsitora using a simple fixed-dose ladder can achieve HbA1c reductions and fasting glucose control comparable to daily glargine, with potential advantages in adherence and reduced injection burden.
- Lower hypoglycemia and dose burden.
- Weight gain was modest but slightly higher with efsitora, and major CV events were infrequent and similar; longer and larger outcome trials would be needed before extrapolating to high-risk cardiorenal populations.

Knowledge Gaps and Future Research

Long-term outcomes; Broader and specific populations; Evaluation in diverse ethnicities and body mass index (BMI) profiles [e.g., lean Asian Indians, elderly, chronic kidney disease (CKD) stages 3–4, hepatic impairment] to refine dosing and safety; Pediatric and pregnancy data are absent; Comparative effectiveness versus newer basals and continuous glucose monitoring (CGM)-guided regimens; Studies integrating efsitora with GLP-1RA/dual incretin or SGLT-2i in fixed-ratio or co-pack strategies to define its role within modern multi-agent injectable pathways.

11. Effects of GLP-1 Receptor Agonists on Incidence and Outcomes of Ischemic Stroke and Myocardial Infarction: A Systematic Review and Meta-analysis

Ref: Alammari N, Alshehri A, Al Khalaf A, Alamri RA, Alhalal N, Sultan MA, et al. Effects of GLP-1 receptor agonists on incidence and outcomes of ischemic stroke and myocardial infarction: A systematic review and meta-analysis. Diabetes Obes Metab. 2025;27(8):4387-400.

ABSTRACT

Introduction: Beyond glycemic control, glucagon-like peptide-1 receptor agonists (GLP-1 RAs) show cardiovascular advantages; nevertheless, the literature has not fully examined the benefits of protection across cerebrovascular and cardiovascular areas. Our goal is to determine if GLP-1 RAs offer balanced protection against myocardial infarction (MI) and stroke, as well as to pinpoint the variables that alter this protection.

Techniques: We carried out a comprehensive review and meta-analysis of randomized controlled trials that reported cardiovascular and cerebrovascular outcomes and compared GLP-1 RAs with placebo. To measure relative cerebrovascular versus coronary protection, we computed the hazard ratios (HRs) for stroke and MI and created a unique Territorial Benefit Ratio (TBR = HR stroke/HR MI). Factors influencing territorial protection were found by meta-regression analysis.

Results: Eleven studies with 85,373 individuals satisfied the requirements for inclusion. With an overall balanced TBR of 1.01 (95% CI 0.89–1.15), GLP-1 RAs significantly decreased stroke (HR 0.88, 95% CI 0.80–0.96), and MI (HR 0.87, 95% CI 0.79–0.97). Patient subgroups showed substantial differences in protection patterns: prior stroke experience was associated with better stroke protection [HR 0.73, number needed to treat (NNT) 54], whereas prior MI history was associated with better MI protection (HR 0.79, NNT 55). While stroke protection was stronger with time (over 24 months: HR 0.80), MI protection appeared earlier during the first six months (HR 0.81). While dyslipidemia offered superior MI protection, renal failure, atrial fibrillation, and hypertension pushed protection toward stroke.

Conclusion: With significant temporal findings and translated outcomes, GLP-1 RAs exhibit a protection-in-territory-at-risk pattern. These results lend credence to a personalized strategy to GLP-1 RA treatment that takes individuals' risk profiles and vascular histories into account. Significant highlights for clinical expectations and treatment persistence are provided by the earlier development of MI protection and the later strengthening of stroke protection.

CRITICAL APPRAISAL

What was Known Prior to this Study?

GLP-1 RAs had been established as cardiovascular protective agents beyond their glucose-lowering effects, with demonstrated benefits in reducing major adverse cardiovascular events (MACE) in patients with type 2 diabetes. The cerebrovascular and coronary circulations were known to have different pathophysiological vulnerabilities despite sharing common risk factors. However, the pattern, timing, and territorial distribution of protection across cerebrovascular and cardiovascular systems remained incompletely understood.[35-37]

What this Study Adds?

This meta-analysis introduces the novel concept of the territorial benefit ratio (TBR), providing the first systematic quantification of relative cerebrovascular versus coronary protection offered by GLP-1 RAs. The study demonstrates a "protection-in-territory-at-risk" pattern, where GLP-1 RAs provide preferential protection in vascular territories with prior involvement. It characterizes differential temporal dynamics, showing MI protection emerges within 6 months while stroke protection strengthens progressively beyond 24 months. Additionally, the study reveals that combination therapy with sodium-glucose cotransporter-2 (SGLT-2) inhibitors significantly enhances stroke protection (HR 0.77) compared to GLP-1 RA monotherapy.

Strengths

The study's primary strength lies in its novel analytical framework using the TBR metric, which allows direct quantification of territorial protection patterns. High-quality evidence assessment using both the modified Newcastle-Ottawa Scale (8–9 stars for all studies) and GRADE approach ensures reliability. Meta-regression analyses identifying biomarkers and risk factors that modify territorial protection enable personalized therapeutic approaches.

Limitations

Some subgroup analyses involved smaller sample sizes, reducing precision of estimates as reflected in GRADE assessments downgrading evidence quality to moderate for certain subgroups. Time-to-benefit analysis relied on aggregated data from trial publications rather than individual participant data, limiting detailed time-dependent modeling.

Clinical Implications

The findings support a personalized approach to GLP-1 RA therapy based on individual vascular risk profiles. For secondary stroke prevention, GLP-1 RAs demonstrate substantial benefit (NNT 54). The earlier emergence of MI protection (within 6 months) suggests prompt cardiovascular benefit for patients at high immediate coronary risk. The delayed but strengthening stroke protection (beyond 24 months) emphasizes the importance of treatment adherence and long-term persistence. Combination therapy with SGLT2 inhibitors may optimize stroke protection, offering synergistic vascular benefits. The protection-in-territory-at-risk pattern indicates that physicians should prioritize GLP-1 RAs for patients with specific vascular histories matching the predominant protective benefit.

Knowledge Gap and Scope for Future Research

Extended follow-up studies are required to determine whether strengthening stroke protection continues beyond current trial durations. Development of risk prediction models integrating territorial vulnerability concepts could identify patients most likely to benefit from GLP-1 RA therapy for specific vascular outcomes.

12. The Effect of Once-weekly Insulin Icodec versus Once-daily Basal Insulin on Physical Activity-attributed Hypoglycemia in Type 2 Diabetes: A Post Hoc Analysis of ONWARDS 1–5

Ref: Riddell MC, Heller S, Carstensen L, Rocha TMP, Kehlet Watt S, Woo VC. The effect of once-weekly insulin icodec vs once-daily basal insulin on physical activity-attributed hypoglycaemia in type 2 diabetes: a post hoc analysis of ONWARDS 1–5. Diabetologia. 2025;68:1416-22.

ABSTRACT

Aim/hypothesis: When basal or basal-bolus insulin therapy is used, physical exercise raises the risk of hypoglycemia in people with type 2 diabetes. Because the injected levels cannot be lowered in anticipation of greater physical activity, once-weekly basal insulins may increase the risk of hypoglycemia linked to physical activity compared to other basal insulins. Examining physical activity-attributed hypoglycemic episodes in persons with type 2 diabetes receiving either once-weekly basal insulin icodec (henceforth referred to as "icodec") or once-daily basal insulins was the goal of this post hoc analysis of five distinct randomized studies (ONWARDS 1–5).

Methods: The ONWARDS 1–5 Phase 3a randomized controlled trials examined the safety and effectiveness of once-weekly basal icodec against once-daily basal insulin in persons with type 2 diabetes who were either insulin-naive (ONWARDS 1, 3, and 5) or insulin-experienced (ONWARDS 2 and 4). Using a digital journal and a blood glucose meter, participants self-monitored their blood glucose levels. Additional self-measured blood glucose readings were prompted by suspected hypoglycemia symptoms in each trial, and values suggestive of hypoglycemia were noted in the participants' digital diaries. Individuals who had hypoglycemic episodes were asked to record any connection between each episode and physical activity. Hypoglycemic events were categorized as severe (level 3: cognitive impairment requiring outside assistance), clinically significant (level 2: blood glucose < 3.0 mmol/L), or alert value (level 1: blood glucose < 3.9 but ≥ 3.0 mmol/L). For each of the five trials, the percentages of hypoglycemic episodes linked to physical activity and the odds of experiencing a hypoglycemic episode linked to physical activity were computed for the two basal insulin types (once-weekly vs. once-daily).

Results: The percentages of hypoglycemic episodes that were linked to physical activity did not consistently differ between icodec and the once-daily insulin comparators across all studies; these occurrences were primarily alert value or clinically significant hypoglycemic episodes. The incidence of clinically significant or severe hypoglycemic episodes related to physical activity was consistently $\leq 3.0\%$ in ONWARDS 1, 2, 3, and 5 in both insulin-naive and insulin-experienced subjects. As anticipated given the basal-bolus insulin regimen, the incidence of physical activity-attributed hypoglycemic episodes in ONWARDS 4 was quantitatively greater in both treatment groups [18.6% (icodec) vs. 17.9% (insulin glargine U100)]. The risks of having a clinically significant or severe hypoglycemic episode linked to physical activity did not differ statistically significantly between icodec and once-daily insulin comparators in any of the trials. There were few repeated occurrences of clinically significant or severe hypoglycemia in the 24 hours following an incident linked to physical activity; ONWARDS 1, 3, and 5 did not have any such episodes. On the other hand, in ONWARDS 2 and 4, the frequency of recurrent clinically significant hypoglycemic episodes in the 24 hours following a clinically significant or severe hypoglycemic episode linked to physical activity was numerically higher with icodec compared to the once-daily insulin comparators, and no additional severe episodes were reported in any of the trial participants.

Conclusion/interpretation: These results do not imply that physical activity with once-weekly basal icodec versus once-daily basal insulins increases the incidence of hypoglycemia in persons with type 2 diabetes.

CRITICAL APPRAISAL

What was Known Prior to this Study?

Physical activity increases hypoglycemia risk in individuals with type 2 diabetes on insulin therapy due to increased glucose requirements and enhanced insulin sensitivity. The ONWARDS 1–5 trials had previously demonstrated that insulin icodec achieved noninferior (and in some trials, superior) HbA1c reduction compared to once-daily basal insulins, with clinically significant or severe hypoglycemia rates below one episode per person-year in most trials. A meta-analysis suggested that once-weekly icodec may increase the rate of clinically significant hypoglycemia compared with once-daily basal insulins, particularly if not carefully titrated.[38-40]

What this Study Adds?

This is the first systematic examination of physical activity-attributed hypoglycemia with once-weekly versus once-daily basal insulin in type 2 diabetes. The analysis demonstrates that 10–23% of hypoglycemic episodes across the ONWARDS trials were attributed to physical activity, with no consistent differences between icodec and once-daily comparators. The study provides reassurance that the increased overall hypoglycemia rates observed with icodec in meta-analyses are not specifically driven by physical activity. It establishes that the incidence of physical activity-attributed clinically significant or severe hypoglycemia remains low (≤ 3% in most trials) regardless of insulin frequency. Additionally, the analysis shows that recurrent hypoglycemia within 24 hours after a physical activity-attributed episode was infrequent, with no severe recurrent episodes reported.

Strengths

The study leverages data from five large, well-designed Phase 3a randomized controlled trials encompassing diverse patient populations including both insulin-naive and insulin-experienced participants. The substantial sample size and long trial durations provide robust statistical power and real-world applicability.

Limitations

Several important limitations constrain the interpretation of findings. The absence of a specific definition for "physical activity" in the ONWARDS trials may have led to inconsistent participant reporting and attribution of hypoglycemic episodes. No data were collected on participants' baseline physical activity levels, exercise intensity, duration, or type, precluding analysis of dose-response relationships or activity-specific risk assessment.

Clinical Implications

These findings provide important reassurance for clinicians prescribing once-weekly insulin icodec to physically active patients with type 2 diabetes. The data suggest that the theoretical concern about inability to reduce once-weekly insulin doses before exercise does not translate into increased physical activity-attributed hypoglycemia risk in practice. Patients can be counseled that once-weekly insulin does not appear to require special precautions beyond standard hypoglycemia prevention strategies used with daily basal insulins. However, the higher incidence in ONWARDS 4 (18.6% with basal-bolus regimen) underscores that patients on intensive insulin therapy require continued vigilance regardless of basal insulin frequency. Clinicians should still emphasize standard exercise management strategies including blood glucose monitoring before and after activity, appropriate carbohydrate intake, and awareness of hypoglycemia symptoms. The flexibility of icodec to adjust injection day by up to 3 days (with minimum 4-day intervals) may allow some accommodation for unusual activity patterns.

Knowledge Gap and Scope for Future Research

Future studies should prospectively define and categorize physical activity by intensity, duration, and type (aerobic vs. resistance vs. mixed) to enable activity-specific risk stratification. Continuous glucose monitoring would provide more comprehensive assessment of hypoglycemia patterns during and after exercise, capturing asymptomatic episodes missed by self-monitoring.

13. Once-weekly IcoSema versus Once-weekly Insulin Icodec in Type 2 Diabetes Management (COMBINE 1): An Open-label, Multicentre, Treat-to-target, Randomized, Phase 3a Trial

Ref: Mathieu C, Giorgino F, Kim SG, Larsen JH, Philis-Tsimikas A, Ramachandran A, et al. Once-weekly IcoSema versus once-weekly insulin icodec in type 2 diabetes management (COMBINE 1): An open-label, multicentre, treat-to-target, randomised, phase 3a trial. Lancet Diabetes Endocrinol. 2025;13:568-79.

ABSTRACT

Background: IcoSema is a once-weekly combination treatment that consists of semaglutide, a glucagon-like peptide 1 (GLP-1) analogue, and basal insulin icodec (icodec). COMBINE 1 examined the safety and effectiveness of IcoSema against once-weekly icodec alone in persons with poorly managed type 2 diabetes receiving daily basal insulin treatment.

Techniques: A 52-week open-label, treat-to-target, randomized, phase 3a trial called COMBINE 1 was conducted at 192 outpatient clinics and hospital departments in 20 different nations and regions. Using a randomization and trial supply management system, individuals 18 years of age or older with type 2 diabetes [glycated hemoglobin (HbA1c) 7.0–10.0% (53.0–85.8 mmol/mol)] treated with daily basal insulin with or without oral glucose-lowering medications were randomly assigned (1:1) to either IcoSema (700 U/mL plus 2 mg/mL) or icodec (700 U/mL), both given as subcutaneous injections on the same day every week, at any time of day. Based on the baseline characteristics of the subjects, there was no segmentation. The main outcome, which was assessed in the entire study set (all randomly assigned subjects), was the change in HbA1c from baseline to week 52. The trial has been finished and is registered with ClinicalTrials.gov with the number NCT05352815.

Findings: 1,671 people were tested between June 1, 2022, and March 13, 2023. Of them, 1,291 {mean age 60.6 years [standard deviation (SD) 10.3]; 799 (62%)} males and 492 (38%) females] were randomly assigned to either icodec (n = 645) or IcoSema (n = 646). At week 52, the estimated mean change in HbA1c was −1.55 percentage points [standard error (SE) 0.03; −16.9 mmol/mol (0.4)] with IcoSema and −0.89 percentage points [(SE 0.03); −9.7 mmol/mol (0.4)] with icodec {estimated treatment difference (ETD) −0.66 percentages points [95% confidence interval (CI) −0.76 to −0.57]; −7.3 mmol/mol (−8.3 to −6.2); $p < 0.0001$; superiority confirmed}. IcoSema significantly reduced the rate of combined clinically significant or severe hypoglycemia from baseline to week 57 compared to icodec [0.14 vs. 0.63 episodes per person-year of exposure; estimated rate ratio 0.22 (95% CI 0.14–0.36); $p < 0.0001$; superiority verified]. Infections and infestations in the icodec group [275 (43%) of 644 participants had 466 occurrences] and gastrointestinal problems in the IcoSema group [303 (47%) of 644 participants had 1,033 events during the study] were the most commonly reported side effects. A major adverse event occurred in 59 (9%) of the IcoSema group and 69 (11%) of the icodec group. There were no treatment-related deaths.

Interpretation: Once-weekly IcoSema outperformed once-weekly icodec alone in terms of HbA1c improvements and the overall decreased rate of combined clinically significant or severe hypoglycemia in people with poorly managed type 2 diabetes receiving daily basal insulin treatment. For individuals with type 2 diabetes, IcoSema may offer a way to intensify insulin therapy.

This study is financed by Novo Nordisk.

CRITICAL APPRAISAL

What was Known Prior to this Study?

Prior to COMBINE 1, several important therapeutic principles were established in type 2 diabetes management. Once-daily fixed-ratio combinations of basal insulin with glucagon-like peptide-1 (GLP-1) receptor agonists (IDegLira and IGlarLixi) had demonstrated improved glycemic control compared to basal insulin alone with comparable or numerically lower hypoglycemia rates. The ONWARDS 1–5 trials had established the efficacy and safety profile of once-weekly insulin icodec. The SUSTAIN clinical program had extensively evaluated once-weekly semaglutide. Current guidelines recommended combining insulin with GLP-1 receptor agonists for improved glycemic control, beneficial effects on weight, and reduced hypoglycemia risk compared to basal insulin alone.[41-43]

What this Study Adds?

COMBINE 1 represents the first phase 3a trial demonstrating superiority of a once-weekly fixed-ratio combination (IcoSema) over once-weekly basal insulin alone in adults with inadequately controlled type 2 diabetes on daily basal insulin. The study achieved a remarkable estimated treatment difference in glycated hemoglobin (HbA1c) of –0.66 percentage points (–7.3 mmol/mol), with 71.7% of IcoSema participants reaching HbA1c < 7.0% versus 35.5% with icodec alone. IcoSema demonstrated a 78% reduction in clinically significant or severe hypoglycemia risk compared to icodec. The combination showed insulin-sparing effects, requiring a mean weekly dose of 182 U versus 355 U with icodec during weeks 50–52. IcoSema achieved 75.9% time in range during weeks 48–52.

Strengths

Strengths include large multicentric population and robust long-term efficacy and safety data, with high completion rates (90% IcoSema, 93% icodec). Continuous glucose monitoring data collection during weeks 48–52 provided objective glycemic metrics including time in range, time below range, and time above range. The treat-to-target design with standardized titration algorithms reflected real-world clinical practice, enhancing applicability.

Limitations

The open-label design; only 41% of participants in the IcoSema group received semaglutide doses ≥0.5 mg at week 52, suggesting many participants may not have reached optimal GLP-1 receptor agonist dosing. Continuous glucose monitoring was limited to a 5-week period (weeks 47–52). Postprandial glucose data were not captured, limiting comprehensive understanding of glycemic profiles. The predominantly white and Asian population (96% combined) limits generalizability to other ethnic groups.

Clinical Implications

IcoSema offers a compelling therapeutic option for insulin therapy intensification in adults with type 2 diabetes inadequately controlled on daily basal insulin, addressing multiple unmet clinical needs simultaneously. The combination achieves superior glycemic control while reducing injection burden from daily to weekly administration, potentially improving treatment adherence and patient satisfaction. The significant weight reduction of 3.70 kg with IcoSema versus weight gain of 1.89 kg with icodec addresses a major barrier to insulin intensification. The 78% reduction in hypoglycemia risk provides substantial clinical and psychological benefits. Clinicians should anticipate transient early hyperglycemia during IcoSema initiation and provide appropriate patient education.

Knowledge Gaps and Scope for Future Research

Long-term cardiovascular and renal outcomes; optimal starting dose and titration algorithm;

comparative effectiveness studies against basal-bolus insulin regimens in real-world settings; the efficacy and safety of IcoSema in diverse populations including different ethnic groups, elderly patients, and those with renal impairment require specific study.

14. Once-weekly IcoSema versus Once-Weekly Semaglutide in Adults with Type 2 Diabetes: The COMBINE 2 Randomized Clinical Trial

Ref: Lingvay I, Benamar M, Chen L, Fu A, Jódar E, Nishida T, et al. Once-weekly IcoSema versus once-weekly semaglutide in adults with type 2 diabetes: The COMBINE 2 randomised clinical trial. Diabetologia. 2025;68:739-51.

ABSTRACT

Aim/hypothesis: COMBINE 2 evaluated the safety and effectiveness of once-weekly semaglutide [a glucagon-like peptide-1 (GLP-1) analogue] 1.0 mg versus once-weekly IcoSema (a combination therapy of basal insulin icodec and semaglutide) in people with type 2 diabetes who were not well controlled with GLP-1 receptor agonist (GLP-1 RA) therapy, with or without additional oral glucose-lowering drugs.

Techniques: This 52-week Phase IIIa, randomized, multicenter, open-label, parallel group study was carried out at 121 locations throughout 13 nations and regions. Once-weekly IcoSema or once-weekly semaglutide 1.0 mg was randomly assigned 1:1 to adults with type 2 diabetes [glycated hemoglobin (HbA1c) 53.0–85.8 mmol/mol (7.0–10.0%)] receiving GLP-1 RA treatment with or without other oral glucose-lowering medicines. Change in HbA1c from baseline to week 52 was the main outcome, and IcoSema's superiority to semaglutide 1.0 mg was evaluated. Changes in fasting plasma glucose and body weight (from baseline to week 52) and combined clinically significant (level 2; <3 mmol/L) or severe (level 3; associated with severe cognitive impairment requiring external assistance for recovery) hypoglycemia (from baseline to week 57) were secondary endpoints.

Results: A randomization and trial supply management system was used to randomly assign 683 subjects to either semaglutide 1.0 mg (n = 341) or IcoSema (n = 342). The following were the mean ± standard deviation (SD) baseline characteristics: Body mass index (BMI) 31.1 ± 4.7 kg/m^2, diabetes duration 12.6 ± 6.9 years, and HbA1c 64.0 ± 8.2 mmol/mol (8.0 ± 0.7%). The mean change in HbA1c from baseline to week 52 was –14.7 mmol/mol (–1.35% points) in the IcoSema group and –9.88 mmol/mol (–0.90% points) in the semaglutide group; the estimated treatment difference (ETD) was –4.85 [95% confidence interval (CI) –6.13, –3.57] mmol/mol [–0.44 (95% CI –0.56, –0.33) % points], indicating that IcoSema was superior to semaglutide (p < 0.0001). IcoSema versus semaglutide significantly decreased the estimated mean change in fasting plasma glucose from baseline to week 52 [–2.48 mmol/L vs. –1.41 mmol/L, respectively; ETD –1.07 (95% CI –1.37, –0.76) mmol; p < 0.0001]. There was a statistically significant difference between the groups' mean body weight changes from baseline to week 52: +0.84 kg for IcoSema and –3.70 kg for semaglutide [ETD 4.54 kg (95% CI 3.84, 5.23); p < 0.0001]. IcoSema and semaglutide did not significantly vary in the risk of combined clinically significant or severe hypoglycemia [0.042 vs. 0.036 episodes per person-year of exposure; estimated rate ratio 1.20 (95% CI 0.53, 2.69); p = 0.66]. Between treatment groups, the percentage of participants who experienced gastrointestinal side events was comparable (IcoSema 31.4%; semaglutide 34.4%).

Conclusion/interpretation: When compared to once-weekly semaglutide 1.0 mg, switching to once-weekly IcoSema showed superiority in HbA1c reduction, similar rates of clinically significant or severe hypoglycemia, and similar frequency of gastrointestinal adverse events in individuals with type 2 diabetes who were not adequately managed with GLP-1 RA therapy, with or without additional oral glucose-lowering medications. However, there was a statistically significant difference in weight between baseline and week 52 in favor of semaglutide 1.0 mg.

Registration for a trial NCT05259033 on ClinicalTrials.gov.

Finance Novo Nordis provided funding for this trial.

CRITICAL APPRAISAL

What was Known Prior to this Study?

- Fixed-ratio combinations of basal insulin and glucagon-like peptide-1 receptor agonists (GLP-1 RAs) (IDegLira, IGlarLixi) demonstrated efficacy in improving glycemic control with reduced weight gain and hypoglycemia risk compared to basal-bolus insulin.
- Once-daily combination products reduced glycated hemoglobin (HbA1c) more than monotherapy with either GLP-1 RA or insulin alone, while maintaining favorable weight and hypoglycemia profiles.
- GLP-1 RAs as monotherapy demonstrated comparable or slightly superior HbA1c reduction compared to basal insulin, with additional benefits of weight loss and minimal hypoglycemia risk.
- Insulin icodec demonstrated noninferiority to daily basal insulins.
- Semaglutide established efficacy in the SUSTAIN trials with robust HbA1c reduction and weight loss benefits.[42,44,45]

What this Study Adds?

- Once-weekly IcoSema is superior to once-weekly semaglutide 1.0 mg for HbA1c reduction.
- Glycemic benefit without unacceptable weight gain (only 0.84 kg gain)
- Evidence that once-weekly combination therapy can address treatment intensification needs in a population already on GLP-1 RAs.
- Comparable gastrointestinal tolerability despite previous GLP-1 RA exposure, with similar proportions experiencing gastrointestinal (GI) adverse events (31.4% vs. 34.4%).

Strengths

- Large sample size, multicenter trial enhancing generalizability
- 52-week treatment period provides adequate long-term efficacy and safety data.
- Lesser dropout rates
- Intention-to-treat approach handling intercurrent events appropriately, reflecting real-world effectiveness

Limitations

Limitations include open-label design; significant weight gain with IcoSema (+0.84 kg) versus loss with semaglutide (–3.70 kg) may limit acceptability in obesity-predominant populations [baseline body mass index (BMI) 31.1 kg/m^2]; no cardiovascular outcome assessment or patient-reported quality of life measures; and absence of continuous glucose monitoring.

Clinical Implications

- IcoSema represents a viable treatment intensification option for patients inadequately controlled on GLP-1 RA therapy, offering superior glycemic control with once-weekly dosing convenience.
- The 73.5% achievement of HbA1c < 7.0% with IcoSema suggests this combination can effectively address the therapeutic gap in GLP-1 RA partial responders.

- Modest weight gain (0.84 kg) with IcoSema is substantially less than typically expected with insulin initiation, representing successful mitigation by the semaglutide component.
- Similar hypoglycemia rates between groups (no severe episodes in either arm)
- The once-weekly formulation addresses adherence challenges and reduces injection burden compared to daily basal insulin or separate administration of components.

Knowledge Gaps and Scope for Future Research

- Cardiovascular outcome trial (CVOT) data needed to establish cardiovascular safety and potential benefits, particularly given baseline cardiovascular risk factors in this population
- Head-to-head comparison with once-daily combinations
- Continuous glucose monitoring substudy
- Long-term retinopathy outcomes

15. Once-weekly IcoSema versus Multiple Daily Insulin Injections in Type 2 Diabetes Management (COMBINE 3): An Open-label, Multicentre, Treat-to-target, Non-inferiority, Randomized, Phase 3a Trial

Ref: Billings LK, Andreozzi F, Frederiksen M, Gourdy P, Gowda A, Ji L, et al. Once-weekly IcoSema versus multiple daily insulin injections in type 2 diabetes management (COMBINE 3): an open-label, multicentre, treat-to-target, non-inferiority, randomised, phase 3a trial. Lancet Diabetes Endocrinol. 2025;13:556-67.

ABSTRACT

Background: IcoSema is a once-weekly combination medication for type 2 diabetes that consists of semaglutide, a glucagon-like peptide-1 (GLP-1) analogue, and basal insulin icodec. In persons with type 2 diabetes who are not properly controlled on daily basal insulin, we sought to compare the safety and effectiveness of IcoSema versus basal–bolus treatment (BBT).

Techniques: 109 outpatient clinics and hospital departments in 14 countries participated in COMBINE 3, a 52-week, open-label, treat-to-target, noninferiority, randomized, phase 3a trial. People with type 2 diabetes [glycated hemoglobin (HbA1c) 7.0–10.0% (53.0–85.8 mmol/mol)] who were 18 years of age or older and receiving daily basal insulin (20–80 U) were randomly assigned (1:1) to receive either BBT (once-daily insulin glargine U100 with two to four daily insulin aspart injections) or once-weekly IcoSema injection using a pen device. Change in HbA1c from baseline to week 52 was the main outcome, and it was assessed for noninferiority (0.3 percentage-point margin). Change in bodyweight from baseline to week 52, weekly total insulin dose during weeks 50–52, and a combination of clinically significant hypoglycemic episodes [<3.0 mmol/L (<54 mg/dL), verified by blood glucose meter] or severe hypoglycemic episodes (associated with severe cognitive impairment requiring external assistance for recovery) from baseline to week 57 were all considered confirmatory secondary endpoints. The entire analytic set (all randomly assigned participants) was used to assess the primary and confirmatory secondary outcomes. The safety analysis set (participants exposed to a trial product) served as the basis for descriptive statistics for safety endpoints, while the complete analysis set served as the basis for statistical analyses. This trial is finished and has been registered with ClinicalTrials.gov (NCT05013229).

Results: 844 participants were screened between November 30, 2021, and September 28, 2022; 679 [mean age 59.6 years (SD 10.4); 399 (59%) males and 280 (41%) females] were randomly assigned to either BBT ($n = 339$) or IcoSema ($n = 340$). The estimated mean change in HbA1c at week 52 was −1.47 percentage points [standard error (SE) 0.05; −16.0 mmol/mol (0.6)] with IcoSema and −1.40 percentage points [0.06; −15.3 mmol/mol (0.7)] with BBT, indicating that IcoSema was not inferior to BBT {estimated treatment difference (ETD) −0.06 percentage points [95% confidence interval (CI) −0.22 to 0.09; −0.70 mmol/mol (−2.39 to 0.99)]; $p < 0.0001$}. IcoSema was found to be superior to BBT in terms of bodyweight change from baseline to week 52 [ETD −6.72 kg (95% CI −7.58 to −5.86); $p < 0.0001$], weekly total insulin dose during weeks 50–52 [ETD −270 U (−303 to −236); $p < 0.0001$], and overall rate of clinically significant or severe hypoglycemia from baseline to week 57 [0.21 vs. 23 episodes per person-year of exposure; estimated rate ratio 0.12 (0.08–0.17); $p < 0.0001$]. During the experiment, gastrointestinal disorders with IcoSema [148 (44%) of 340 participants had 443 occurrences] and infections and infestations with BBT [116 (35%) of 328 participants had 193 incidents] were the most commonly reported adverse events.

Interpretation: When compared to daily BBT, once-weekly IcoSema produced noninferior HbA1c reduction and superiority in bodyweight change, weekly total insulin dose, and hypoglycemia rates, indicating that there may be a useful treatment intensification alternative for individuals with type 2 diabetes.

Funding is provided by Novo Nordisk.

CRITICAL APPRAISAL

What was Known Prior to this Study

Prior to COMBINE 3, treatment intensification for type 2 diabetes inadequately controlled on basal insulin traditionally involved basal–bolus therapy (BBT) and is associated with treatment complexity, hypoglycemia risk, weight gain, and high injection burden (up to 1,460 injections annually). Fixed-ratio combinations of once-daily basal insulin with glucagon-like peptide 1 (GLP-1) receptor agonists (IDegLira and IGlarLixi) demonstrated efficacy in reducing glycated hemoglobin (HbA1c) with favorable weight profiles and lower hypoglycemia rates compared to BBT.[43,46-48]

What this Study Adds?

COMBINE 3 is the first trial to evaluate a once-weekly fixed-ratio combination of basal insulin and GLP-1 receptor agonist versus BBT in adults with type 2 diabetes. The study demonstrates that IcoSema achieves noninferior glycemic control to BBT while requiring only 52 injections annually versus up to 1,460 with BBT. Key novel findings include superior weight outcomes, markedly lower hypoglycemia rates, and significantly improved treatment satisfaction scores. The study also identified a transient increase in prebreakfast glucose during the first 10 weeks of IcoSema therapy due to the conservative initiation dose strategy, which subsequently normalized without impacting long-term outcomes.

Strengths

Multicenter recruitment, adequate sample size, high completion rates (92% IcoSema, 86% BBT); the study addresses a critical unmet need in diabetes management by evaluating a practical intensification strategy that dramatically reduces injection burden while addressing the key concerns of hypoglycemia and weight gain that limit BBT adoption. The trial included continuous glucose monitoring (CGM) data during weeks 0–8 and 48–52.

Limitations

Limitations include open-label design, different titration algorithms, limited diversity, short-duration safety assessment, and absence of adherence data.

Clinical Implications

IcoSema represents a compelling alternative to BBT for insulin intensification in type 2 diabetes, offering comparable glycemic efficacy with superior profiles for weight management, hypoglycemia risk reduction, and treatment satisfaction. The dramatic reduction in injection frequency (96% fewer injections annually) addresses a major barrier to treatment intensification and may improve long-term adherence in real-world settings. Clinicians should anticipate transient glucose elevations during the first 10 weeks when transitioning patients from established basal insulin to IcoSema, and consider temporary adjustments to existing glucose-lowering medications, particularly for patients with higher baseline insulin requirements or HbA1c levels. The conservative semaglutide dose escalation strategy minimizes gastrointestinal adverse events. The 58% lower insulin dose requirement with IcoSema may also offer cost advantages and reduce insulin-related weight gain concerns.

Knowledge Gaps and Scope for Future Research

- Long-term outcomes
- Optimal transition strategies
- Real-world effectiveness
- Pediatric applicability

16. Risk Factors for Bone Fractures in Type 2 Diabetes and the Impact of Once-weekly Exenatide: Insights from An EXSCEL Post Hoc Analysis

Ref: Maddaloni E, Coleman RL, Holman RR. Risk factors for bone fractures in type 2 diabetes and the impact of once-weekly exenatide: Insights from An EXSCEL post-hoc analysis. Diabetes Res Clin Pract. Diabetes Res Clin Pract . 2025;223:112125.

ABSTRACT

Aim: We examined the impact of once-weekly exenatide (EQW) on incident bone fractures and looked into bone fracture predictors in type 2 diabetes (T2D) participants in the EXenatide Study of Cardiovascular Event Lowering (EXSCEL).

Techniques: With a median follow-up of 3.2 years, EXSCEL randomly assigned 14,752 participants to either EQW 2 mg or a placebo. In this post-hoc study, multivariable Cox proportional hazard regression models were used to assess baseline characteristics linked to incident bone fractures while taking sex and age into consideration as confounders. Cox-proportional hazard models were used for time-to-event analyses and incidence rates were compared between study arms.

Results: 168 participants (1.1%) experienced the main result. While taking metformin at baseline was linked to a 47% lower risk of incident bone fractures [hazard ratio (HR) 0.53, 95% confidence interval (CI) 0.39–0.73, $p < 0.001$], the presence of neuropathy at baseline was linked to a 50% greater risk [HR 1.50, 95% CI 1.10–2.05, $p = 0.010$]. The EQW group and the placebo group had comparable incidence rates of bone fractures (HR 1.11, 95% CI 0.82–1.51, $p = 0.49$).

Conclusion: In individuals with type 2 diabetes, bone fractures are more common in those with diabetic neuropathy, although they are less common in those on metformin. There was no proof that EQW therapy had any effect on bone fractures.

CRITICAL APPRAISAL

What was Known Prior to this Study?

Type 2 diabetes (T2D) is associated with increased risk of hip and nonvertebral fractures compared with nondiabetic populations. Prior observational work suggested links between neuropathy and fracture and an increased fracture risk with thiazolidinediones and possibly sodium-glucose cotransporter-2 (SGLT-2) inhibitors, while data on glucagon-like peptide-1 receptor agonists (GLP-1 RAs) and metformin were inconsistent and largely from meta-analyses or registries.[49-52]

What this Study Adds?

- In this large cardiovascular outcome trial (CVOT) cohort, incident fractures were independently associated with older age and prevalent diabetic neuropathy, and were less frequent among baseline metformin users, after adjustment for age and sex.
- Once-weekly exenatide 2 mg had no detectable effect on overall or major osteoporotic fracture incidence over a median 3.8 years, suggesting a neutral effect on clinical fractures in this context.

Strengths

Strengths include large, double-blind, randomized, placebo-controlled trial with rigorous data collection, long follow-up, and balanced baseline characteristics by treatment, supporting internal validity for treatment comparisons; usage of age- and sex-adjusted multivariable Cox models.

Limitations

Fractures were not a primary or key secondary EXSCEL endpoint; ascertainment relied on adverse event reporting, raising risks of under-ascertainment and reporting bias. Confounding effect by healthier phenotype, shorter disease duration, or competing risks cannot be excluded despite multivariable adjustment. Limited generalizability across GLP-1 RAs and populations.

Clinical Implications

- Presence of clinically evident diabetic neuropathy and advancing age should prompt explicit assessment of skeletal risk and fall risk in T2D, with a lower threshold for dual-energy X-ray absorptiometry (DXA), vertebral fracture assessment, and initiation of bone-protective strategies.
- The association between metformin use and lower fracture risk provides some reassurance about its skeletal safety and supports its continued role as foundational therapy.
- Neutral fracture risk with exenatide in this large trial suggests that bone safety should not be a primary concern.

Knowledge Gaps and Scope for Future Research

- Studies integrating detailed neuropathy phenotyping, fall metrics, bone mineral density (BMD), microarchitecture [high-resolution peripheral quantitative computed tomography (HR-pQCT)], and bone turnover markers
- Head-to-head or harmonized analyses across CVOTs (exenatide, liraglutide, semaglutide, etc.) with standardized fracture adjudication would help determine whether observed differences in bone markers/BMD translate into clinically meaningful, agent-specific fracture effects.
- Inclusion of broader T2D populations

17. Efficacy of Imeglimin Treatment versus Metformin Dose Escalation on Glycemic Control in Subjects with Type 2 Diabetes Treated with a Dipeptidyl Peptidase-4 Inhibitor Plus Low-dose Metformin: A Multicenter, Prospective, Randomized, Open-label, Parallel-group Comparison Study (MEGMI Study)

Ref: Takahashi A, Nomoto H, Yokoyama H, Yokozeki K, Furusawa S, Oe Y, et al. Efficacy of imeglimin treatment versus metformin dose escalation on glycemic control in subjects with type 2 diabetes treated with a dipeptidyl peptidase-4 inhibitor plus low-dose metformin: A multicenter, prospective, randomized, open-label, parallel-group comparison study (MEGMI study). Diabetes Obes Metab. 2025;27(3):1466-76.

ABSTRACT

Aim: Aim of the study is to evaluate the effects of increasing the dosage of metformin versus adding imeglimin on glycemic control in individuals with type 2 diabetes receiving low-dose metformin (500–1,000 mg/day) and a dipeptidyl peptidase-4 inhibitor.

Supplies and procedures: Imeglimin (2,000 mg/day) or metformin escalation was administered for 24 weeks to eligible participants in this multicenter, open-labeled, prospective, randomized, parallel-group comparison research. The mean change in glycated hemoglobin (HbA1c) throughout a 24-week period was the main outcome. The occurrence of adverse events, modifications in metabolic parameters, biomarkers, and variables linked to HbA1c improvement were examined as secondary objectives.

Results: There were 73 subjects who met the eligibility requirements. The entire analysis set was comprised of 65 people. At 24 weeks, imeglimin (n = 33) improved HbA1c more than metformin dose escalation (n = 32) [from 7.61 ± 0.48% to 6.93 ± 0.49% in imeglimin and from 7.56 ± 0.61% to 7.09 ± 0.56% in metformin escalation; change difference: 0.21% (95% confidence interval: 0.41–0.01%) (p = 0.038)]. Nevertheless, seven subjects in the imeglimin group stopped taking the medication due to severe gastrointestinal side effects. Imeglimin therapy lowered liver enzyme increase and significantly decreased body weight in intragroup pre/post-comparisons. Indicators of fatty liver disease and HbA1c improvement levels were significantly correlated in the imeglimin group.

Conclusion: In contrast to metformin dose escalation, imeglimin in conjunction with a dipeptidyl peptidase-4 inhibitor and low-dose metformin improved HbA1c.

CRITICAL APPRAISAL

What was Known Prior to this Study?

- Metformin is the established first-line agent in type 2 diabetes (T2D), with dose-dependent glycated hemoglobin (HbA1c) lowering but limited by gastrointestinal (GI) intolerance, lactic acidosis risk.
- Dipeptidyl peptidase 4 inhibitors (DPP-4i) are widely used in East Asian populations, with good safety, low hypoglycemia risk, and weight neutrality, and are often combined with metformin.
- Imeglimin, a tetrahydrotriazine oral agent, had shown HbA1c reduction as monotherapy and in combination (including with metformin or DPP-4i) in phase II/III trials, with generally favorable short-term safety.

- Prior evidence suggested complementary mechanisms for imeglimin but no head-to-head, prospective interventional trial examined imeglimin add-on versus intensifying metformin in patients already on both DPP-4i and metformin.[53-55]

What this Study Adds?

- It provides the first randomized, multicenter, pragmatic-style comparison of imeglimin add-on versus metformin dose escalation in DPP-4i + low-dose metformin-treated T2D, reflecting a common Japanese prescribing pattern.
- It demonstrates a statistically significant but small incremental HbA1c benefit of imeglimin over metformin escalation at 24 weeks (–0.21% difference).
- It shows imeglimin is associated with modest weight loss and potential hepatic/metabolic pleiotropy effects beyond glycemia.
- 18.9% of imeglimin-treated participants discontinued due to GI symptoms.

Strengths

Strengths include randomized, multicentric design, and prespecified protocol and registration.

Limitations

Limitations include open-label design, small sample and limited power, short duration, metformin dosing context and external validity, no postprandial or continuous glucose monitoring (CGM) data in this main trial, potential selection bias and limited generalizability and conflict of interest.

Clinical Implications

In Japanese-style regimens where metformin is already near or at tolerated doses and DPP-4i is in place, adding imeglimin yields an additional ≈0.2% HbA1c reduction on average, with possibly greater benefit in those with higher baseline HbA1c.

The hepatic enzyme and Fatty Liver Index (FLI) improvements suggest imeglimin might be preferable in patients with coexistent fatty liver or mild transaminitis, provided GI tolerability is acceptable.

The relatively high rate of GI discontinuation mandates careful patient selection, counseling and possibly slower uptitration although the trial used a fixed 2,000 mg dose.

Knowledge Gaps and Scope for Future Research

Long-term efficacy and safety; cardiovascular and renal outcomes; GI tolerability management; given the enzyme and FLI signals, dedicated imaging and biopsy-based NAFLD/NASH (Nonalcoholic Fatty Liver Disease/Nonalcoholic Steatohepatitis) studies could elucidate hepatic histological effects and potential use in metabolic-associated steatotic liver disease.

REFERENCES [Drugs and Therapeutics (Part 2)]

1. Newsome PN, Buchholtz K, Cusi K, Linder M, Okanoue T, Ratziu V, et al. A placebo-controlled trial of subcutaneous semaglutide in nonalcoholic steatohepatitis (phase 2). N Engl J Med. 2021;384:1113-24.
2. Harrison SA, Bedossa P, Guy CD, Schattenberg JM, Loomba R, Taub R, et al. A phase 3, randomized trial of resmetirom in NASH with liver fibrosis. N Engl J Med. 2024;390(6):497-509.
3. Sanyal AJ, Van Natta ML, Clark J. Prospective study of outcomes in adults with NAFLD, highlighting fibrosis stage as a key prognostic determinant. N Engl J Med. 2021;385(17):1559-69.
4. Rinella ME, Neuschwander-Tetri BA, Siddiqui MS, Abdelmalek MF, Caldwell S, Barb D, et al. AASLD practice guidance on clinical assessment and management of NAFLD/MASLD. Hepatology. 2023;77(5):1797-835.
5. Aronne LJ, Horn DB, le Roux CW, Ho W, Falcon BL, Gomez Valderas E, et al. Tirzepatide vs Semaglutide for Obesity. N Engl J Med. 2025;393(1):26-36.
6. Rodriguez PJ, Goodwin Cartwright BM, Gratzl S, Brar R, Baker C, et al. Semaglutide vs Tirzepatide for Weight Loss. JAMA Intern Med. 2024;184(9):1056-64.
7. Garvey WT, Batterham RL, Bhatta M, Buscemi S, Christensen LN, Frias JP, et al. STEP 5: Two-year Semaglutide Effects. Nat Med. 2022;28(10):2083-91.
8. Jastreboff AM, Aronne LJ, Ahmad NN, Wharton S, Connery L, Alves B, et al. Tirzepatide for Obesity (SURMOUNT-1). N Engl J Med. 2022;387(3):205-16.

9. Loomba R, Hartman ML, Lawitz EJ, Vuppalanchi R, Boursier J, Bugianesi E, et al. Tirzepatide for metabolic dysfunction-associated steatohepatitis with liver fibrosis. N Engl J Med. 2024;391(4):299-310.
10. Sanyal AJ, Newsome PN, Kliers I, Østergaard LH, Long MT, Kjær MS, et al. Phase 3 trial of semaglutide in metabolic dysfunction-associated steatohepatitis. N Engl J Med. 2025;392(22):2089-99.
11. European Association for the Study of the Liver, European Association for the Study of Diabetes, European Association for the Study of Obesity. EASL-EASD-EASO Clinical Practice Guidelines on the management of metabolic dysfunction-associated steatotic liver disease (MASLD). J Hepatol. 2024;81(3):492-542.
12. Heerspink HJL, Sattar N, Pavo I, Haupt A, Duffin KL, Yang Z, et al. Effects of tirzepatide versus insulin glargine on kidney outcomes in type 2 diabetes in the SURPASS-4 trial: post-hoc analysis of an open-label, randomised, phase 3 trial. Lancet Diabetes Endocrinol. 2022;10(11):774-85.
13. Perkovic V, Tuttle KR, Rossing P, Mahaffey KW, Mann JFE, Bakris G, et al. Effects of semaglutide on chronic kidney disease in patients with type 2 diabetes. N Engl J Med. 2024;391(2):109-21.
14. Heerspink HJL, Wheeler DC, Pasko DA, Miao S, Tighiouart H, Appel GB, et al. A meta-analysis of albuminuria as a surrogate endpoint for kidney failure. Nat Med. 2025;32(1): 281-7.
15. Brown RJ, Araujo-Vilar D, Cheung PT, Dunger D, Garg A, Jack M, et al. The diagnosis and management of lipodystrophy syndromes: a multi-society practice guideline. J Clin Endocrinol. Metab. 2016;101:4500-11.
16. Oral EA, Simha V, Ruiz E, Andewelt A, Premkumar A, Snell P, et al. Leptin-replacement therapy for lipodystrophy. N Engl J Med. 2002;346(8):570-8.
17. Jastreboff AM, Aronne LJ, Ahmad NN, Wharton S, Connery L, Alves B, et al. Tirzepatide once weekly for the treatment of obesity. N Engl J Med. 2022;387(3):205-16.
18. Roumane A, Nolan JJ, Sherlock M, Han W, Heisler LK, Rochford JJ, et al. GLP-1 receptor agonist improves metabolic disease in a pre-clinical mouse model of lipodystrophy. Sci Rep. 2024;14:9967.
19. Thomas MK, Nikooienejad A, Bray R, Cui X, Wilson J, Duffin K, Milicevic Z, et al. Dual GIP and GLP-1 receptor agonist tirzepatide improves beta-cell function and insulin sensitivity in type 2 diabetes. J Clin Endocrinol Metab. 2021;106(2): 388-96.
20. Heise T, Mari A, DeVries JH, Urva S, Li J, Pratt EJ, Coskun T, et al. Effects of subcutaneous tirzepatide versus placebo or semaglutide on pancreatic islet function and insulin sensitivity in adults with type 2 diabetes: a multicentre, randomised, double-blind, parallel-arm, phase 1 clinical trial. Lancet Diabetes Endocrinol. 2022;10(6):418-29.
21. Jastreboff AM, Aronne LJ, Ahmad NN, Wharton S, Connery L, Elves B, et al.; SURMOUNT-1 Investigators. Tirzepatide once weekly for the treatment of obesity. N Engl J Med. 2022;387(3):205-16.
22. Eldor R, Avraham N, Rosenberg O, Shpigelman M, Golan-Cohen A, Cukierman-Yaffe T, et al. Gradual Titration of Semaglutide Results in Better Treatment Adherence and Fewer Adverse Events: A Randomized Controlled Open-Label Pilot Study Examining a 16-Week Flexible Titration Regimen Versus Label-Recommended 8-Week Semaglutide Titration Regimen. Diabetes Care. 2025;48(9):1607-11.
23. Mody R, Manjelievskaia J, Marchlewicz EH, Malik RE, Zimmerman NM, Irwin DE, et al. Greater adherence and persistence with injectable dulaglutide compared with injectable semaglutide at 1-year follow-up: data from US clinical practice. Clin Ther. 2022;44(4):537-54.
24. Zhang X, Wang L, Qin G, Liu Y, Ding Y, Zhang Q, et al. Gastrointestinal adverse events associated with semaglutide: A pharmacovigilance study based on FDA adverse event reporting system. Front Public Health. 2022;10:996179.
25. Neal B, Perkovic V, Mahaffey KW, de Zeeuw D, Fulcher G, Erondu N, et al. Canagliflozin and cardiovascular and renal events in type 2 diabetes. N Engl J Med. 2017;377:644-57.
26. Sendor R, Stürmer T. Core concepts in pharmacoepide-miology: confounding by indication and the role of active comparators. Pharmacoepidemiol Drug Saf 2022;31:261-9.
27. Mahendraraj K, Lau D, Sampson UK. Exploration of residual confounding in analyses of associations of metformin in a type 2 diabetes population. JAMA Health Forum. 2022;3(10):e223742.
28. Verma S, Mazer CD, Al-Omran M, Inzucchi SE, Fitchett D, Hehnke U, et al. Cardiovascular outcomes and safety of empagliflozin in patients with type 2 diabetes mellitus and peripheral artery disease: a subanalysis of EMPA-REG OUTCOME. Circulation. 2018;137(4):405-7.
29. Sacre JW, Wentworth JM, Magliano DJ, Shaw JE. Incidence of Type 2 Diabetes With Verapamil Compared With Other Calcium Channel Blockers. Diabetes Care. 2025;48(12):2111-8.
30. Malayeri A, Zakerkish M, Ramesh F, Galehdari H, Hemmati AA, Angali KA. The Effect of Verapamil on TXNIP Gene Expression, GLP1R mRNA, Fasting Blood Glucose, and Postprandial Blood Glucose in Patients With Type 2 Diabetes. Front Endocrinol (Lausanne). 2021;12:704063.
31. Forlenza GP, McVean J, Beck RW, Bauza C, Bailey R, Buckingham B, et al. Effect of verapamil on pancreatic beta cell function in newly diagnosed pediatric type 1 diabetes: a randomized clinical trial. JAMA. 2023;329(12):990-9.
32. Rosenstock J, Bailey T, Connery L, Miller E, Desouza C, Wang Q, et al. Weekly fixed-dose insulin efsitora in type 2 diabetes without previous insulin therapy (QWINT-1). N Engl J Med. 2025;393:325-35.
33. Wysham C, Bajaj HS, Del Prato S, Franco DR, Kiyosue A, Dahl D, et al. Insulin efsitora versus degludec in insulin-naïve type 2 diabetes (QWINT-2). N Engl J Med. 2024;391: 2201-11.
34. Rosenstock J, Bain SC, Gowda A, Jódar E, Liang B, Lingvay I, et al. Weekly insulin icodec vs daily glargine U100 in insulin-naïve type 2 diabetes (ONWARDS 1). N Engl J Med. 2023;389:297-308.

35. Badve SV, Bilal A, Lee MMY, Sattar N, Gerstein HC, Ruff CT, et al. Effects of GLP-1 receptor agonists on kidney and cardiovascular disease outcomes: a meta-analysis of randomised controlled trials. Lancet Diabetes Endocrinol. 2025;13(1):15-28.
36. Lin YM, Wu JY, Lee MC, Su CL, Toh HS, Chang WT, et al. Comparative cardiovascular effectiveness of glucagon-like peptide-1 receptor agonists and sodium-glucose cotransporter-2 inhibitors in atherosclerotic cardiovascular disease phenotypes: a systematic review and meta-analysis. Eur Heart J Cardiovasc Pharmacother. 2025;11:174-89.
37. Neuen BL, Fletcher RA, Heath L, Perkovic A, Vaduganathan M, Badve SV, et al. Cardiovascular, kidney, and safety outcomes with GLP-1 receptor agonists alone and in combination with SGLT2 inhibitors in type 2 diabetes: a systematic review and meta-analysis. Circulation. 2024;150(22):1781-90.
38. Riddell MC, Heller S, Carstensen L, Pagliaro Rocha TM, Kehlet Watt S, Woo VC. The effect of once-weekly insulin icodec vs once-daily basal insulin on physical activity-attributed hypoglycaemia in type 2 diabetes: a post hoc analysis of ONWARDS 1–5. Diabetologia. 2025;68(7): 1416-22.
39. Bajaj HS, Ásbjörnsdóttir B, Bari TJ, Begtrup K, Vilsbøll T, Rosenstock J. Once-weekly insulin icodec compared with daily basal insulin analogues in type 2 diabetes: participant-level meta-analysis of the ONWARDS 1–5 trials. Diabetes Obes Metab. 2024;26(9):3810-20.
40. Younk LM, Mikeladze M, Tate D, Davis SN. Exercise-related hypoglycemia in diabetes mellitus. Expert Rev Endocrinol Metab. 2011;6(1):93-108.
41. Mathieu C, Giorgino F, Kim SG, Larsen JH, Philis-Tsimikas A, Ramachandran A, et al. Once-weekly IcoSema versus once-weekly insulin icodec in type 2 diabetes management (COMBINE 1): An open-label, multicentre, treat-to-target, randomised, phase 3a trial. Lancet Diabetes Endocrinol. 2025;13:568-79.
42. Lingvay I, Benamar M, Chen L, Fu A, Jódar E, Nishida T, et al. Once-weekly IcoSema versus once-weekly semaglutide in adults with type 2 diabetes: the COMBINE 2 randomised clinical trial. Diabetologia. 2025;68:739-51.
43. Billings LK, Andreozzi F, Frederiksen M, Gourdy P, Gowda A, Ji L, et al. Once-weekly IcoSema versus multiple daily insulin injections in type 2 diabetes management (COMBINE 3): an open-label, multicentre, treat-to-target, non-inferiority, randomised, phase 3a trial. Lancet Diabetes Endocrinol. 2025;13(7):556-67.
44. Nauck MA, Quast DR, Wefers J, Meier JJ. GLP-1 receptor agonists in the treatment of type 2 diabetes - state-of-the-art. Mol Metab. 2021;46:101102.
45. Billings LK, Doshi A, Gouet D, Oviedo A, Rodbard HW, Tentolouris N, et al. Efficacy and safety of IDegLira versus basal-bolus insulin therapy in patients with type 2 diabetes uncontrolled on metformin and basal insulin: the DUAL VII randomized clinical trial. Diabetes Care. 2018;41(5): 1009-16.
46. Owens DR, Luzio SD, Sert-Langeron C, Riddle MC. Effects of initiation and titration of a single pre-prandial dose of insulin glulisine while continuing titrated insulin glargine in type 2 diabetes: a 6-month 'proof-of-concept' study. Diabetes Obes Metab. 2011;13(11):1020-7.
47. Meece J. Basal Insulin Intensification in Patients with Type 2 Diabetes: A Review. Diabetes Ther. 2018;9(3): 877-90.
48. Kalra S, Das AK, Sahay RK, Baruah MP, Tiwaskar M, Das S, et al. Consensus Recommendations on GLP-1 RA Use in the Management of Type 2 Diabetes Mellitus: South Asian Task Force. Diabetes Ther. 2019;10(5):1645-717.
49. Maddaloni E, Coleman RL, Holman RR. Risk factors for bone fractures in type 2 diabetes and the impact of once-weekly exenatide: Insights from an EXSCEL post-hoc analysis. Diabetes Res Clin Pract. 2025;223:112125.
50. Vilaca T, Schini M, Harnan S, Sutton A, Poku E, Allen IE, et al. The risk of hip and non-vertebral fractures in type 1 and type 2 diabetes: a systematic review and meta-analysis update. Bone. 2020;137:115457.
51. Starup-Linde J, Gregersen S, Frost M, Vestergaard P. Use of glucose-lowering drugs and risk of fracture in patients with type 2 diabetes. Bone. 2017;95:136-42.
52. Cheng L, Hu Y, Li YY, Cao X, Bai N, Lu TT, et al. Glucagon-like peptide-1 receptor agonists and risk of bone fracture in patients with type 2 diabetes: A meta-analysis of randomized controlled trials. Diabetes Metab Res Rev. 2019;35(7):e3168.
53. Takahashi A, Nomoto H, Yokoyama H, Yokozeki K, Furusawa S, Oe Y, et al. Efficacy of imeglimin treatment versus metformin dose escalation on glycemic control in subjects with type 2 diabetes treated with a dipeptidyl peptidase-4 inhibitor plus low-dose metformin (MEGMI study). Diabetes Obes Metab. 2025;27(3):1466-76.
54. Dubourg J, Fouqueray P, Quinslot D, Grouin JM, Kaku K. Long-term safety and efficacy of imeglimin as monotherapy or in combination with existing antidiabetic agents in Japanese patients with type 2 diabetes (TIMES 2): A 52-week, open-label, multicentre phase 3 trial. Diabetes Obes Metab. 2022;24:609-19.
55. Nomoto H, Takahashi A, Nakamura A, Kurihara H, Takeuchi J, Nagai S,et al. Add-on imeglimin versus metformin dose escalation: study protocol for the MEGMI study. BMJ Open Diabetes Res Care. 2022;10:e002815.

Section 6: TYPE 1 DIABETES

Section Editor: Sumit Kumar Chakrabarti

1. Clinical Characteristics in Swedish Children with and without Autoantibodies at the Time of Type 1 Diabetes Diagnosis

Ref: Hedlund E, Maziarz M, Lindahl T, Elding-Larsen H, Forsander G, Persson M, et al. Clinical characteristics in Swedish children with and without autoantibodies at the time of type 1 diabetes diagnosis. Diabetes Care. 2025;48(12):2067-73.

ABSTRACT

Objective: Although autoantibodies have long been identified as biomarkers of islet autoimmunity in type 1 diabetes, it is unclear how they contribute to the pathophysiology of the disease. This study examined the clinical and genetic features of children diagnosed with type 1 diabetes, both with and without autoantibodies.

Methods and research design: As part of Sweden's nationwide Better Diabetes Diagnosis study, data were gathered from children (<0.001) compared at the time of diabetes diagnosis. Participants were divided into groups according to whether or not they had autoantibodies. Age at diagnosis, sex, glycated hemoglobin (HbA1c), diabetic ketoacidosis (DKA), parental inheritance of type 1 and type 2 diabetes, C-peptide level, body mass index standard deviation score (BMI-SDS), and human leukocyte antigen (HLA) genotype were all compared. For comparisons, we employed logistic regression, *t*-tests, and χ^2 tests.

Results: At the time of type 1 diabetes diagnosis, 169 (6.1%) of the 2,753 children were autoantibody negative. Compared to 56% of children with autoantibodies, 66% of those were boys ($p = 0.009$). Additionally, children lacking autoantibodies were more likely to have a parental history of type 2 diabetes (8% vs. 2%), had a higher HbA1c at diagnosis [11.3% vs. 10.8% (100 vs. 94 mmol/mol), $p = 0.003$], and were less likely to present with DKA (9% vs. 15%, $p = 0.039$). The children with and without autoantibodies did not differ in terms of age at diagnosis, C-peptide levels, BMI-SDS, or HLA genotype.

Conclusion: When comparing children with and without autoantibodies at type 1 diabetes diagnosis, we found differences in clinical features, suggesting possible heterogeneity in the pathophysiology of the disease across subgroups.

CRITICAL APPRAISAL

What was Known Prior to this Study?

Genetic predisposition and environmental factors are known to contribute to the disease pathogenesis. The immune system drives β-cell destruction through autoantibody production. There are activation and interaction of T and B cells also. The presence of at least two antibodies, combined with an human leukocyte antigen (HLA) risk profile, leads to a 10-year risk of 70% for developing type 1 diabetes and a lifetime risk approaching 100%. According to the new staging criteria, positive autoantibody combined with normoglycemia is considered stage 1 diabetes, whereas clinical diabetes is viewed as stage 3.

However, the role of autoantibodies in the type 1 diabetes pathogenesis remains unclear, and ~10% of patients have been shown to present without autoantibodies at the time of type 1 diabetes diagnosis. Children without autoantibodies at the time of type 1 diabetes diagnosis have been referred to as "type 1b diabetes".

What does this Study Add?

- This study investigated potential clinical differences at diagnosis of type 1 diabetes children with and without autoantibodies. Data were collected from children (<18 years) at the time of diabetes diagnosis as part of Sweden's National Better Diabetes Diagnosis study.
- The mean age at type 1 diabetes diagnosis for the 2,753 children was 10.0 (SD 4.3) years; with 57% ($n = 1,557$) were boys.
- Autoantibody negative at the time of diagnosis was 6.1% ($n = 169$).
- Among children without autoantibodies, 66% ($n = 112$ of 169) were boys.
- Among children with autoantibodies 56% ($n = 1,445$ of 2,584) were boys ($p = 0.009$).
- The glycated hemoglobin (HbA1c) level was higher among those without autoantibodies compared with those with autoantibodies at the time of diagnosis [11.3% vs. 10.8% (100 vs. 94.2 mmol/mol), $p = 0.003$].
- Subjects without autoantibody were less likely to present with diabetic ketoacidosis (DKA) (9% vs. 15%, $p = 0.039$).
- Regarding parental history of type 1 diabetes, the study did not find any difference between the group with and without autoantibodies.
- It was more common for children without autoantibodies to have a parent with type 2 diabetes than for children with autoantibodies (8% vs. 2%, $p < 0.001$).
- The study did not find any statistically significant differences for age at diagnosis, C-peptide levels, body mass index standard deviation score (BMI-SDS), or HLA risk group between the two groups.

Major Strengths of the Study

It was a large study of type 1 diabetes subjects with >2,700 patients enrolled when they were first diagnosed. Trial design was elaborate to find assessments of multiple characteristics. There was high rate of participant retention. These allowed for robust data analyses, including comparison between two subgroups. The outcome elaborated different differences in the characteristics between auto antibody positive versus negative subjects.

Limitations of the Study

The study population belonged to one country only, Sweden. It remains speculative whether data of one European country could be applicable and comparable to population of other geographic regions like our part of country, southeast Asia, or Africa or other places.

Also, the characteristics were studied only at the time of diagnosis. The possibility of any change in some of them over time, as children age, was not followed up.

Implications of the Findings for the Clinicians

Clinicians should be aware of the heterogeneity of the clinical characteristics as well as pathogenesis of type 1 diabetes. Autoantibody was negative in about 6% of the study population, so antibody negativity by no means excludes type 1 diabetes diagnosis.

Knowledge Gaps Identified and Scope for Future Research

Reasonable explanation of the findings underlying the heterogenous characters remains largely speculative. Autoantibody negative children showed more HbA1c but less events of DKA. These areas need more study to gather in depth knowledge.

2. Repeated OGTT versus Continuous Glucose Monitoring for Predicting Development of Stage 3 Type 1 Diabetes: A Longitudinal Analysis

Ref: Desouter AK, Keymeulen B, Van de Velde U, Van Dalem A, Lapauw B, De Block C, et al. Repeated OGTT Versus Continuous Glucose Monitoring for Predicting Development of Stage 3 Type 1 Diabetes: A Longitudinal Analysis. Diabetes Care. 2025;48(4):528-36.

ABSTRACT

Objective: The majority of the evidence supporting the use of continuous glucose monitoring (CGM) in place of oral glucose tolerance tests (OGTTs) in people with type 1 diabetes who are not yet symptomatic comes from cross-sectional studies. In order to forecast the progression to stage 3 type 1 diabetes, we compared the diagnostic performance of repeated CGM, glycated hemoglobin (HbA1c), and OGTT measurements using longitudinal data.

Methods and research design: In a multicenter trial, 34 multiple autoantibody-positive first-degree relatives (FDRs) [body mass index standard deviation score (BMI-SDS) <2] were monitored for a median of 3.5 [interquartile range (IQR) 2.0–7.5] years using semiannual 5-day CGM recordings, HbA1c, and OGTT. Progression status was used to compare longitudinal patterns. Receiver operating characteristic (ROC) areas under the curve (AUC), the Kaplan–Meier method, baseline Cox proportional hazards models (concordance), and extended Cox proportional hazards models with time-varying covariates were used to predict rapid (<3 years) and overall progression to stage 3 in multiple record data (n = 197 OGTTs and concurrent CGM recordings), adjusted for intraindividual correlations [corrected Akaike information criterion (AICc)].

Results: 17 out of 34 FDRs (baseline median age 16.6 years) developed stage 3 type 1 diabetes after a median of 40 (IQR: 20–91) months. With significant intra- and interindividual variability, CGM measurements rose near onset in tandem with OGTT changes. The best OGTT and CGM measurements predicted both quick (ROC AUC = 0.86–0.92) and overall progression (concordance = 0.73–0.78) cross-sectionally. OGTT-derived AUC glucose (AICc = 71) performed better in longitudinal models than the best CGM measure (AICc = 75) and HbA1c (AICc = 80) (all $p < 0.001$). While OGTT-based multivariable models continued to be superior (AICc = 59), HbA1c complemented repeated CGM metrics (AICc = 68).

Conclusion: Repeated CGM and HbA1c were almost as successful in predicting stage 3 type 1 diabetes in longitudinal models as OGTT, and they might be more practical for long-term clinical monitoring.

CRITICAL APPRAISAL

What was Known Prior to this Study?

Presymptomatic type 1 diabetes is defined by the presence of multiple (two or more) islet autoantibodies (mAAbs). It confers a 90% 20-year risk of developing symptomatic T1 diabetes both in children and adults. This presymptomatic phase starts with normoglycemia (stage 1) but progresses to dysglycemia (stage 2) and later when clinical onset approaches, it is called stage 3. Screening for presymptomatic type 1 diabetes has gained momentum with the US Food and Drug Administration approval of teplizumab, the first therapy that can delay insulin initiation. Presymptomatic disease staging is currently based on findings from oral glucose tolerance tests (OGTTs) and increasing glycated hemoglobin (HbA1c) values. A 10% rise in

HbA1c is a specific indicator of impending clinical onset of diabetes.

Several continuous glucose monitoring (CGM) metrics, particularly time out of range during the daytime, have been shown to predict disease progression in cross-sectional studies in at-risk children.

A large TrialNet study found that OGTT-derived metrics outperformed CGM.

What does this Study Add?

The current study compared the diagnostic performance of serial CGM, HbA1c, and OGTT metrics in predicting clinical onset. The study was based on longitudinal data collected by the Belgian Diabetes Registry (BDR).

This study showed that longitudinal analysis with repeated intermittent CGM metrics, especially when combined with HbA1c, were nearly as effective as repeated OGTTs for predicting progression to stage 3 type 1 diabetes in first-degree relatives (FDRs) who are mAAb1 positive. Both CGM and OGTT showed considerable intra- and interindividual variability over time.

The study followed longitudinal prediction models. Observations indicated that repeated CGM recordings alone provide less predictive information compared with repeated OGTTs. This observation was similar to the TrialNet's primarily cross-sectional report.

Major Strengths of the Study

Novel concept of the study. Backed by robust statistical analysis.

Limitations of the Study

- Predominant European-Caucasian descent of the cohort
- The start of metabolic follow-up did not align with the moment of seroconversion.

Implications of the Findings for the Clinicians

The message to the clinicians implies that intermittent CGM, especially when combined with HbA1c, may serve as a minimally invasive alternative to OGTTs for long-term monitoring of individuals with presymptomatic diabetes.

Knowledge Gaps Identified and Scope for Future Research

Further validation is needed for longitudinal studies incorporating newer CGM technologies. Increased CGM frequency is also needed. There should be direct comparisons of psychological impact, user acceptance, practical implementation, and cost-effectiveness.

3. The Efficacy of Islet Autoantibody Screening with or without Genetic Prescreening Strategies for the Identification of Presymptomatic Type 1 Diabetes

Ref: Bonifacio E, Coelho R, Ewald DA, Gemulla G, Hubmann M, Jarosz-Chobot P, et al. The efficacy of islet autoantibody screening with or without genetic pre-screening strategies for the identification of presymptomatic type 1 diabetes. Diabetologia. 2025;68(6):1101-7.

ABSTRACT

Treatment that can postpone the start of the disease delay the onset of the disease is one of the many clinical benefits of early identification of type 1 diabetes in its presymptomatic stage. The goal of current screening is to detect islet autoantibody positivity. Ideal testing is suggested at ages 2, 6, and 10 years, with a possible sensitivity of up to 80%. However, participation rates and the expenses of multiple screenings present difficulties. Although genetic prescreening has been proposed as an additional tactic to identify high-risk patients before autoantibody testing, its practical advantages are still unknown. Subsets of the population at increased risk can be identified using broad genetic selection techniques based on human leukocyte antigen (HLA) typing, family history, or polygenic risk scores. These methods, however, have problems with low recall rates, socioeconomic biases, and limited applicability across a variety of ancestries. The infrastructure needs and cost-effectiveness of incorporating genetic testing into standard medical treatment continue to be major obstacles. Predictive value may be increased by combining autoantibody and genetic testing, particularly with advancements like point-of-care genetic testing. However, maximizing public and healthcare provider engagement, guaranteeing high participation, and addressing socioeconomic and demographic gaps are more important for the eventual success of any screening program than particular tactics. In order to sustain follow-up adherence and increase recall rates, digital health infrastructure may be essential. In conclusion, genetic screening before islet autoantibody testing may be feasible in some situations, if adequate resources and fair tactics are used, even if repeated islet autoantibody screening is still the most successful standalone method. To fully realize the potential of early type 1 diabetes detection programs, public involvement and strong infrastructure are crucial.

CRITICAL APPRAISAL

What was Known Prior to this Study?

Optimal time for islet autoantibody screening is at 3 years of age if screening is performed once. It can identify around 35% of individuals who will develop clinical type 1 diabetes by the time they are 18 years old.

Increased frequency of screening tests done at ages 2 and 6 years increases the sensitivity of screening to approximately 65%. A further screen at 10 years of age, if available, captures the majority of individuals who will develop type 1 diabetes by 18 years of age. Additional screening will incur additional costs and increase the risk of drop out.

What does this Study Add?

This study provides the idea of incorporating a prior genetic screening test. It aims to pick up the selected subjects susceptible to develop type 1 diabetes by genetic testing. For type 1 diabetes, selection can be achieved through use of family history, human leukocyte antigen (HLA) typing, and polygenic risk scores in children and adolescents. This could include all youth with a first-degree relative with type 1 diabetes or with HLADR3 or HLA-DR4-DQ8 haplotypes positivity. After that they are to be subjected into islet autoantibody screening programs. The idea is to reduce the number and, consequently, the cost of islet autoantibody testing.

Major Strengths of the Study

If one is working in a developed and digitally advanced healthcare infrastructure, prior genetic testing can identify the susceptible individuals. Subsequent autoantibody testing can detect the patient in presymptomatic phase. The patient can be identified for treatment with teplizumab which can often prevent the subsequent development of diabetes.

Limitations of the Study

Genetic risk determination for type 1 diabetes by genetic testing in itself is not a diagnosis of type 1 diabetes or its presymptomatic stage. It necessitates further testing for islet autoantibody to confirm the diagnosis. The more number the patient is recalled for testing increases the budget as well as the risk of participation loss.

Implications of the Findings for the Clinicians

Clinicians have to advise tests in a potential real-world setting, where rate of participant turning up for subsequent tests is of utmost importance. Asking to come once for genetic testing and then again for autoantibody testing at 2, 6, and 10 years of age bound to increase the loss to follow-up share. Economic burden of the tests is to be kept in mind too. Clinicians have to be decisive in choosing the tests.

Knowledge Gaps Identified and Scope for Future Research

How to choose patients for genetic testing from general population needs further input. These tests are costly and of limited availability. Follow-up adherence is also another issue.

4. Combination SGLT-2 Inhibitor and Glucagon Receptor Antagonist Therapy in Type 1 Diabetes: A Randomized Clinical Trial

Ref: Boeder SC, Thomas RL, Le Roux MJ, Giovannetti ER, Gregory JM, Pettus JH. Combination SGLT-2 inhibitor and glucagon receptor antagonist therapy in type 1 diabetes: A randomized clinical trial. Diabetes Care. 2025;48(1):52-60.

ABSTRACT

Objective: To investigate how insulin-adjunctive treatment with a glucagon receptor antagonist (GRA) and a sodium-glucose cotransporter-2 (SGLT-2) inhibitor affects glycemia, insulin usage, and ketogenesis in type 1 diabetes.

Methods and research design: We evaluated the effects of adjunctive SGLT-2 inhibitor medication (dapagliflozin 10 mg daily) alone and in combination with the GRA volagidemab (70 mg weekly) in 12 persons with type 1 diabetes in a randomized, double-blind, placebo-controlled, crossover experiment. During the insulin-only (baseline), SGLT-2 inhibitor, and combination (SGLT-2 inhibitor + GRA) therapy periods, continuous glucose monitoring, insulin dosage, and insulin withdrawal tests (IWT) were performed to evaluate glucose and ketogenesis during insulinopenia.

Results: In comparison to baseline with SGLT-2 inhibitor, combination therapy improved average glucose and the percentage of time with glucose in the range (70–180 mg/dL) [131 vs. 150 and 138 mg/dL ($p < 0.001$ and $p = 0.01$) and 86% vs. 70% and 78% ($p < 0.001$ and $p = 0.03$), respectively] without increasing hypoglycemia. Combination therapy reduced total daily insulin consumption compared to baseline with SGLT-2 inhibitor [0.41 vs. 0.56 and 0.52 units/kg/day ($p < 0.001$ and $p = 0.002$)]. Peak β-hydroxybutyrate levels during insulin withdrawal test (IWT) were comparable to those attained during the baseline testing period (2.1 mmol/L) and were lower with combination therapy than with SGLT-2 inhibitor (2.0 vs. 2.4 mmol/L; $p = 0.048$). Combination therapy improved treatment acceptance and satisfaction, according to participants.

Conclusion: In type 1 diabetes, glucagon antagonism amplifies the therapeutic benefits of SGLT-2 inhibition. Combination therapy lowers insulin dosage, enhances glycemic control, and offers a way to maximize the advantages of SGLT-2 inhibitors while lowering the risk of diabetic ketoacidosis.

CRITICAL APPRAISAL

What was Known Prior to this Study?

The sodium-glucose cotransporter-2 (SGLT-2) inhibitor medications have revolutionized the treatment of type 2 diabetes, heart failure, and chronic kidney disease. However, their use in type 1 diabetes has been limited due to an increased risk of diabetic ketoacidosis (DKA). The major barrier to approval by the United States Food and Drug Administration (US FDA) was three- to fourfold increased risk of DKA.

Research showed that SGLT-2 inhibitor therapy in patients with type 1 diabetes leads to a 37% increase in fasting glucagon levels. The increased glucagon increases endogenous glucose production as well as ketone production, especially under insulinopenic conditions.

So, hypothetically, if a glucagon antagonist could be used in these situations, possible benefit would have been increased to a great extent.

What does this Study Add?

This study used the glucagon receptor antagonist (GRA), volagidemab—a fully human monoclonal antibody that inhibits glucagon receptor (GCGR).

This study analyzed the impact of GRA therapy on ketogenesis, particularly in combination with an SGLT-2 inhibitor.

The study showed blocking glucagon led to significant improvements in metabolic control, decreasing average glucose by 20 mg/dL and increasing absolute percent time in target range by 16%, without increasing hypoglycemia. Additionally, combination therapy reduced total insulin requirements by 27% and reduced peak β-hydroxybutyrate (BHB) during periods of insulinopenia.

The study also showed that combination therapy with SGLT-2 inhibitor and GRA therapy was associated with increased patient reported treatment acceptability and satisfaction in comparison with baseline and SGLT-2 inhibitor alone.

The study did not show significant elevations in bilirubin or alkaline phosphatase which are signs of severe drug-induced liver injury.

Major Strengths of the Study

- This includes a 100% retention rate.
- The randomized, double-blind, placebo-controlled trial design and the crossover format, which removes interparticipant variability and increases the power to detect differences between treatment.
- All participants used automated insulin delivery systems, the gold standard therapy for people with T1D.

Limitations of the Study

- The study included a modest sample size ($n = 12$)
- A moderate treatment duration—4 weeks for each treatment with a 6-week washout phase

Implications of the Findings for the Clinicians

The study demonstrates the potential of combination SGLT-2 inhibitor and GRA therapy as an effective adjunct to insulin in type 1 diabetes. This approach has shown to improve glycemic control and reduce insulin dosing. Also, it suggests a means to minimize the risk of DKA associated with SGLT-2 inhibitor use.

Knowledge Gaps Identified and Scope for Future Research

Scope of further research always remains. A more long-term study may be able to focus on the effects of the combination of SGLT-2 inhibitors and GRAs on the different complications of T1 diabetes.

5. A Randomized Trial Comparing Inhaled Insulin Plus Basal Insulin versus Usual Care in Adults with Type 1 Diabetes

Ref: Hirsch IB, Beck RW, Marak MC, Kudva Y, Akturk HK, Bhargava A, et al. A randomized trial comparing inhaled insulin plus basal insulin versus usual care in adults with type 1 diabetes. Diabetes Care. 2025;48(3):353-60.

ABSTRACT

Objective: To assess an inhaled technosphere insulin (TI) with insulin degludec regimen in persons with type 1 diabetes who were primarily receiving multiple daily insulin injections (MDIs) with continuous glucose monitoring or an automated insulin delivery (AID) system prior to the research.

Methods and design of research: Adults with type 1 diabetes were randomly randomized at 19 sites to either TI with insulin degludec (n = 62) or usual care (UC) with continuation of prestudy insulin administration technique (n = 61) for a period of 17 weeks.

Results: 48% of participants in the research used AID and 45% used MDI. The TI group's mean ± SD glycated hemoglobin (HbA1c) was 7.57% ± 0.97% at baseline and 7.62% ± 1.06% at 17 weeks, while the UC group's was 7.59% ± 0.80% and 7.54% ± 0.77%, respectively [adjusted difference 0.11%; 95% confidence interval (CI) 20.10–0.33; p-value for noninferiority = 0.01]. In 12 (21%) of the TI group and 3 (5%) of the UC group, HbA1c improved by >0.5% (5.5 mmol/mol) from baseline to 17 weeks, but in 15 (26%) of the TI group and 2 (3%) of the UC group, it worsened by >0.5% (5.5 mmol/mol). A short cough was the most frequent side effect of TI, and eight subjects stopped taking it as a result.

Conclusion: After 17 weeks on a TI and degludec regimen, HbA1c in persons with type 1 diabetes was noninferior to UC, which was mostly composed of either AID or MDI. For persons with type 1 diabetes, especially those who need to lower postprandial hyperglycemia, TI should be taken into consideration.

CRITICAL APPRAISAL

What was Known Prior to this Study?

Glycemic targets set by the American Diabetes Association are met in only 20% of adults with type 1 diabetes even with automated insulin delivery (AID) systems.

Inhaled Technosphere insulin (TI) (Afrezza; MannKind, Danbury, CT) is a dry-powder formulation of recombinant human insulin absorbed onto Technosphere microparticles for oral inhalation. TI was approved by the US Food and Drug Administration (FDA) 10 years ago.

But it was not frequently prescribed despite its potential benefits. Most likely the limited use was due to the limited clinical trial data available.

What does this Study Add?

Glycated hemoglobin (HbA1c) improved from baseline to 17 weeks by >0.5% (5.5 mmol/mol) in 12 (21%) in the TI group versus 3 (5%) in the usual care (UC) group. HbA1c worsened by >0.5% (5.5 mmol/mol) in 15 (26%) in the TI group versus 2 (3%) in the UC group. Among participants with baseline HbA1c >7.0% (53 mmol/mol), 8 (21%) in the TI group compared with 0 in the UC group had a 17-week HbA1c level < 7.0% (53 mmol/mol).

Continuous glucose monitoring (CGM)-measured hypoglycemia was observed to be low at baseline and showed little change at 17 weeks in both groups, meeting the pre-specified criterion for noninferiority. Other CGM parameters reflective of hyperglycemia also showed no meaningful differences between the two groups.

There were no cases of DKA.

The current US guideline of TI use is to base initial dosing on an approximate 1:1 conversion of the usual rapid-acting analog (RAA) dose for a patient. However, this is based on the amount of powdered insulin in a cartridge and not on the amount that is actually absorbed in the lungs. Thus, the appropriate, bioequivalent dose of TI should be at least twofold higher than the RAA dose.

The most common side effect was a brief cough associated with TI inhalation.

Major Strengths of the Study

It was a multicenter study. The study design was also different.

Previous trial from Bode et al. indicates that the starting initial TI dose should be 1.0–1.3 times the RAA dose, for most of the dose range, but clinical experience showed that this dose is too low and a higher dose is needed. The initial TI conversion dose in the current trial was much higher than in the earlier trial.

Continuous glucose monitoring was a key component of the current trial unlike that of previous trials. In the current trial CGM was used to monitor for hyperglycemia and hypoglycemia during the daytime and nighttime, which were not available in the previous trial.

The cohorts in the trials were quite different, with just multiple daily insulin injection (MDI) users in the prior trial and both MDI and AID users in the current trial. The inclusion of AID users provided the ability in the current study to compare the TI-degludec regimen with AID.

Limitations of the Study

- The cohort being predominantly of white population
- The length of the follow-up period for the randomized controlled trial (RCT) being only 17 weeks

Implications of the Findings for the Clinicians

Postmeal hyperglycemia is common with type 1 diabetes. Inhaled TI has a more rapid onset of action than RAA insulin. Clinicians can use this property to improve glycemic control in a noninjectable fashion.

Overall, eight participants discontinued TI due to side effect like cough and bronchospasm. So, a clinician must choose his patients wisely and monitor for respiratory side effects.

Knowledge Gaps Identified and Scope for Future Research

Patient selection is very important with respect to prescribing TI.

Future work is needed for better identification of the profile of patients who may be ideal candidates for TI. This will also help us to know for whom a switch to TI is unlikely to be successful.

Establishment of best clinical practices for optimal titration of TI dosing is still awaited.

6. Cardiovascular Outcomes and Efficacy of the PCSK9 Inhibitor Evolocumab in Individuals with Type 1 Diabetes: Insights from the FOURIER Trial

Ref: Kang YM, Giugliano RP, Ran X, Deedwania P, De Ferrari GM, George JT, et al. Cardiovascular outcomes and efficacy of the PCSK9 inhibitor evolocumab in individuals with type 1 diabetes: Insights from the FOURIER trial. Diabetes Care. 2025;48(9):1512-6.

ABSTRACT

Objective: To assess the therapeutic effectiveness of intensive low-density lipoprotein cholesterol (LDL-C) reduction in people with type 1 diabetes mellitus (T1DM).

Methods and research design: Participants with atherosclerotic cardiovascular disease (ASCVD) taking statins were randomized to either evolocumab or a placebo in Further Cardiovascular Outcomes Research With PCSK9 Inhibition in Subjects With Elevated Risk (FOURIER) (median follow-up 2.2 years). Cardiovascular death, myocardial infarction, stroke, hospitalization for unstable angina, or coronary revascularization were the primary endpoints (PEP).

Results: Of the 27,564 individuals, 197 (0.7%) had type 1 diabetes and 10,834 (39.3%) had type 2 diabetes. The 2.5-year PEP Kaplan–Meier rate increased gradually in the placebo arm from 11.0% to 15.2% to 20.4% in individuals without diabetes, type 2 diabetes mellitus (T2DM), and T1DM, respectively ($p < 0.0001$). In the groups with no diabetes, T2DM, and T1DM, the hazard ratios for PEP with evolocumab were 0.87 [95% confidence interval (CI) 0.79–0.96], 0.84 (0.75–0.93), and 0.66 (0.32–1.38), and the absolute risk decrease was 1.3%, 2.5%, and 7.3%, respectively.

Conclusion: People with T1DM and ASCVD may benefit significantly from intensive low-density lipoprotein cholesterol (LDL-C) reduction. In this cohort, more randomized controlled cardiovascular outcome trials are required.

CRITICAL APPRAISAL

What was Known Prior to this Study?

Atherosclerotic cardiovascular disease (ASCVD) is the leading cause of death in people with type 1 diabetes mellitus (T1DM). To reduce this risk, clinical guidelines emphasized the importance of optimal glycemic control and suggested optimization of cardiovascular (CV) risk factors such as dyslipidemia and hypertension. However, these guidelines mostly gathered evidence from observations conducted in individuals with type 2 diabetes mellitus (T2DM), largely because of the limited availability of T1DM-dedicated randomized trials. The data was then extrapolated to the T1DM subjects. This raises concerns about applicability of the recommendations to those with T1DM.

A decline in mortality was observed among people with T1DM over the past decade along with the rising prevalence of T1DM in older adults (≥65 years of age). These observations further stress upon the importance of effective CV risk reduction strategies. We have observed the effects of many glucose-lowering and lipid-modifying therapies that have demonstrated CV benefits primarily in T2DM patients. Whether these benefits extend to people with T1DM remains unclear.

Proprotein convertase subtilisin/kexin type 9 (PCSK9) inhibitors, such as evolocumab, have been shown to significantly lower low-density lipoprotein cholesterol (LDL-C) and reduce the risk of major adverse cardiovascular events (MACEs) in adults with ASCVD. However, its efficacy in individuals with T1DM has not been well-studied. To address this knowledge gap, the Further Cardiovascular Outcomes Research With PCSK9 Inhibition in Subjects With Elevated Risk (FOURIER) study assessed the efficacy of evolocumab in individuals with T1DM.

What does this Study Add?

- Of the 27,564 participants, 16,533 (60.0%) did not have diabetes at baseline, 10,834 (39.3%) had T2DM, and 197 (0.7%) had T1DM. Participants with T1DM were younger, were more likely to be female, and had higher LDL-C and high-sensitivity C-reactive protein levels, compared with those without diabetes or with T2DM.
- Risk of MACE increases with any diabetes type
- In the placebo group, the Kaplan–Meier (KM) event rates at 2.5 years for primary endpoint increased stepwise by diabetes status: 11.0% in participants without diabetes, 15.2% in those with T2DM, and 20.4% in those with T1DM (p trend < 0.0001)
- Evolocumab consistently led to marked reductions in LDL-C concentration irrespective of the presence and type of diabetes
- The observed relative risk reduction for the primary outcome with evolocumab was 13% [hazard ratio (HR) 0.87; 95% confidence interval (CI) 0.79–0.96] for participants without diabetes, 16% for those with T2DM (HR 0.84; 95% CI 0.75–0.93), and 34% (HR 0.66; 95% CI 0.32–1.38) for those with T1DM.

- The efficacy of evolocumab in reducing the risk of MACE was numerically greater for those with T1DM.

Major Strengths of the Study

- More than 27,000 participants, a good number for proper statistical analysis
- Included people without diabetes, with T2DM and T1 diabetes, so the effects of evolocumab can be assessed across the spectrum.
- Robust study design—event-driven, randomized, double-blind, placebo-controlled study
- *Endpoint assessment:* Multiple endpoints were taken into account. The primary endpoint of the FOURIER study was the composite of CV death, myocardial infarction (MI), stroke, hospitalization due to unstable angina, and coronary revascularization when needed.

Limitations of the Study

The proportion of participants with T1DM in the FOURIER trial (0.7%) is almost equal to its prevalence in the general adult population (0.5%). This inherently limits the statistical power to detect significant interactions by diabetes type. Therefore, future studies with a larger number of individuals with T1DM are warranted.

Implications of the Findings for the Clinicians

Type 1 diabetes mellitus is associated with a substantial risk of premature death compared with the general population. CV mortality is more commonly detected in the older subjects, later in life. Robust preventive measures apart from statin in T1DM subjects were lacking. After this FOURIER trial, clinicians will be able to use evolocumab in T1DM patients as an additional preventive measure against ASCVD.

Knowledge Gaps Identified and Scope for Future Research

The current analysis cannot identify any specific mechanisms responsible for the potentially greater CV benefit of PCSK9 inhibition in T1DM despite the comparable degree of LDL-C reduction in all groups.

7. Statin Therapy and Neuropathy in Type 1 Diabetes: A Cross-sectional Study

Ref: Pasha R, Kamath A, Linn Z, Kalteniece A, Bashir B, Schofield JD, et al. Statin therapy and neuropathy in type 1 diabetes: A cross-sectional study. Diabetes Obes Metab. 2025;27(10):5675-82.

ABSTRACT

Aim: The pathophysiology of diabetic peripheral neuropathy (DPN) is influenced by dyslipidemia. Although statins enhance cardiovascular outcomes in diabetics, there is ongoing discussion regarding their possible neurotoxic consequences. The effect of statin use on neuropathy in people with type 1 diabetes mellitus (T1DM) was investigated in this study.

Supplies and procedures: Corneal confocal microscopy (CCM), cardiac autonomic neuropathy (CAN), and DPN symptoms and clinical evaluations were performed on participants with T1DM ($n = 160$) and healthy controls ($n = 64$). Statin use was used to stratify T1DM patients (nonstatin: $n = 68$; statin treated: $n = 92$).

Results: There were notable variances among nonstatin patients, statin patients with T1DM, and healthy controls regarding the diabetic neuropathy symptom score (DNS) (0.49 ± 0.14 vs. 0.90 ± 0.13

vs. 0.15 ± 0.13, $p < 0.001$), neuropathy disability score (NDS) (2.55 ± 0.29 vs. 3.67 ± 0.26 vs. 0.44 ± 0.28, $p < 0.001$), vibration perception threshold (13.68 ± 1.16 vs. 16.03 ± 1.03 vs. 6.05 ± 1.08, $p < 0.001$), corneal nerve fiber density (19.61 ± 1.04 vs. 19.02 ± 0.92 vs. 28.48 ± 0.97, $p < 0.001$), branch density (20.40 ± 2.21 vs. 21.39 ± 1.94 vs. 37.31 ± 2.05, $p < 0.001$), fiber length (11.97 ± 0.51 vs. 11.51 ± 0.45 vs. 16.55 ± 0.47, $p < 0.001$), DB-HRV (26.27 ± 1.76 vs. 24.21 ± 1.51 vs. 30.18 ± 1.67, $p = 0.033$), and 30:15 ratio (1.32 ± 0.04 vs. 1.21 ± 0.03 vs. 1.15 ± 0.07, $p = 0.033$). With the exception of DNS ($p = 0.04$), NDS ($p = 0.009$), and 30:15 ratio ($p = 0.04$), statin-treated patients did not exhibit significant differences in most neuropathy parameters, despite the statin group being substantially older ($p < 0.001$), having a higher body mass index (BMI) ($p = 0.001$), and having had diabetes for a longer period of time ($p < 0.001$).

Conclusion: This study shows that people with T1DM have neuropathic symptoms and impairment, elevated vibration perception thresholds, loss of corneal nerve fibers, and CAN. Despite statin-treated individuals having a greater BMI and a longer duration of diabetes, statin medication was linked to similar levels of DPN and CAN.

CRITICAL APPRAISAL

What was Known Prior to this Study?

Diabetic peripheral neuropathy (DPN) and cardiac autonomic neuropathy (CAN) affect at least 50% of patients with diabetes mellitus. Older age, diabetes duration, and metabolic and vascular factors are also associated with DPN. Statins (HMG-CoA reductase inhibitors) are the most widely prescribed lipid-lowering agents that increased clearance of low-density lipoprotein (LDL) particles and lowering of triglyceride levels.

The impact of statin therapy on DPN remains controversial. It is attributed to reduced production of farnesyl pyrophosphates, particularly ubiquinone, a key enzyme in the mitochondrial respiratory chain. Statin use has been linked with the onset of peripheral neuropathy in some patients, but this appears to be reversible upon discontinuation of the statin.

Previous studies have produced conflicting results ranging from potential neurotoxicity to neuroprotection.

What does this Study Add?

This study tried to address the important clinical question using detailed structural and functional assessments in cases with small and large fiber neuropathy.

The study observed there were no significant differences in the neuropathy symptom profile (2.74 ± 0.66 vs. 4.55 ± 0.61, $p = 0.067$) and McGill pain questionnaire [3.60 ± 1.05 vs. 4.16 ± 0.93, $p = 0.713$] analog score in the type 1 diabetes mellitus (T1DM) statin versus nonstatin group.

The neuropathy disability score (0.44 ± 0.28 vs. 2.55 ± 0.29 vs. 3.67 ± 0.26, $p < 0.001$) and vibration perception threshold (6.05 ± 1.08 vs. 13.68 ± 1.16 vs. 16.03 ± 1.03, $p < 0.001$) were significantly lower in the control group compared to the T1DM nonstatin and statin user group.

Corneal nerve fiber length (16.55 ± 0.47 vs. 11.97 ± 0.51 vs. 11.51 ± 0.45, $p < 0.001$) was denser and more had a longer length in the healthy control group compared with the T1DM nonstatin and statin user group.

Assessment of CAN also did not differ significantly between the control and T1DM nonstatin and statin user groups. They observed deep breathing heart rate variability, the 30:15 ratio and Valsalva ratio.

This study showed that older and heavier patients with a longer duration of T1DM, and therefore, with major risk factors for DPN treated with statins have a comparable degree of neuropathy to patients with T1DM who are younger, of less weight and have a shorter duration of diabetes. The study showed that statin use was associated with a reduced odds for developing idiopathic sensory neuropathy.

Major Strengths of the Study

This is the first large study to conduct a detailed assessment of both neuropathic symptoms and objective functional and structural measures of large and small fiber neuropathy.

Limitations of the Study

Limitation is its cross-sectional design. This restricts the ability to draw definitive conclusions about the long-term effects of statin therapy on the development or progression of neuropathy.

The study may be underpowered to detect smaller or subgroup-specific differences across measures of corneal nerve fiber density analysis.

The sample sizes for individual statins were too small to allow for meaningful subgroup analyses. The study was unable to explore potential differences in neuropathy outcomes between different statins, if any.

Implications of the Findings for the Clinicians

Clinicians should continue to use statins in T1DM as per indication. Statin provides cardioprotection and this study showed that statin use may afford protection from DPN and CAN in patients with T1DM.

Knowledge Gaps Identified and Scope for Future Research

Study population was not large future studies with larger and more balanced groups may be in a better position to investigate whether different statins exert distinct effects on peripheral and autonomic neuropathy.

8. Verapamil and Low-dose Anti-mouse Thymocyte Globulin Combination Therapy Stably Reverses Recent-onset Type 1 Diabetes in NOD Mice by Acting on the Beta Cell and Immune Axes

Ref: Degroote L, Martens PJ, Viaene M, Heremans Y, Leuckx G, Geukens N, et al. Verapamil and low-dose anti-mouse thymocyte globulin combination therapy stably reverses recent-onset type 1 diabetes in NOD mice by acting on the beta cell and immune axes. Diabetologia. 2025;68(10):2263-76.

ABSTRACT

Aim/Hypothesis: Both low doses of antithymocyte globulin (ATG) and the calcium channel blocker verapamil have demonstrated effectiveness in maintaining β-cell activity in individuals with newly diagnosed symptomatic type 1 diabetes (stage 3). We postulated that treatments with distinct targets and complementing mechanisms of action would be more effective in halting β-cell death and fostering disease recovery.

Methods: The potential to promote disease remission and mechanism of action of verapamil administered continuously by drinking water in conjunction with a brief course of low-dose rabbit-anti-mouse ATG (mATG) was investigated in female nonobese diabetic (NOD) mice with recent-onset diabetes.

Results: By day 56 following the start of treatment, verapamil had successfully cured diabetes in 3 out of 15 mice (20%). By day 7 after therapy began, low-dose mATG corrected diabetes in 7 out of 18 mice (39%), but by day 56, the impact had diminished to 3 out of 18 animals (17%). By day 56, 9 out of 20 mice (45%) showed persistent diabetes reversal when verapamil and mATG were combined. This was linked to less severe insulitis, higher pancreatic insulin content, and retained β-cell activity. On day 3 following the commencement of therapy, mATG alone or in combination caused a brief decrease in peripheral blood lymphocytes. However, by day 14, when naive cells had changed to a memory phenotype in both CD4+ and CD8+ T cells, this depletion had mostly subsided. The ratio of CD4+ regulatory T cells to CD8+ effector memory T cells in the pancreatic draining lymph nodes was only greater in combination-treated mice. Regardless of whether the reversed mice got verapamil or not, the expression of the glucose-induced gene producing thioredoxin-interacting protein (TXNIP), a crucial regulator of β-cell death and malfunction, was decreased in the pancreatic β-cells.

Conclusion and interpretation: In NOD mice with recent-onset type 1 diabetes, the combination of verapamil and low-dose mATG was more effective than monotherapy. This concept suggests a promising method for reversing type 1 diabetes in humans by focusing on both the immunological and β-cell axes.

CRITICAL APPRAISAL

What was Known Prior to this Study?

Verapamil, the orally active calcium channel blocker reduced the expression of the thioredoxin-interacting protein (TXNIP), a ubiquitously expressed cellular redox regulator. TXNIP overexpression promoted mitochondria-dependent β-cell apoptosis and TXNIP deficiency stimulated β-cell survival and protected against streptozotocin-induced diabetes.

Polyclonal antithymocyte globulin (ATG) has a unique disease-modifying profile. It depletes conventional T cells, effector memory, and central memory T cells through complement-dependent lysis and T cell apoptosis.

Monotherapy with either of the two agents was effective in reversing stage 3 of type 1 diabetes but the effects waned off subsequently. Long-term effectiveness was lacking. Experience with combination therapy was lacking too.

What does this Study Add?

In the group that received verapamil monotherapy, hyperglycemia reversal was observed in 20% of mice (3 out of 15 mice), which was sustained throughout the 56-day follow-up period.

Similarly, Low dose ATG (antithymocyte globulin) monotherapy resulted in 17% reversal (3 out of 18 mice).

In contrast, the combination of verapamil and low-dose ATG-induced immediate hyperglycemia reversal in 20% of the mice. The efficacy increased progressively, up to 45% (9 out of 20 mice) by the end of the follow-up period. Notably, by day 14 after therapy started, only combination therapy-treated mice demonstrated significantly better preservation of C-peptide secretion compared with untreated control.

The present study pointed out that combination therapy with verapamil and low-dose mATG together also reduced pancreatic insulitis severity. Verapamil treatment reduced *TXNIP* expression in pancreatic β-cells, supporting improved β-cell function.

Major Strengths of the Study

This study is the first to demonstrate the combined efficacy of verapamil and low-dose mATG in reversing type 1 diabetes in recent-onset diabetic nonobese diabetic (NOD) mice.

The combination therapy stably reversed type 1 diabetes in nearly half of the mice.

It was associated with both immune-modulatory and β-cell protective effects, suggesting a synergistic interaction between the two interventions.

Limitations of the Study

Technically, it is a challenging study. It may not be possible to be done in resource poor setting.

Implications of the Findings for the Clinicians

This is not a study conducted on humans. Clinicians need to understand that animal model may be showing promising result, but it needs to be reflected on human population before practically using the model.

Knowledge Gaps Identified and Scope for Future Research

Study was conducted on NOD mice, whether the beneficial results can be observed on humans remains to be explored through future research.

9. Treatment Regimens and Glycemic Outcomes in More than 100,000 Children with Type 1 Diabetes (2013–2022): A Longitudinal Analysis of Data from Pediatric Diabetes Registries

Ref: Zimmermann AT, Lanzinger S, Kummernes SJ, Lund-Blix NA, Holl RW, Fröhlich-Reiterer E, et al. Treatment regimens and glycaemic outcomes in more than 100,000 children with type 1 diabetes (2013-22): a longitudinal analysis of data from paediatric diabetes registries. Lancet Diabetes Endocrinol. 2025;13(1):47-56. Erratum in: Lancet Diabetes Endocrinol. 2025; 13(4):e7.

ABSTRACT

Background: Glycemia has improved, the risk of severe hypoglycemia has decreased, and quality of life has enhanced as a result of advancements in pediatric type 1 diabetes care and increased use of diabetes technology. Glycated hemoglobin (HbA1c) targets have been gradually lowered since 1993. This study used data from eight national and one international juvenile diabetes registry to conduct a longitudinal analysis of HbA1c, treatment plans, and acute complications between 2013 and 2022.

Methods: The Australasian Diabetes Data Network, the Czech National Childhood Diabetes Register, the Danish Registry of Childhood and Adolescent Diabetes, the Norwegian Childhood Diabetes Registry, the Diabetes Prospective Follow-up Registry, the National Paediatric Diabetes Audit of England and Wales, the Swedish Childhood Diabetes Registry, the T1D Exchange Quality Improvement Collaborative, and the SWEET initiative provided the data used in this longitudinal analysis. All youngsters (under 18 years old) who had type 1 diabetes for >3 months were included. Researchers compared data from 2013 to 2022; each registry's analysis of the data was predetermined and carried out independently. Demographic information, HbA1c, treatment plan, and event rates of severe hypoglycemia and diabetic ketoacidosis were gathered. To compare means between registries and years, ANOVA (analysis of variance) was used. Significant breakpoints in temporal patterns were examined using join point regression analysis.

Results: 35,590 children from SWEET and 109,494 children from the national registries had data accessible in 2022. The aggregate mean HbA1c dropped from 8.2% [95% confidence interval (CI) 8.1–8.3%; 66.5 mmol/mol (65.2–67.7)] to 7.6% [7.5–7.7; 59.4 mmol/mol (58.2–60.5)] between 2013 and 2022, whereas the percentage of participants who met HbA1c objectives of <7% (<53 mmol/mol) rose from 19.0 to 38.8% ($p < 0.0001$). The overall rate of severe hypoglycemia was 3.0 occurrences per 100 person-years (95% CI 2.0–4.9) in 2013 and 1.7 events per 100 person-years (1.0–2.7) in 2022. The overall incidence of diabetic ketoacidosis was 3.1 events per 100 person-years (95% CI 2.0–4.8) in 2013 and 2.2 events per 100 person-years (1.4–3.4) in 2022. The percentage of participants using insulin pumps rose from 42.9% (95% CI 40.4–45.5) in 2013 to 60.2% (95% CI 57.9–62.6) in 2022 [mean difference 17.3% (13.8–20.7); $p < 0.0001$]. Similarly, the percentage of participants using continuous glucose monitoring (CGM) increased from 18.7% (95.5–28.0) in 2016 to 81.7% (73.0–90.4) in 2022 [mean difference 63.0% (50.3–75.7); $p < 0001$].

Interpretation: Glycemic outcomes have improved between 2013 and 2022, coinciding with a rise in the usage of diabetes technologies. The International Society for Pediatric and Adolescent Diabetes (ISPAD) 2022 target for HbA1c was exceeded by many children. It is encouraging to note that severe hypoglycemia event rates are declining despite efforts to decrease HbA1c. Further advancements in diabetes management are necessary to help achieve ISPAD glycemic targets, even for children with type 1 diabetes who have access to specialized diabetes care and diabetes technology.

CRITICAL APPRAISAL

What was Known Prior to this Study?

It was estimated that about 1.5 million children and adolescents younger than 20 years have type 1 diabetes across the world. Last decade has witnessed increase in the use of newer devices in diabetes management like continuous subcutaneous insulin infusion (CSII) pumps and monitoring with continuous glucose monitor (CGM) devices. Small trials were done to assess the impact of these inductions. Real world data of the global scenario on the impact of these devices were scarce.

What does this Study Add?

This is the largest study spanning over a decade that presented real-world data on glycemic outcomes, changes in treatment regimen, use of technology in managing diabetes and its impact on acute metabolic complications.

The study showed an improvement in diabetes outcome. The event rate of acute metabolic complications was low. Glycemic improvements were accompanied by lower rates of diabetic ketoacidosis and severe hypoglycemia which was observed consistently.

This study observed that between 2013 and 2022, the mean glycated hemoglobin (HbA1c) decreased from 8.2% [95% confidence interval (CI) 8.1–8.3%; 66.5 mmol/mol (65.2–67.7)] to 7.6% (7.5–7.7; 59.4 mmol/mol (58.2–60.5)], and the proportion of participants who had achieved HbA1c targets of <7% (<53 mmol/mol) increased from 19.0 to 38.8% ($p < 0.0001$).

In 2013, the event rate of severe hypoglycemia was 3.0 events per 100 person-years (95% CI 2.0–4.9), in 2022 it came down to 1.7 events per 100 person-years (1.0–2.7).

In 2013, the complication diabetic ketoacidosis was 3.1 events per 100 person-years (95% CI 2.0–4.8). In 2022, the figure came down to 2.2 events per 100 person-years (1.4–3.4).

The use of insulin pump has increased from 42.9% (95% CI 40.4–45.5) in 2013 to 60.2% (95% CI 57.9–62.6) in 2022 [mean difference 17.3% (13.8–20.7); $p < 0.0001$].

Last but not the least, the proportion of participants using CGM increased to a great extent. It was 18.7% (95% CI 9.5–28.0) in 2016 and the value increased to 81.7% (73.0–90.4) in 2022 [mean difference 63.0% (50.3–75.7); $p < 0.0001$].

Major Strengths of the Study

The major strength of the study was that it included a large number of participants and it was followed up over about 10 years.

It was an international collaborative study, and the study investigators were able to examine data from the large number of participants.

There was prospective registration of participants into registries, and high population coverage was there.

Limitations of the Study

The study data were not pooled. This was due to multinational data privacy regulations. Data were analyzed separately.

Each registry provided aggregated data from within their own registries. As a result of that, data for comparison were not analyzed by an independent party.

All of the national registries actually originated in high-income countries. So, the results cannot be assumed to be representative of a global pattern of changes in glycemia.

Implications of the Findings for the Clinicians

The study findings confirmed improved glycemic outcomes in children on an international scale. Application of modern technology obviously facilitated the improvement. Clinicians should be able to connect themselves to the technical advancements such as using insulin pumps and CGM devices.

Knowledge Gaps Identified and Scope for Future Research

Scope for future research always remains. How the improvements in outcome can be translated into actuality in resource poor countries remains the sacred challenge. Also, the so called "not so developed" countries should be motivated to log up the data in their own registries which can later be analyzed to guide future strategies.

10. Systematic Review and Meta-analysis Corrected for History of Smoking Tobacco Identifies Type 1 Diabetes as a Possible Risk Factor for Bladder Cancer

Ref: Bennett HO, Bogumil D, Kysh L, van den Brandt P, Watanabe RM, Siegmund KD, et al. Systematic review and meta-analysis corrected for history of smoking tobacco identifies type 1 diabetes as a possible risk factor for bladder cancer. Diabetes Res Clin Pract. 2025;230:112976.

ABSTRACT

Although type 2 diabetes is known to increase the incidence of bladder cancer, it is yet unknown how type 1 diabetes may contribute to the disease. We looked for published estimates of the relationship between type 1 diabetes and incidence bladder cancer in humans, evaluated them critically, and synthesized them quantitatively. Nine independent studies with pertinent data were obtained through a systematic review; however, eight of these studies could not account for confounding caused by a history of tobacco use, which is a significant risk factor for bladder cancer. Thus, in order to discover and quantify residual confounding caused by tobacco smoking, the quantitative synthesis of the original data was implemented in this study using meta-regression. Smoking-controlled estimates were then combined using synthetic meta-analysis. According to this research, people with type 1 diabetes had a fourfold increased risk of bladder cancer [summary estimate 4.29 (95% confidence interval 2.45–7.47), 9 studies]. Therefore, type 1 diabetes looks to be a significant risk factor for bladder cancer, and it appears likely that smoking has severe negative confounding, which previously masked this link. To further understand the role of type 1 diabetes in bladder cancer etiology and to guide patient therapy, studies addressing identified risk factors for bladder cancer along with the duration and severity of type 1 diabetes are now necessary.

CRITICAL APPRAISAL

What was Known Prior to this Study?

Bladder cancer is the ninth most common malignancy worldwide. Urothelial carcinoma is the predominant histologic type of bladder cancer seen in the United States and Western Europe, where it accounts for over 90% of all bladder cancers. The case fatality rate is approximately 50%. This malignancy is prone to recurrence. It increases healthcare cost and morbidity.

A history of diabetes is a well identified risk factor for bladder carcinoma. As type 2 diabetes is far more prevalent than type 1 diabetes, most efforts to characterize diabetes-associated risk stratification of specific cancers have examined type 2 diabetes alone.

Therefore, characterization of the type 1 diabetes-bladder cancer association remains a largely unexplored area requiring further research.

What does this Study Add?

Studies included in this meta-analysis had surveilled over 190,000 individuals with type 1 diabetes. Total 372 incident cases of bladder cancer were diagnosed between 1972 and 2016. This shows a strong association between type 1 diabetes and bladder cancer development.

Major Strengths of the Study

Strengths of this work depend on the fact that the study included a complete set of relevant data for analysis. The data was free of redundancies.

Complete information on prevalence of smoking in source populations was gathered and analyzed to address previously unaddressed confounding factors.

The researchers in this study anticipated that individuals with type 1 diabetes may have been disinclined to smoke, owing to the characteristically young age at type 1 diabetes diagnosis. This could result in negative confounding by smoking and thus underestimation of any type 1 diabetes-bladder cancer association.

The use of meta-regression analysis on the nonredundant data formulated the quantitative bias analysis and thereby helped to identify the positive association between type 1 diabetes and bladder cancer that had previously been obscured by negative confounding of original studies by smoking history.

Limitations of the Study

This study is entirely based on statistical analysis. Completeness of data availability may influence the study results.

Implications of the Findings for the Clinicians

Clinicians need to be aware of the credible associations that could plausibly be causal in nature for both forms of diabetes. Accordingly, not just the medications used to treat type 2 diabetes, clinicians need to consider background common feature of both types of the disease to fully understand and investigate bladder carcinogenesis.

Knowledge Gaps Identified and Scope for Future Research

The study observed approximately fourfold occurrence of bladder cancer reported for type 1 diabetes and this is far stronger than the 20–30% greater occurrence characteristically reported for type 2 diabetes.

New studies should be designed to understand reasons that underlie this difference in occurrence of the bladder cancer. We need to address these questions urgently is underscored because of the possibility that those living with type 1 diabetes may experience greatly elevated bladder cancer risk amidst the ongoing epidemic of type 2 diabetes.

Section 7: DIABETES IN PREGNANCY

Section Editor: Indira Maisnam

1. Subtypes of Gestational Diabetes Mellitus are Differentially Associated with Newborn and Childhood Metabolic Outcomes

Ref: Osmulski ME, Yu Y, Kuang A, Josefson JL, Hivert MF, Scholtens DM, et al. Subtypes of Gestational Diabetes Mellitus Are Differentially Associated With Newborn and Childhood Metabolic Outcomes. Diabetes Care. 2025;48(3):390-9.

ABSTRACT

Objective: Based on insulin secretion and sensitivity, subtypes of gestational diabetes mellitus (GDM) have been identified. We investigated the hypothesis that the anthropometric and glycemic outcomes of newborns and children are differently correlated with GDM subtypes.

Methods and research design: In the hyperglycemia and adverse pregnancy outcome (HAPO) study and HAPO follow-up study, 7,970 and 4,160 mother-offspring dyads, respectively, had their newborn and child (ages 11–14 years) outcomes analyzed. GDM was categorized as either insulin-resistant GDM (insulin sensitivity < 25th percentile with preserved insulin secretion), insulin-deficient GDM (insulin secretion < 25th percentile with preserved insulin sensitivity), or mixed-defect GDM (both < 25th percentile). Maternal BMI, field center, and other pregnancy factors were adjusted for in regression models for newborn and child outcomes. Additionally, child models took into account the child's age, sex, and family history of diabetes.

Results: All three GDM subtypes were linked to birth weight and sum of skinfolds > 90th percentile when compared to mother with normal glucose tolerance. Cord C-peptide levels above the 90th percentile were linked to insulin resistance and mixed-defect GDM. An increased incidence of newborn hypoglycemia was linked to insulin-resistant GDM. Neonatal hypoglycemia and childhood obesity were linked to insulin-resistant GDM [odds ratio (OR) 1.53; 95% CI 1.127–2.08). Increased risk of childhood impaired glucose tolerance was seen in insulin resistant GDM (OR 2.21; 95% CI 1.5–3.25) and mixed defect GDM (OR 3.01; 95% CI 1.47–6.19).

Conclusion: Newborn and childhood outcomes are differently correlated with GDM subtypes. In order to provide targeted, preventative interventions early in life, it may be possible to identify at-risk offspring by better defining persons with GDM.

CRITICAL APPRAISAL

What was Known Prior to this Study?

It is known that GDM is associated with increased newborn birth weight, percentage of body fat, and cord C-peptide. GDM is associated with higher 30-min, 1-h, and 2-h glucose along with lower insulin sensitivity, insulin secretion, and disposition index, and a higher risk for childhood obesity and impaired glucose tolerance. GDM subtypes have been identified as insulin resistant, insulin deficient, and mixed defect. However, the differential effects of GDM subtypes on childhood metabolic outcomes are not clear.

What this Study Adds?

There are differential effects on childhood metabolic outcomes according to GDM subtypes. Offspring glucose intolerance is seen in insulin resistant or mixed-defect GDM. Offspring obesity at 5 years is seen in insulin resistant GDM. Increased cord C-peptide was seen in insulin resistant and mixed GDM and neonatal hypoglycemia was increased in insulin resistant GDM. Skin fold thickness was increased in all types. Thus, the effects of different subtypes on childhood metabolic outcomes are different and not homogeneous.

Major Strengths

The longitudinal nature of the study allowed a comprehensive picture of long-term outcomes on the effect of GDM subtypes on newborn and subsequent child metabolic outcomes. This allows for identification of at-risk offspring for better care.

Limitations

Some of the subtypes were of limited number to sufficiently identify childhood metabolic outcomes. Some cases of GDM did not fit into a single subtype.

Clinical Implications

The current study helps to offspring with metabolic risk. This will help to provide better prevention strategy.

Scope for Future Research

The influence of genetic factors, intrauterine environment including maternal metabolomics need to be studied to explain the association between subtypes and differential childhood metabolic outcomes.

2. Gestational Diabetes Mellitus Recurrence Rate and Risk Factors: A Systematic Review and Meta-analysis

Ref: Pan Y, Gu R, Wang J, Li Q, Zhang Y, Xu Y, et al. Gestational diabetes mellitus recurrence rate and risk factors: a systematic review and meta-analysis. Diabetes Res Clin Pract. 2025;230:112949.

ABSTRACT

There are substantial short-term and long-term metabolic hazards associated with gestational diabetes mellitus (GDM). Concerns regarding GDM recurrence have increased due to changing fertility patterns, but the evidence is highly heterogeneous, which makes it difficult to identify modifiable predictors and limits evidence-based counseling. In order to address this, we searched nine electronic databases for a systematic review and meta-analysis. We found 30 trials with 30,524 women, 13,610 of whom had recurrences. There was significant heterogeneity (I^2 = 97.7%; $p < 0.001$, range: 30.87–73.75%), primarily caused by variations in diagnostic criteria, the pooled recurrence rate was 50.7% [95% confidence interval (CI) 46.6–55.2]. Ten important risk factors were found in the metabolic, obesity-related, and maternal domains. The best predictors were advanced mother age [subsequent pregnancy ≥ 35 years: odds ratio (OR) = 3.408; 95% CI 2.591–4.482] and prepregnancy obesity (BMI ≥ 30 kg/m^2 BMI ≥ 25 kg/m^2 in index pregnancy: OR = 3.248; 95% CI 1.838–5.742; in subsequent pregnancy: OR = 2.273; 95% CI 1.463–3.530). The risk was considerably elevated by prior macrosomia (OR = 2.064; 95% CI 1.820–2.341), index-pregnancy insulin therapy (OR = 2.353; 95% CI 1.351–4.098), early subsequent-pregnancy hyperglycemia (OR = 2.665; 95% CI 2.022–3.513), and hypertriglyceridemia (OR = 2.022; 95% CI 1.548–2.641). Initial diagnostic criteria and patient-specific characteristics must be integrated in risk-stratified prevention.

CRITICAL APPRAISAL

What was Known Prior to this Study?

There is recurrence in GDM. However, the rate of recurrence and the risk factors for recurrence have not been exactly identified.

What this Study Adds?

The study found that the risk of recurrence was very high though heterogeneous. The study specifically identified 10 risk factors which were robust predictors of recurrence. This study therefore adds to our knowledge about the specific factors which increase the risk of GDM recurrence which include age, BMI, elevated 1-h and 2-h glucose levels, and insulin therapy among others. This information will help in preventive and counseling measures regarding recurrence. However, though the study did not find family history of DM, weight gain during pregnancy, inter-pregnancy weight gain, gestational hypertension, etc., as risk factors for recurrence, these factors cannot be entirely ruled out and further studies are needed.

Major Strengths

There were stringent inclusion/exclusion criteria coupled with multivariable adjustment, with effect sizes obtained after controlling for potential confounders in the original studies. The risk of confounding bias was low.

Limitations

Racial and geographical generalizability is not possible. The difference in the diagnostic criteria was a challenge, which affected the rates of recurrence. Protective factors against recurrence were not adequately analyzed though duration and exclusivity of breast feeding were identified as protective factors.

Clinical Implications

Recurrence of GDM is high. Some robust risk factors have been identified. Focus is on counselling and prevention in those at risk.

Scope for Future Research

Diagnostic criteria need to be uniform. However, it is not clear whether uniform criteria would apply across all racial groups. More research on this is needed. Larger, heterogeneous population is needed to study the risk factors. Protected factors need to be identified. Factors which were found not to be associated with risk but are conceptually supposed to increase the risk need to be studied in more greater detail.

3. Real-time Continuous Glucose Monitoring in Pregnancies with Gestational Diabetes Mellitus: A Randomized Controlled Trial

Ref: Valent AM, Rickert M, Pagan CH, Ward L, Dunn E, Rincon M. Real-Time Continuous Glucose Monitoring in Pregnancies With Gestational Diabetes Mellitus: A Randomized Controlled Trial. Diabetes Care. 2025;48(9):1581-8.

ABSTRACT

Objective: To determine whether real-time continuous glucose monitoring (CGM; intervention) or capillary blood glucose monitoring (CBG; control) alone is more effective in increasing the percent glucose time in range (%TIR) in pregnant patients with gestational diabetes mellitus (GDM).

Methods and research design: Pregnant women with GDM who were at least 20 weeks pregnant participated in an open-label, single-center, randomized controlled trial. The use of real-time CGM plus adjunctive CBG versus CBG alone for glucose monitoring was randomly assigned (2:1) to the subjects. The intervention group received training on how to use the Dexcom G6 CGM system continuously from enrollment until delivery admission. During the course of the trial, the control group received blinded CGM roughly every 20 days and employed CBG monitoring four times a day. The CGM %TIR, which was defined as 60–140 mg/dL (3.3–7.8 mmol/L) from trial enrollment until hospital admission during delivery, was the main outcome.

Results: Between February 2021 and June 2023, 111 participants were enrolled (n = 74 in the intervention group and n = 37 in the control group). There were no statistically significant variations in the groups' demographics. At 60–140 mg/dL, the CGM group's %TIR ±SD was considerably higher (93 ± 6 minutes vs. 88 ± 14 minutes; $p = 0.027$). Key secondary CGM measure outcomes showed that, in comparison to the control group, the intervention group had significantly higher daytime TIR with lower 24-hour and daytime mean glucose and percent time > 140 mg/dL.

Conclusion: Among GDM patients, we showed a significantly greater %TIR using real-time CGM as opposed to CBG glucose monitoring. To find out if lowering CGM glucose levels can enhance prenatal and neonatal outcomes, more research is required.

CRITICAL APPRAISAL

What was Known Prior to this Study?

The Continuous Glucose Monitoring in Women With Type 1 Diabetes in Pregnancy Trial (CONCEPTT) in pregnant type 1 diabetes (T1D) showed that RT-CGM improved glycemic and neonatal outcomes. However, the evidence of benefit with RT-CGM use in GDM is scarce.

What this Study Adds?

CGM metrics like TIR, mean blood glucose concentration, better daytime TIR and lower daytime and 24-h TAR was better with the use of RT-CGM and CBG compared to CBG use alone. However, as there was no difference in the rate of perinatal, delivery and neonatal outcomes, it needs to be determined in larger studies if this better glycemic metrics translate into better outcomes.

Major Strengths

One of the few studies comparing combined RT-CGM and CBG; with CBG monitoring. The CBG and CGM data were well-characterized in the study.

Limitations

This was a single center study. The study was not powered to assess pregnancy and neonatal outcomes.

Clinical Implications

It needs to be seen if the large amount of data that is provided by CGM is actually required to favorably affect pregnancy outcomes in GDM; or whether such excess data is redundant. Based on current evidences, it appears the use of CBG monitoring is sufficient in GDM.

Scope for Future Research

It needs to be seen if the better CGM metrics with use of RT-CGM along with CBG; compared to only CBG monitoring actually translates to favorable pregnancy outcome.

4. Lack of Validity of the Glucose Management Indicator in Type 1 Diabetes in Pregnancy

Ref: Meek CL, Feig DS, Scott EM, Corcoy R, Murphy HR; CONCEPTT Collaborative Group. Lack of Validity of the Glucose Management Indicator in Type 1 Diabetes in Pregnancy. Diabetes Care. 2025;48:1323-8.

ABSTRACT

Objective: Although the glucose management indicator (GMI) is frequently employed in place of HbA1c, very little is known about its use during pregnancy. We evaluated GMI accuracy and correlations with pregnancy outcomes in individuals with type 1 diabetes.

Methods and research design: We used logistic/linear regression and Bland–Altman plots to examine HbA1c, continuous glucose monitoring (CGM) measures, GMI at 12, 24, and 34 weeks' gestation, and outcomes in 220 women from the Continuous Glucose Monitoring in Women With Type 1 Diabetes in Pregnancy Trial (CONCEPTT).

Results: During pregnancy, GMI equations were less accurate and more biased, especially during the first and third trimesters. The ability of GMI and mean CGM glucose to predict pregnancy outcomes was comparable. Over time in range (63–140 mg/dL; 3.5–7.8 mmol/L), time above range (> 140 mg/dL; > 7.8 mmol/L), and average CGM glucose concentrations, GMI did not provide any additional predictive potential.

Conclusion: In pregnant women with type 1 diabetes, GMI is not a reliable substitute for HbA1c.

CRITICAL APPRAISAL

What was Known Prior to this Study?

Glucose management indicator (GMI) has been used as an approximation of HbA1c in nonpregnant individuals. Earlier study of GMI in type 1 diabetes (T1D) pregnancy had shown that, it is not suitable to be a replacement with HbA1c; but its association with outcomes was not studied.

What this Study Adds?

GMI performed less accurately as an approximation of HbA1c in pregnancy; associations and bias varied according to trimester. GMI did not predict additional outcomes over average glucose. Pregnancy outcomes at 34 weeks were better predicted with HbA1c than GMI. HbA1c or alternative CGM metrics, such as time in range or time above range, offer similar or better predictive capability for pregnancy outcomes compared to GMI.

Major Strengths

Study population was well characterized and was longitudinally followed up during pregnancy.

Limitations

GMI was calculated based on shorter (6 days) CGM data. Whether longer CGM data would provide additional information is not known. There was less ethnic diversity.

Clinical Implications

CGM metrics and HbA1c are the best currently available options for monitoring and outcome prediction in GDM.

Scope for Future Research

There is a need to identify the pregnancy-related factors that determine GMI in pregnancy before it can be used safely in pregnancy to assess glycemic control and pregnancy outcomes.

5. Metformin Safety during Pregnancy in Women with Gestational Diabetes Mellitus: A Systematic Review and Meta-analysis of Maternal, Neonatal, and Long-term Outcomes

Ref: Brinkmann MLS, Krasilnikoff NJ, Chaaban MA, Luef BM, Newman C, Dunne F, et al. Metformin safety during pregnancy in women with gestational diabetes mellitus: A systematic review and meta-analysis of maternal, neonatal and long-term outcomes. Diabet Med. 2025:e70173.

ABSTRACT

Aim: This systematic review and meta-analysis assessed the safety and efficacy of metformin in managing gestational diabetes mellitus (GDM), focusing on maternal, neonatal, and long-term outcomes. While lifestyle changes are first-line treatment, pharmacological therapy is often required. Insulin, the standard treatment, has drawbacks including weight gain, neonatal hypoglycemia, and maternal anxiety. Metformin is a promising alternative due to its insulin-sensitizing effects, but concerns remain about placental transfer and long-term effects on offspring.

Methods: A systematic search was conducted in PubMed and Embase up to 29 August 2024, including randomized controlled trials (RCTs) and follow-up studies. Primary outcomes were neonatal hypoglycemia, birthweight, and long-term metabolic outcomes. Study quality was assessed using risk of bias (RoB) 2.0 and ROBINS-I. Data were synthesized using the inverse variance heterogeneity (IVhet) model.

Results: Ten RCTs were included. Metformin was associated with a statistically significant reduction in neonatal hypoglycemia [odds ratio (OR) 0.65; 95% CI 0.46–0.92] and lower birthweight [MD −68.96 g; 95% confidence interval (CI) −108.34 to −29.57]. A nonsignificant trend toward reduced LGA risk was observed. No significant differences in prediabetes, diabetes, or insulin resistance were found. Long-term outcomes in children remain uncertain due to limited and heterogeneous follow-up data.

Conclusion: Metformin appears safe and effective in GDM management, but more data are needed on long-term outcomes.

CRITICAL APPRAISAL

What was Known Prior to this Study?

Balsells et al., in a systematic review and meta-analysis, provided evidence supporting metformin as a viable alternative to insulin in pregnancy. Farrar et al., in a systematic review and meta-analysis incorporated newer trials and reaffirmed metformin's benefits across a spectrum of pregnancy outcomes. Although no teratogenic effects have been reported, concerns regarding use of metformin during pregnancy persist. Metformin crosses the placenta, resulting in comparable maternal and fetal concentrations. Studies also indicated that metformin may influence fetal metabolic programming, with potential long-term consequences for offspring. In utero exposure to metformin has also been linked to a greater prevalence of obesity and increased waist to height ratios in children.

What this Study Adds?

Metformin use in pregnancy showed statistically significant reduction in neonatal hypoglycemia and a modest reduction in birthweight.

Metformin appears to be safe and effective in gestational diabetes.

Major Strength

This systematic review focused exclusively on GDM and did not combine with type 2 diabetes in pregnancy, which enhances clinical specificity.

Independent screening was performed by two blinded reviewers, with third reviewer resolved any disagreements or uncertainties. Involvement of multiple-blinded reviewers in data extraction helped to reduce potential bias and improve the consistency of results.

Use of Inverse variance heterogeneity model (IVhet model) offers more robust confidence intervals than the traditional random effects model and reduces the risk of underestimating uncertainty, in presence of low or moderate heterogeneity.

In this systematic review, effect estimates were expressed as OR rather than risk ratios (RRs). Logittorisk module was used to convert ORs into absolute risk differences and numbers needed to treat or harm (NNT/NNH) across assumed baseline risks.

Limitations

Long-term outcomes for mothers and offspring remain uncertain due to limited and heterogeneous follow-up data.

A threshold of > 100 patients in RCTs were kept as inclusion criteria in this systematic review. As a result, potentially meaningful effects observed in smaller trials were not captured.

The analysis was further complicated by variability in study populations, treatment protocols, definitions of outcomes, variations in glycemic targets, dosage regimens, and maternal baseline characteristics across the included trials.

Clinical Implications

This systematic review supports metformin as a viable treatment option for managing GDM, specially in patients who refuse to take insulin.

But clinical management should remain individualized, considering patient preferences, clinical context, and resource availability.

Scope for Future Research

Future studies should focus on standardizing outcome definitions, especially birthweight, gestational weight gain.

Adoption of the recently developed core outcome set (COS) for reporting of studies on prevention and treatment of GDM, which includes 14 key short-term maternal and neonatal outcomes, can improve consistency.

Large-scale, multicenter trials with diverse populations to improve generalizability are needed.

Longitudinal studies are needed to assess the long-term health of mothers and their offspring, including metabolic, developmental, and cardiovascular outcomes.

Section 8: NEWER TECHNOLOGIES IN DIABETES

Section Editor: Mainak Banerjee

1. Adults with Type 2 Diabetes Benefit from Automated Insulin Delivery Irrespective of C-peptide Level

Ref: Hirsch IB, Kudva YC, Ahn DT, Blevins T, Rickels MR, Raghinaru D, et al. Adults with type 2 diabetes benefit from automated insulin delivery irrespective of C-peptide level. Diabetes Care. 2025;48:2061-6.

ABSTRACT

Objective: Many persons with type 2 diabetes cannot receive coverage for automated insulin delivery (AID) systems because the Centers for Medicare and Medicaid Services (CMS) demands a low C-peptide level for insulin pump coverage unless the person is beta-cell autoantibody positive.

Methods and research design: Adults with insulin-treated type 2 diabetes were divided into high C-peptide ($n = 195$) and low C-peptide ($n = 59$) groups according to CMS criteria in the Randomized Trial Evaluating the Efficacy and Safety of Control-IQ+ Technology in Adults With Type 2 Diabetes Using Basal-Bolus Insulin Therapy study evaluating the t:slim X2 insulin pump with Control-IQ+ technology.

Results: With both high ($p < 0.001$) and low ($p = 0.02$) C-peptide levels, the AID group's mean glycated hemoglobin (HbA1c) dropped from baseline by 0.8%, which was considerably higher than that of the control group. The outcomes for those over 65 years old were comparable.

Conclusion: Both high and low C-peptide levels benefit from AID. Therefore, it is not justified to make a low C-peptide level as a requirement for AID therapy.

CRITICAL APPRAISAL

What was Known Prior to the Study?

- Automated insulin delivery (AID) systems significantly improve glycemic control in insulin-treated type 2 diabetes.
- Payers, including the Centers for Medicare and Medicaid Services (CMS), often require a low C-peptide level (≤110% of the lower limit of normal) to authorize insulin pump therapy.
- This requirement assumes that only those with severe endogenous insulin deficiency benefit from automated delivery technology.

What this Study Adds?

- It provides definitive evidence that the magnitude of glycated hemoglobin (HbA1c) reduction and "*time in range*" (TIR) improvement is nearly identical for patients with high versus low C-peptide levels.
- The research demonstrates that AID effectively manages the high insulin demands and resistance characteristic of type 2 diabetes, even when significant endogenous insulin is present.
- It identifies that baseline HbA1c, rather than C-peptide level, is the primary predictor of the degree of improvement with AID.
- The study directly challenges existing insurance policies, suggesting they unfairly exclude a large population of type 2 diabetes patients who could derive significant clinical benefit.

Major Strengths

- Utilization of high-quality data from a large-scale, multicenter randomized controlled trial (2IQP).

- Robust stratification of C-peptide levels reflecting a broad clinical spectrum of type 2 diabetes.
- Consistency of findings across multiple glycemic metrics [TIR, time above range (TAR), and HbA1c].

Limitations

- As a post hoc analysis, the study was not originally powered specifically for these subgroups.
- Fasting C-peptide was used as a proxy for beta-cell function rather than stimulated C-peptide.
- The study period (26 weeks) may not capture very long-term differences in therapy adherence between subgroups.

Clinical Implications

- C-peptide testing should not be used as a clinical or administrative barrier to AID access in type 2 diabetes.
- Clinicians can expect robust improvements in glycemic control when prescribing AID to type 2 patients regardless of their degree of insulin deficiency.
- Standardizing access based on clinical need (e.g., suboptimal HbA1c on intensive insulin) rather than biochemical thresholds could improve population-level diabetes outcomes.

Knowledge Gaps and Scope for Future Research

Future research should investigate whether C-peptide levels influence the long-term durability of AID benefits or the rate of "technology fatigue" over several years. Additionally, prospective studies are needed to determine if AID can preserve residual beta-cell function in type 2 diabetes by reducing glucotoxicity. Evaluating the cost-effectiveness of removing C-peptide barriers within different healthcare systems is also essential to support policy changes. Finally, research into algorithms specifically optimized for high-resistance, high-C-peptide phenotypes could further enhance the precision of automated delivery.

2. Now is the Time to Remove Barriers to AID Treatment for Those with Detectable C-peptide (Commentary)

Ref: Lumb AN. Now is the time to remove barriers to AID treatment for those with detectable C-peptide (commentary). Diabetes Care. 2025;48:2007-9.

ABSTRACT

An automated insulin delivery (AID) system modulates insulin delivery via an insulin pump by feeding data from a person's continuous glucose monitor (CGM) into a mathematical algorithm. AID systems are linked to increases in quality of life and have been shown to protect against both low and high glucose levels in type 1 diabetes. A crucial component of guaranteeing access to therapies for individuals who stand to gain is the evaluation of clinical efficacy and cost-effectiveness by organizations with the power to shape policy. For instance, the National Institute for Health and Care Excellence (NICE) conducts assessments in England and Wales. The nationwide provision of AID systems for individuals with type 1 diabetes who satisfy well-defined prespecified criteria is currently being driven by their publishing of a supportive evaluation (Technology Appraisal 943). This is one instance of how AID systems are becoming the global standard of care for individuals with type 1 diabetes. Significant improvements in the treatment of type 2 diabetes have resulted from the increasing use of sodium-glucose cotransporter-2 inhibitors (SGLT-2i) and glucagon-like peptide-1 receptor agonists (GLP-1 RA), which can provide both glycemic and cardiorenal benefits. Despite the availability of these medications, a significant portion of type 2 diabetics still fail to meet glycemic objectives, and insulin therapy is still a viable treatment choice. This may be especially pertinent to those who are diagnosed with type 2 diabetes at a younger age, whose life expectancy is disproportionately impacted by the diagnosis, and for whom meeting treatment goals may be more crucial. A growing body of research supports the safety and effectiveness of AID systems in individuals with type 2 diabetes who are receiving insulin.

CRITICAL APPRAISAL

What was Known Prior to the Study?

- Automated insulin delivery (AID) systems significantly improve glycemia in type 1 diabetes.
- Many healthcare payers require a "detectable" or "low" C-peptide level to justify the cost of insulin pump technology.
- There was a prevailing clinical assumption that patients with high residual insulin (high C-peptide) would not benefit from automated algorithmic delivery.

What this Study Adds?

- It reinforces evidence that AID efficacy in type 2 diabetes is independent of endogenous insulin production.
- The paper identifies a significant disconnect between modern clinical evidence and outdated national reimbursement policies.
- It clarifies that C-peptide levels are a poor predictor of who will achieve glycemic success with AID.
- The work advocates for a shift in policy toward "clinical-need-based" access rather than "biomarker-based" restriction.

Major Strengths

- Critically bridges the gap between primary clinical data and healthcare policy
- Uses high-quality trial data (2IQP) to debunk long-standing physiological myths
- Provides a clear, global perspective on administrative barriers to technology

Limitations

- As a commentary, it does not provide new experimental data.
- It focuses primarily on high-income healthcare systems (USA and UK).
- It does not extensively address the specific economic cost–benefit ratios of removing these barriers.

Clinical Implications

- Clinicians should advocate for AID in type 2 diabetes based on a patient's inability to reach targets, regardless of C-peptide status.
- Removing C-peptide requirements would likely lead to a significant increase in technology uptake and improved population-level glycated hemoglobin (HbA1c).
- Standardizing access could reduce health disparities among type 2 diabetes patients who are currently excluded by arbitrary administrative rules.

Knowledge Gaps and Scope for Future Research

Future research should focus on the long-term economic impact of expanding AID access to the broader type 2 diabetes population, particularly regarding the prevention of costly chronic complications. Additionally, there is a need to investigate whether earlier introduction of AID in patients with high C-peptide levels can preserve remaining beta-cell function. Studies exploring the psychosocial benefits and reduction in caregiver burden in this specific subgroup would also provide a more holistic justification for policy changes.

3. Continuous Glucose Monitoring Metrics Predict All-cause Mortality in Diabetes: A Real-world Long-term Study

Ref: Okuno T, Macwan SA, Norman GJ, Miller DR, Reaven PD, Zhou JJ. Continuous glucose monitoring metrics predict all-cause mortality in diabetes: A real-world long-term study. Diabetes Care. 2025;48:1794-802.

ABSTRACT

Objective: Examine the relationship between all-cause mortality in individuals with type 1 or type 2 diabetes (T1D or T2D) and glucose measurements generated from continuous glucose monitoring (CGM).

Methods and research design: Data from 2,752 persons (≥21 years old) with diabetes (65% T2D) who got Dexcom CGM between 2015 and 2020 from the Veterans Affairs Healthcare System were evaluated. Every participant had at least 10 days of CGM data combined with electronic health records during landmark (LM) periods (14 days, 3 months, and 6 months). Five years after the start of CGM, all-cause mortality was evaluated. Mean glucose (MG, mg/dL), time in range (TIR,%), time above range (TAR,%), coefficient of variation (CV), and glycemic risk index (GRI,%) were all assessed as correlations between mortality and CGM parameters by Cox models.

Outcomes: The median duration of CGM use was over 3 years, and the mean age at CGM commencement was 64. About 407 people died. Higher MG, TAR, CV, and GRI as well as lower TIR during the 6-month LM were linked to 5-year mortality in separate multivariable Cox models (adjusting for mortality-related variables) (hazard ratios: MG 1.18, TAR 1.20, GRI 1.23, CV 1.18, and TIR 0.83; all $p \leq 0.01$). These associations persisted even after controlling for LM glycated hemoglobin (HbA1c). Shorter CGM LM observation windows produced comparable results. The correlation between CV and mortality seemed to be highest in people with lower HbA1c levels and was independent of other CGM parameters.

Conclusion: Compared to HbA1c, CGM-derived metrics were linked to all-cause mortality in diabetic individuals and may more accurately reflect long-term risk related to glucose variations and times of hypo- and hyperglycemia.

CRITICAL APPRAISAL

What was Known Prior to the Study?

- Glycated hemoglobin (HbA1c) is the standard predictor for long-term diabetes complications and mortality.
- Continuous glucose monitoring (CGM) metrics like time in range (TIR) are validated markers for microvascular risk.
- Short-term studies suggest glucose variability impacts cardiovascular health, but long-term mortality data linked specifically to CGM metrics remained scarce.

What this Study Adds?

- It establishes that CGM-derived metrics [TIR and time above range (TAR)] are independent predictors of all-cause mortality, regardless of a patient's HbA1c.
- It demonstrates a linear, rather than J-shaped, relationship between hyperglycemia metrics and death in a real-world veteran population.
- It shows that a 10% increase in TIR (~2.4 hours/day) translates to a significant reduction in mortality hazard.
- It provides a 5-year longitudinal validation of CGM metrics as hard clinical endpoints for survival.

Major Strengths

- Large, real-world cohort with a significant 5-year follow-up period

- Robust adjustment for a wide range of clinical covariates and HbA1c
- Use of spline analysis to characterize the nature of the risk relationship

Limitations

- Retrospective design may include inherent selection bias toward patients capable of utilizing CGM technology.
- The study population was predominantly male (90%) and older, limiting generalizability to women and younger populations.
- Cause-specific mortality data (e.g., cardiovascular vs. cancer) was not analyzed.

Clinical Implications

- TIR and TAR should be prioritized alongside HbA1c as primary clinical targets to improve patient survival.
- The prognostic value of CGM allows for more precise risk stratification of patients with diabetes in primary and specialty care.
- Healthcare providers can use CGM data to demonstrate the direct impact of daily glucose stability on long-term life expectancy.

Knowledge Gaps and Scope for Future Research

Future investigations should examine whether these mortality associations hold true for more diverse populations, particularly women and nonveteran cohorts. There is also a need to determine the impact of time below range (hypoglycemia) on mortality, which was less clear in this study. Further research should explore if interventions specifically aimed at improving TIR, independent of lowering HbA1c, result in reduced death rates. Finally, determining the cause-specific mortality associated with CGM metrics will help clarify the biological mechanisms involved.

4. Continuous Glucose Monitor Accuracy for Diabetes Management in Hospitalized Children

Ref: Garg N, Lewis K, White PC, Adhikari S. Continuous glucose monitor accuracy for diabetes management in hospitalized children. Diabetes Care. 2025;48:259-64.

ABSTRACT

Objective: Due to a lack of information regarding the reliability of continuous glucose monitors (CGMs) in hospitalized children, their adoption in pediatric inpatient settings has been sluggish.

Methods and research design: The accuracy of the Dexcom G6 CGM system in juvenile diabetic patients admitted to our university children's hospital between March 2018 and September 2023 was examined retrospectively. To evaluate every child with CGM data who was admitted to the hospital, we cross-referenced the Dexcom Clarity database with an internal database of inpatient admissions. Blood urea nitrogen (BUN), pH, and point-of-care (POC) glucose values were recorded from the electronic medical record, together with sensor glucose readings from Clarity. Clarke Error Grid (CEG) and mean absolute relative difference (MARD) analyses were used to assess CGM accuracy and clinical dependability.

Results: Of the 3,200 children with diabetes who were admitted during this time, 277 (out of 202 kids aged 2–18) had corresponding CGM data. A comparison of paired CGM and POC measurements (n = 2,904) yielded a MARD of 15.9%, with 96.6% of the values in zones A and B of the CEG analysis. About 62% of paired results fell between 15% or 15 mg/dL difference whichever was greater

(15%/15 mg/dL range), 74% between 20%/20, and 88% between 30%/30. CGM results and the absolute relative difference in linear regression analysis were unaffected by serum pH, salt, or BUN.

Conclusion: In children with diabetes who were hospitalized, CGMs showed respectable accuracy. To maximize management, CGM data should be included into hospital electronic records.

CRITICAL APPRAISAL

What was Known Prior to the Study?

- Continuous glucose monitor (CGM) is highly accurate and widely utilized for outpatient pediatric type 1 diabetes management.
- Hospitalized children often face physiological stress and medication changes that may impact interstitial glucose sensor performance.
- Data regarding the accuracy of CGM specifically in noncritically ill hospitalized children remained sparse compared to adult inpatient data.

What this Study Adds?

- It establishes a real-world inpatient mean absolute relative difference (MARD) of 15.9% for CGM in a pediatric population, which is slightly higher than reported in controlled outpatient trials.
- The study confirms high clinical safety, with over 96% of readings residing in clinically acceptable Clarke Error Grid zones, supporting its utility in reducing painful fingersticks.
- It identifies that CGM accuracy in the hospital is significantly compromised during hypoglycemia (glucose <70 mg/dL), where the MARD increases substantially.
- The research demonstrates that while CGM generally overestimates blood glucose slightly, it remains a robust tool for tracking inpatient glycemic trends.

Major Strengths

- Large dataset featuring nearly 3,000 paired glucose points from diverse pediatric encounters
- Evaluation conducted in a real-world clinical environment rather than a controlled research unit.
- Use of rigorous statistical metrics, including Bland–Altman and Clarke Error Grid analysis

Limitations

- Retrospective design prevents control over the timing and technique of point-of-care (POC) blood glucose checks.
- Single-center study may limit generalizability to other pediatric facilities with different protocols.
- Potential interference from medications common in inpatient settings was not specifically analyzed.

Clinical Implications

- CGM can be integrated into pediatric inpatient workflows to provide continuous trend data and reduce the frequency of capillary testing.
- Clinicians must continue to mandate POC verification for hypoglycemic readings or before making significant insulin dose adjustments due to sensor lag.
- The adoption of CGM in hospitals can improve patient and caregiver satisfaction by minimizing the burden of frequent nocturnal fingersticks.

Knowledge Gaps and Scope for Future Research

Future research should focus on prospective trials to determine if CGM use in hospitalized children improves outcomes, such as length of stay or time in target range. Investigating the impact of common inpatient medications, like acetaminophen or vitamin C, on sensor accuracy in this specific population is also required. Furthermore, studies should explore the implementation of "hybrid" protocols that combine automated CGM data alerts with standardized nursing responses to enhance safety during acute illness.

5. Intersystem Accuracy in Continuous Glucose Monitoring: When Does this Matter? (Commentary)

Ref: Kim SJ, Hirsch IB. Intersystem accuracy in continuous glucose monitoring: When does this matter? (Commentary). Diabetes Care. 2025;48:1161-3.

ABSTRACT

Continuous glucose monitoring, or CGM, has been a mainstay of diabetes care since its inception in 1999. For all diabetic patients who need insulin, CGMs are now considered the gold standard of care. There are many options available to patients for using CGM. However, a number of variables, including price, insurance coverage, ease of use, compatibility with other technology [such automated insulin delivery (AID) systems, smart insulin pens, or smartwatches], and patient preferences, can modify the choice of device. Even though CGM accuracy has increased with time, problems still exist. When compared to the numbers listed on the labels of Food and Drug Administration (FDA)-approved CGMs, CGM accuracy in real-world situations is frequently lower. Glycemic measurements may be impacted by the variety in accuracy across systems that has evolved as a result of various firms developing CGMs. Therefore, the question to address is whether treatment choices and safety are affected by these variations in accuracy. According to this article in Diabetes Care, Freckmann et al. examined the performance of three popular CGM systems: Medtronic Simplera (MSP), Dexcom G7 (DG7), and FreeStyle Libre 3 (FL3). They discovered variations in important glycemic parameters. Although the extent of these variations has been objectively evaluated, it may not always be evident how they affect safety and treatment choices. Numerous earlier research involving older CGMs have emphasized intersystem variances. Hanson et al. performed a head-to-head examination comparing the point accuracy of the FL3 and DG7 systems with respect to currently available devices. The percentage and quantity of sensor glucose readings in this investigation fell between ±15, ±20, and ±40 mg/dL of the glucose reference for glucose values <0.0001. However, these findings by themselves do not address the potential effects on safety or treatment choices.

CRITICAL APPRAISAL

What was Known Prior to the Study?

- Continuous glucose monitoring (CGM) is the recognized standard for insulin-requiring diabetes, significantly improving glycemic outcomes.
- Regulatory approval is based on mean absolute relative difference (MARD) compared to laboratory standards, but real-world performance often lags behind label claims.
- International consensus guidelines treat CGM metrics [time in range (TIR), glucose management indicator (GMI)] as universal values, assuming high interoperability between different sensor brands.

What this Study Adds?

- It clarifies that the same patient wearing different sensors will receive conflicting glycemic reports, potentially affecting insurance coverage and treatment eligibility.
- The analysis points out that proprietary algorithms handle "noise" and interstitial-to-blood glucose lags differently, leading to systematic over- or under-estimation of hypoglycemia.
- It highlights the "GMI-HbA1c (glycated hemoglobin) gap", where different sensors produce varying GMI values for the same laboratory-measured HbA1c.
- The work advocates for a shift in how clinicians view CGM data—moving from seeing them as absolute numbers to brand-specific trends.

Major Strengths

- Provides a high-level critical synthesis of the latest head-to-head sensor trials
- Directly addresses the practical risks of device-driven clinical bias
- Authored by prominent experts in diabetes technology and clinical practice

Limitations

- As a commentary, it relies on external data rather than original experimental findings.
- It focuses heavily on high-end, latest-generation sensors, which may not be accessible in all global markets.
- It does not offer a specific mathematical formula to "correct" for interdevice discrepancies.

Clinical Implications

- Providers should maintain the same CGM brand for a patient when evaluating the success of a therapeutic intervention to avoid "device-switching" artifacts.
- Decisions regarding hypoglycemia management must be verified with blood glucose if the sensor used is known for low-range bias.
- Administrative bodies and insurers should be educated that a "failure" to meet TIR targets may be due to sensor selection rather than patient nonadherence.

Knowledge Gaps and Scope for Future Research

There is an urgent need for the international standardization of CGM algorithms to ensure that metrics like *TIR* are equivalent across all manufacturers. Future research should investigate how these intersystem discrepancies impact the safety and efficacy of automated insulin delivery (AID) systems, which rely heavily on these inputs. Additionally, long-term studies are required to determine if choosing a specific CGM brand over another leads to better microvascular outcomes or reduced acute complications over several years.

---

6. A Comparative Analysis of Glycemic Metrics Derived from Three Continuous Glucose Monitoring Systems

Ref: Freckmann G, Wehrstedt S, Eichenlaub M, Pleus S, Link M, Jendrike N, et al. A comparative analysis of glycemic metrics derived from three continuous glucose monitoring systems. Diabetes Care. 2025;48:1213-7.

ABSTRACT

Objective: This study examined how three current-generation systems differed in metrics produced from continuous glucose monitoring (CGM) and assessed how these differences affected therapeutic decision-making.

Methods and research design: For 14 days in parallel, 23 subjects used the Medtronic Simplera CGM, Dexcom G7, and FreeStyle Libre 3. CGM measurements were computed independently for each CGM system and participant.

Outcomes: The used CGM system had an impact on the apparent glucose profile, leading to significantly differing glycemic measurements between the three systems. Compared to Medtronic Simplera, which generally displayed lower glucose levels, FreeStyle Libre 3 and Dexcom G7 exhibited more agreement. There were significant intraparticipant differences that could have led to differing treatment recommendations.

Conclusion: The CGM systems revealed inconsistent glucose measurements, which ought to be taken into account while treating diabetes. When utilized by the same individual, various CGM systems ought to yield identical glucose readings and CGM-derived measures.

CRITICAL APPRAISAL

What was Known Prior to the Study?

- Continuous glucose monitoring (CGM) systems are essential for managing diabetes, with metrics like *time in range* (TIR) guiding clinical adjustments.
- While mean absolute relative difference (MARD) is used to measure accuracy against blood glucose, it does not account for how different algorithms interpret interstitial fluid data.
- International guidelines assume CGM metrics are universal, regardless of the hardware or software brand used.

What this Study Adds?

- It demonstrates that wearing different CGM brands simultaneously results in markedly different glycemic profiles and reported metrics for the same patient.
- The study reveals that the Medtronic Simplera tends to report higher TIR and lower hyperglycemia compared to its competitors.
- It highlights that FreeStyle Libre 3 may report significantly more time in hypoglycemia than the other systems.
- The findings prove that therapeutic decisions, such as insulin dose adjustments, would vary in approximately one-third of cases depending on the specific CGM system used.

Major Strengths

- Prospective, head-to-head design utilizing simultaneous wear to eliminate physiological interday variability.
- Use of latest-generation sensors (Libre 3, G7, Simplera) ensures contemporary relevance.
- Focus on clinical decision-making impact rather than just technical accuracy.

Limitations

- Small sample size of 23 participants may limit the breadth of glycemic variability observed.
- Lack of a continuous reference (like YSI) prevents determining which system was most "correct".
- Short 14-day duration may not account for sensor performance changes over months of use.

Clinical Implications

- Clinicians should exercise caution when comparing CGM reports from different manufacturers, as the "success" of a treatment may be an artifact of the device.
- Therapeutic targets may need to be contextualized based on the specific sensor's known biases toward over- or under-reporting hypoglycemia.

- Patients switching between systems should be monitored closely, as their TIR and time below range (TBR) may shift significantly without any change in actual metabolic control.

Knowledge Gaps and Scope for Future Research

Future research must determine if these interdevice discrepancies lead to different long-term outcomes, such as glycated hemoglobin (HbA1c) reduction or complication rates. There is a critical need for the standardization of CGM algorithms to ensure that "70% TIR" represents the same physiological state across all platforms. Studies with larger cohorts should investigate whether specific patient factors, such as skin temperature or hydration, disproportionately affect one algorithm over another, further complicating the interoperability of CGM-derived data in automated insulin delivery systems.

7. Automated Insulin Pump in Type 2 Diabetes (Editorial)

Ref: Hatipoglu B. Automated insulin pump in type 2 diabetes (Editorial). N Engl J Med . 2025;392(18):1862-3.

ABSTRACT

In the United States, about 10% of people have type 2 diabetes, and the percentage is rising among kids, teens, and young adults. Only 50% of adults with diabetes have succeeded in lowering their glycated hemoglobin and glucose levels to the recommended range of <7%. Insulin treatment in type 2 diabetes varies; however, it is mainstay of treatment in type 1 diabetes. In addition to alternative therapy choices including glucagon-like peptide-1 receptor agonists and sodium-glucose cotransporter-2 inhibitors, 12.3% of patients with type 2 diabetes are administered insulin within a year after diagnosis, according to the Centers for Disease Control and Prevention. Over the past few decades, technological advancements have improved care and outcomes for people with type 1 diabetes, but its application to patients with type 2 diabetes is only now beginning to catch up. Continuous glucose monitoring (CGM) devices are increasingly more widely accepted and used, particularly by primary care physicians. The type 1 population has benefited from advancements in pump technology, such as the automated suspension of insulin delivery to help prevent hypoglycemia, easier daily management to help with the burden of diabetes, and the achievement of glycemic control to prevent complications. However, Kudva and colleagues present a clinical trial in this journal issue that involves a group that many practitioners would not have considered candidates for automated insulin delivery (AID) in the past. 319 insulin-treated individuals with type 2 diabetes, ages 19-87 years, were enrolled in this experiment by 1,862 scientists at 21 locations. In a 2:1 ratio, the patients were randomized to either continue using their prior insulin delivery regimen or receive AID. The t:slim X2 insulin pump with Control IQ, which has been shown to dramatically lower mean glucose and glycated hemoglobin levels in patients with type 1 diabetes, was given to the patients in the AID group. In the current type 2 diabetes cohort, the AID group's mean glycated hemoglobin level decreased by 0.9 percentage points (from 8.2% at baseline to 7.3% at 13 weeks), and the patients with a baseline glycated hemoglobin level of 9.0% or higher saw an even larger decrease (from 10.3 to 7.9%).

CRITICAL APPRAISAL

What was Known Prior to the Study?

- Automated insulin delivery (AID) systems were primarily developed and validated for type 1 diabetes populations.
- Type 2 diabetes management often faces "therapeutic inertia", where insulin intensification is delayed due to complexity and hypoglycemia fear.

- Preliminary evidence suggested that continuous glucose monitoring (CGM) alone improves outcomes, but its combination with automated dosing in type 2 was less robustly documented.

What this Study Adds?

- This editorial provides a high-level critical appraisal of recent trial data showing that AID is superior to CGM-only management for insulin-treated type 2 diabetes.
- It shifts the focus from purely clinical efficacy to "implementation science", highlighting how software reliability and battery performance (referencing recent recalls) are critical to patient safety.
- The authors argue that AID can overcome the specific challenges of type 2 diabetes, such as varied meal patterns and high insulin requirements, which often lead to manual dosing errors.
- It establishes a framework for selecting candidates for AID, emphasizing those who struggle with high glycated hemoglobin (HbA1c) despite intensive conventional therapy.

Major Strengths

- It provides a balanced view of technological promise versus real-world operational risks.
- It integrates clinical outcomes with the necessity of patient education and healthcare system economics.
- It is authored by experts in both endocrinology and healthcare quality improvement.

Limitations

- As an editorial/perspective piece, it does not provide new primary data.
- The analysis is largely centered on high-income healthcare systems with access to advanced technologies.
- Limited discussion on the specific physiological differences in algorithm performance for insulin-resistant versus insulin-sensitive patients

Clinical Implications

- Clinicians should consider AID as a viable therapeutic escalation for type 2 diabetes patients who are failing multiple daily injections.
- The reduction in "decision fatigue" for patients may lead to higher long-term adherence compared to manual pump therapy or injections.
- Robust patient education programs must accompany technology deployment to ensure users understand the system's limitations and the necessity of basic self-care.

Knowledge Gaps and Scope for Future Research

Future research must focus on long-term cost–benefit analyses to justify the high initial expenditure of AID in type 2 diabetes. There is a need for head-to-head trials comparing different AID algorithms specifically tuned for the high insulin doses required in type 2 diabetes. Furthermore, research should explore "fully" closed-loop systems that eliminate meal announcements, as this would significantly lower the cognitive burden for a population often managing multiple comorbidities and complex medication regimens.

8. A Randomized Trial of Automated Insulin Delivery in Type 2 Diabetes

Ref: Kudva YC, Raghinaru D, Lum JW, Graham TE, Liljenquist D, Spanakis EK, et al. A randomized trial of automated insulin delivery in type 2 diabetes. N Engl J Med. 2025;392:1801-12.

ABSTRACT

Background: Data from randomized, controlled studies are required to determine the relevance of automated insulin delivery (AID) systems in the management of insulin-treated type 2 diabetes; advantages of AID in type 1 diabetes have already been established.

Techniques: Adults with insulin-treated type 2 diabetes were randomly assigned in a 2:1 ratio to either receive AID or continue using their previous insulin administration method (control group) during this 13-week multicenter trial; both groups received continuous glucose monitoring (CGM). The glycated hemoglobin level at 13 weeks was the main outcome.

Results: Randomization was performed on 319 patients in total. Glycated hemoglobin levels decreased by 0.3 percentage points (from 8.1 ± 1.2% to 7.7 ± 1.1%) in the control group and by 0.9 percentage points (from 8.2 ± 1.4% at baseline to 7.3 ± 0.9% at week 13) in the AID group [mean adjusted difference, −0.6 percentage points; 95% confidence interval (CI) −0.8 to −0.4; $p < 0.001$]. In the AID group, the mean percentage of patients in the target glucose range of 70–180 mg/dL rose from 48 ± 24% to 64 ± 16%, whereas in the control group, it grew from 51 ± 21% to 52 ± 21% (mean difference, 14 percentage points; 95% CI 11–17; $p < 0.001$). The AID group outperformed the control group in every other multiplicity-controlled CGM outcome that was measured and indicative of hyperglycemia. Both groups had modest rates of hypoglycemia as determined by the CGM. One patient in the AID group experienced a severe hypoglycemic episode.

Conclusion: AID was linked to a higher decrease in glycated hemoglobin levels than CGM alone in this 13-week randomized, controlled study of persons with insulin-treated type 2 diabetes. Tandem Diabetes Care provided funding; the 2IQP ClinicalTrials.gov code is NCT05785832.

CRITICAL APPRAISAL

What was Known Prior to the Study?

- AID systems significantly improve outcomes in type 1 diabetes.
- Type 2 diabetes management often struggles with insulin titration and glycemic variability.
- Previous evidence for AID in type 2 diabetes was largely limited to small-scale or nonrandomized studies.

What this Study Adds?

- It provides definitive randomized controlled evidence that AID systems substantially increase time in range (by over 3 hours daily) compared to standard care in type 2 diabetes.
- It demonstrates a robust glycated hemoglobin (HbA1c) reduction in a diverse patient population, including those on complex insulin regimens.
- It validates that automated algorithms can safely manage the high insulin requirements and insulin resistance characteristic of type 2 diabetes.
- It shows that the benefits of AID are consistent across various demographic subgroups and baseline treatment modalities.

Major Strengths

- Randomized, multicenter design with a clinically relevant 26-week duration
- Inclusion of a representative type 2 diabetes population with various comorbidities
- High adherence rates and rigorous monitoring of safety events

Limitations

- Lack of blinding, which is inherent to device-based trials
- The 26-week follow-up may not fully reflect lifetime durability or "technology fatigue".
- Results may not be generalizable to patients with very low literacy or limited access to technology.

Clinical Implications

- AID should be considered a first-line intensification option for type 2 diabetes patients who fail to meet glycemic targets on standard insulin therapy.
- The reduction in manual dosing decisions may alleviate the psychological burden and "decision fatigue" often associated with type 2 diabetes.
- Improved glycemic stability could potentially reduce long-term microvascular and macrovascular complications, although long-term outcomes require further validation.

Knowledge Gaps and Scope for Future Research

Further research should examine the cost-effectiveness of widespread AID adoption in type 2 diabetes to inform healthcare reimbursement policies. Studies focusing on "fully" closed-loop systems, eliminating the need for meal blousing, are particularly relevant for this population. Additionally, exploring the impact of AID on quality-of-life metrics and treatment satisfaction over several years would clarify its role in long-term disease management. Investigating algorithm performance in patients with extreme insulin resistance or those using noninsulin adjunct therapies also remains a priority.

9. Efficacy and Safety of Automated Insulin Delivery in Children Aged 2–6 Years (LENNY): An Open-label, Multicentre, Randomized, Crossover Trial

Ref: Battelino T, Kuusela S, Shetty A, Rabbone I, Cherubini V, Campbell F, et al. Efficacy and safety of automated insulin delivery in children aged 2–6 years (LENNY): An open-label, multicentre, randomised, crossover trial. Lancet Diabetes Endocrinol. 2025;13:662-73.

ABSTRACT

Background: Glycemic control abnormalities in early life can have a detrimental impact on brain development and plasticity. The purpose of this study was to evaluate the safety and effectiveness of automated insulin delivery (AID) using the MiniMed 780 G system in children with type 1 diabetes who were between the ages of 2 and 6 and needed at least six units of insulin per day.

Techniques: We recruited children from 12 institutions in Finland, Italy, Slovenia, and the UK for this open-label, randomized crossover study. The MiniMed 780 G system was utilized in manual mode with the suspend before low (SBL) function enabled (manual + SBL) for 2 weeks during the run-in phase. This was followed by a 26-week study phase. Participants in the study phase were randomized to either the reverse order sequence (MM-AM) or a sequence consisting of a 12-week auto mode, 2-week washout, and 12-week manual + SBL mode (AM-MM sequence). The main outcome was the difference between auto mode and manual + SBL mode in the percentage of time in range (TIR, 70–180 mg/dL), which was evaluated for noninferiority (margin 7.5 percentage points) and expressed as the least-squares mean difference adjusted for sequence effect and run-in TIR. The adjusted between-treatment difference in mean TIR and glycated hemoglobin (HbA1c) was evaluated for superiority, and the adjusted between-treatment difference in mean HbA1c at the conclusion of each 12-week period was evaluated for noninferiority (margin 0.4 percentage points). The purpose of the primary and secondary analyses was to treat. Every participant who completed an informed consent form had their safety evaluated. The trial is finished and has been filed with ClinicalTrials.gov under the number NCT05574062.

Results: The period of recruitment was March 24 to September 21, 2023. The study phase started with 98 participants (AM-MM: n = 50, with two dropouts during the study phase; MM-AM: n = 48).

Of the 98 individuals, 48 (49%) were female and 50 (51%) were male. The average age was 4.7 years (SD 1.2). The run-in phase's mean TIR was 58.1% (SD 14.3), the auto mode's was 68.3% (6.9), and the manual + SBL mode's was 58.3% (12.5) (adjusted between-treatment difference 9.9 percentage points [95% confidence interval (CI) 8.0–11.7]; noninferiority was fulfilled for the primary endpoint with superiority for auto mode). In the run-in phase, the mean HbA1c was 7·53% [SD 0.96; 58.8 mmol/mol (SD 10.5)], 7.00% [0.53; 53.0 mmol/mol (5.8)] in auto mode, and 7.61% [0.91; 59.7 mmol/mol (9.9)] in manual + SBL mode (between treatment difference: −0·61 percentage points [95% CI −0·76 to −0·46; noninferiority met with superiority for auto mode]. Nine major adverse events, including one of diabetic ketoacidosis during auto mode, occurred (five during auto mode, two during manual + SBL mode, one during run-in, and one after washout; all regarded unrelated to the research device or method). There were no documented cases of severe hypoglycemia.

Interpretation: The TIR using the MiniMed 780 G device in auto mode was not inferior to that in manual + SBL mode in children with type 1 diabetes between the ages of 2 and 6 years. Diabetes-related consequences may be avoided thanks to the markedly improved TIR and HbA1c in favor of auto mode. Furthermore, the safety profile in auto mode was satisfactory.

CRITICAL APPRAISAL

What was Known Prior to the Study?

- Achieving glycemic targets in preschool children is challenging due to unpredictable eating, physical activity, and high insulin sensitivity.
- Previous studies on automated insulin delivery (AID) systems focused primarily on older children, adolescents, and adults.
- Small-scale trials suggested AID is safe in young children, but high-quality crossover data comparing advanced algorithms to SAP (sensor-augmented pump) therapy remained limited.

What this Study Adds?

- It provides definitive evidence that AHCL (Advanced Hybrid Closed Loop) systems significantly increase "*time in range*" by over 2.4 hours per day in children aged 2–6 compared to SAP.
- It demonstrates that AID reduces glycated hemoglobin (HbA1c) levels while simultaneously decreasing time spent in nocturnal hypoglycemia.
- It confirms the safety and technical feasibility of using the MiniMed 780 G system, featuring an 8.3 mmol/L setpoint, in a population with very low total daily insulin doses.
- It highlights that glycemic benefits are achievable regardless of whether the child was a previous pump user or transitioning from multiple daily injections.

Major Strengths

- Robust multicenter, randomized crossover design minimizing interpatient variability
- High participant retention and adherence rates
- Inclusion of diverse European clinical settings, increasing generalizability within high-income regions
- Rigorous assessment of both efficacy and safety endpoints

Limitations

- Open-label design could introduce behavioral bias in meal announcements or bolus doses.
- The 12-week duration may not capture long-term developmental changes or "technology fatigue".
- Limited ethnic diversity among participants, potentially affecting broader global applicability

Clinical Implications

- AID should be considered the standard of care for preschool children with type 1 diabetes to optimize long-term metabolic health.
- The system effectively mitigates the burden of nocturnal glycemic management for caregivers by providing superior overnight stability.

- Healthcare providers can confidently prescribe AHCL systems even for children with very low insulin requirements, provided appropriate algorithm settings are utilized.

Knowledge Gaps and Scope for Future Research

Future research should investigate the long-term psychosocial impact of AID on both children and their caregivers to assess quality-of-life improvements over several years. Additionally, studies are needed to evaluate the cost-effectiveness of early AID initiation in various healthcare systems. Further exploration into fully closed-loop systems, which eliminate the need for meal announcements, would be particularly beneficial for this age-group, given the inherent unpredictability of carbohydrate intake in toddlers and young children.

10. Intermittently Scanned Continuous Glucose Monitoring Compared with Blood Glucose Monitoring is Associated with Lower HbA1c and a Reduced Risk of Hospitalization for Diabetes-related Complications in Adults with Type 2 Diabetes on Insulin Therapies

Ref: Nathanson D, Eeg-Olofsson K, Spelman T, Bülow E, Kyhlstedt M, Levrat-Guillen F, et al. Intermittently scanned continuous glucose monitoring compared with blood glucose monitoring is associated with lower HbA1c and a reduced risk of hospitalisation for diabetes-related complications in adults with type 2 diabetes on insulin therapies. Diabetologia. 2025;68:41-51.

ABSTRACT

Aim/Hypothesis: In people with insulin-treated type 2 diabetes (T2D) in Sweden, we evaluated the effects of starting intermittently scanned continuous glucose monitoring (isCGM) versus capillary blood glucose monitoring (BGM) on glycated hemoglobin (HbA1c) levels and hospitalizations for diabetes-related comorbidities.

Techniques: Adults with T2D whose National Diabetes Register initiation date for isCGM was after June 1, 2017, were included in this retrospective comparative cohort analysis. Subgroups treated with baseline insulin (T2D-B) or multiple daily insulin injections (T2D-MDI), with or without concomitant glucose-lowering medications, are listed in the Prescribed Drug Register. Hospitalization rates were obtained from the National Patient Register.

Outcomes: We matched 33,584 and 43,424 BGM control participants with 2,876 people in the T2D-MDI group and 2,292 in the T2D-B group who had an isCGM index date after June 1, 2017. In the T2D-MDI cohort, the baseline-adjusted difference between the change in mean HbA1c for isCGM users and BGM control participants was −3.7 mmol/mol (−0.34%) at 6 months, and this difference persisted at 24 months. In the T2D-B cohort, the baseline-adjusted difference in the change in HbA1c between isCGM users and BGM control participants was −3.5 mmol/mol (−0.32%) at 6 months, and this difference persisted at 24 months. The RR of admission for severe hypoglycemia [0.51; 95% confidence interval (CI) 0.27, 0.95], stroke (0.54; 95% CI 0.39, 0.73), acute nonfatal myocardial infarction (0.75; 95% CI 0.57, 0.99), or hospitalization for any reason (0.84; 95% CI 0.77, 0.90) was significantly lower than that of BGM control participants. The relative risk (RR) of heart failure admission (0.63; 95% CI 0.46, 0.87) and hospitalization for any reason (0.76; 95% CI 0.69, 0.84) was lower among isCGM users in the T2D-B sample.

Conclusion and interpretation: According to this study, compared to BGM control participants, Swedish individuals with T2D on insulin who use isCGM have a considerably lower HbA1c and fewer hospital admissions for problems related to their diabetes.

CRITICAL APPRAISAL

What was Known Prior to the Study?

- Continuous glucose monitoring (CGM) was well-established as beneficial for type 1 diabetes, but evidence for type 2 diabetes was more limited.
- Randomized trials had shown that intermittently scanned CGM (isCGM) reduces hypoglycemia and improves quality of life in type 2 diabetes.
- The correlation between isCGM use and hard clinical endpoints, such as cardiovascular hospitalizations in real-world type 2 diabetes populations, remained insufficiently explored.

What this Study Adds?

- It provides evidence that isCGM initiation leads to a sustained decrease in glycated hemoglobin (HbA1c) for up to 24 months across different insulin regimens.
- The study establishes a novel association between isCGM use and a reduced risk of major adverse cardiovascular events, specifically stroke and myocardial infarction, in the MDI (multiple daily insulin injections) population.
- It highlights a specific benefit for patients on basal insulin, showing a significant reduction in hospitalizations for heart failure.
- The findings suggest that the clinical utility of isCGM extends beyond simple glucose tracking to potentially modifying long-term macrovascular outcomes.

Major Strengths

- Large-scale, nationwide cohort providing high statistical power and real-world external validity
- Robust methodology using PS-IPTW (propensity score-based inverse probability of treatment weighting) to mitigate selection bias and confounding by indication
- Longitudinal follow-up (24 months) allows for the observation of durable clinical trends rather than transient effects.

Limitations

- Observational nature precludes definitive causal inference between isCGM use and reduced complications.
- Potential residual confounding from unmeasured lifestyle factors, such as diet or physical activity
- The Swedish healthcare context, characterized by high registry coverage and universal access, may limit generalizability to disparate healthcare systems.

Clinical Implications

- Clinicians should prioritize isCGM for patients with type 2 diabetes on insulin to reduce the risk of life-threatening acute complications.
- The technology offers a proactive management strategy that may alleviate the economic and clinical burden of diabetes-related hospitalizations.
- Glycemic benefits are particularly pronounced in patients with high baseline HbA1c, suggesting a clear target population for maximum impact.
- The reduction in cardiovascular events suggests that improved glucose visibility facilitates better overall metabolic stability and risk factor management.

Knowledge Gaps and Scope for Future Research

While this study identifies a clear association with reduced macrovascular events, the exact mechanisms, whether through reduced glucose variability, earlier detection of dysglycemia, or increased patient engagement, require further elucidation. Future research should focus on prospective interventional trials to confirm causality regarding cardiovascular protection. Additionally, the impact of isCGM on microvascular complications like retinopathy or nephropathy over longer durations (5–10 years) remains an area of high priority. Investigating the cost-effectiveness of widespread isCGM adoption in noninsulin-treated type 2 diabetes also represents a critical frontier for healthcare policy research.

11. Islet Transplantation versus Standard of Care for Type 1 Diabetes Complicated by Severe Hypoglycemia from the Collaborative Islet Transplant Registry and the T1D Exchange Registry

Ref: Rickels MR, Ballou CM, Foster NC, Alejandro R, Baidal DA, Bellin MD, et al. Islet transplantation versus standard of care for type 1 diabetes complicated by severe hypoglycemia from the collaborative Islet Transplant Registry and the T1D Exchange Registry. Diabetes Care. 2025;48:737-44.

ABSTRACT

Objective: The US Food and Drug Administration recently approved islet transplantation for persons with type 1 diabetes who have frequent severe hypoglycemia episodes (SHEs). In comparison to continuing standard of care, we aimed to determine the long-term benefits of islet transplantation for glycemic management and the risk of immunosuppression on renal function.

Research design and methods: We conducted a case-control analysis using prospectively collected data from patients in the Collaborative Islet Transplant Registry (CITR) who had at least one SHE in the year (2000–2014) prior to transplantation (case subjects) and compared them with data from patients in the T1D Exchange (T1DX) Registry who had at least one SHE in the year (2010–2012) prior to enrollment (control subjects). Both cohorts were monitored for 5 years. SHEs were limited to those that caused unconsciousness or seizures.

Results: When compared to control subjects from T1DX (n = 213), case subjects from CITR (n = 71) more frequently achieved the primary outcome of HbA1c < 0.001) and the outcome of HbA1c ≤6.5% and absence of a SHE (60–75% vs. 10–20%; $p < 0.001$) while requiring significantly less insulin (the majority in CITR were insulin-independent). Estimated glomerular filtration rate, a marker of kidney function, decreased from baseline more in CITR than in T1DX (–8.8 to 220 vs. –1.3 to –6.5 mL/min/1.73 m^2 over 5 years; $p < 0.001$).

Conclusion: Adults with type 1 diabetes complicated by SHEs who have ITA are more likely than those receiving standard therapy to achieve near-normal glycemic control in the absence of SHEs, but at the expense of a larger decline in kidney function.

CRITICAL APPRAISAL

What was Known Prior to the Study?

- Severe hypoglycemia remains a major burden for type 1 diabetes patients despite advances in pumps and continuous glucose monitoring.
- Islet transplantation (ITA) can achieve insulin independence and glycemic stability in the short term.
- Long-term comparative data between transplantation and contemporary medical

management, especially for those with high hypoglycemic risk, was limited.

What this Study Adds?

- It provides a direct 5-year comparison showing that ITA far outperforms intensive medical therapy [standard of care (SOC)] in preventing life-threatening hypoglycemic events.
- The study demonstrates that a high percentage (70–80%) of ITA recipients can maintain near-normal glycated hemoglobin (HbA1c) levels (<6.5%) without severe hypoglycemia for half a decade.
- It highlights that current diabetes technologies used in SOC are insufficient for eliminating severe hypoglycemia in the most vulnerable patients.
- The findings establish a benchmark for the expected clinical benefit of ITA, assisting in patient selection for cellular replacement therapies.

Major Strengths

- Use of robust registry data for a well-matched case-control design
- Long-term (5-year) follow-up providing insights into durable clinical benefits
- Focus on the most clinically relevant endpoints: HbA1c and severe hypoglycemia involving loss of consciousness

Limitations

- Observational registry-based design lacks the randomization of a clinical trial.
- Potential for selection bias as ITA recipients and SOC controls may differ in ways not captured by registry data.
- ITA requires lifelong immunosuppression, the side effects of which were not the primary focus of this specific comparison.

Clinical Implications

- ITA should be prioritized as a therapeutic option for patients with type 1 diabetes who suffer from recurrent severe hypoglycemia despite optimal use of technology.
- The dramatic reduction in HbA1c and severe hypoglycemia episodes (SHEs) suggests a significant improvement in safety and quality of life for high-risk individuals.
- Clinicians should recognize that for certain patients, biological replacement is currently more effective than technological interventions in restoring glucose sensing and insulin secretion.

Knowledge Gaps and Scope for Future Research

Future research must address the long-term metabolic consequences of chronic immunosuppression in ITA recipients compared to the complications of persistent hyperglycemia in SOC. There is a critical need for randomized controlled trials to confirm these registry findings. Additionally, research into "encapsulation" or other methods to protect islets without systemic immunosuppression would significantly expand the eligible patient population. Investigating why a subset of ITA recipients loses graft function over time remains essential for improving long-term success rates.

12. Stem Cell-derived, Fully Differentiated Islets for Type 1 Diabetes

Ref: Reichman TW, Markmann JF, Odorico J, Witkowski P, Fung JJ, Wijkstrom M, et al. Stem cell-derived, fully differentiated islets for type 1 diabetes. N Engl J Med. 2025;393:858-68.

ABSTRACT

Background: Zimislecel is an islet-cell treatment produced from allogeneic stem cells. Information regarding zimislecel's effectiveness and safety in people with type 1 diabetes is required.

Techniques: We studied Zimislecel in individuals with type 1 diabetes in phases 1–2. Participants in part A were given a single portal vein infusion of a half dosage of zimislecel (0.4×10^9 cells), with the option to receive a second half dose within 2 years. Participants in sections B and C were given a single infusion of the entire dose of zimislecel (0.8×10^9 cells). Additionally, glucocorticoid-free immunosuppressive treatment was administered to each subject. Safety was the main goal of section A. With a glycated hemoglobin level of <7% or a drop of at least one percentage point from baseline at one or more time intervals between days 180 and 365, the main end point in part C was the absence of severe hypoglycemia episodes over days 90 through 365. Safety and insulin independence between days 180 and 365 were secondary end objectives in section C. Participants who received the entire dose of zimislecel as a single infusion in either part B or part C were evaluated for the primary and secondary end goals in part C. Engraftment and islet function were evaluated by measuring blood C-peptide during a 4-hour mixed-meal tolerance test. Every analysis was preliminary and not predetermined.

Results: A total of 14 patients were included in the analyses after completing at least 12 months of follow-up (2 in part A and 12 in parts B and C). In all 14 individuals, C-peptide was not detected at baseline. C-peptide detection showed that all individuals had engraftment and islet function following zimislecel infusion. The most frequent significant adverse event, which affected three subjects, was neutropenia. There were two fatalities, one from cryptococcal meningitis and the other from severe dementia with agitation brought on by the advancement of preexisting neurocognitive impairment. With a glycated hemoglobin level of <7% and no severe hypoglycemia episodes, all 12 participants in sections B and C spent >70% of their time in the target glucose range (70–180 mg/dL). At day 365, 10 out of the 12 individuals (83%) were insulin-independent and did not use exogenous insulin.

Conclusion: The findings of this brief, small-scale trial involving individuals with type 1 diabetes provide credence to the theory that zimislecel can restore physiologic islet function, which calls for additional clinical research. (Vertex Pharmaceuticals provided funding; VX-880-101 FORWARD ClinicalTrials.gov number, NCT04786262.)

CRITICAL APPRAISAL

What was Known Prior to the Study?

- Cadaveric islet transplantation is an established treatment for type 1 diabetes but is severely limited by a scarcity of donor organs.
- Cellular therapy can eliminate severe hypoglycemia and restore metabolic stability.
- Previous attempts at using stem cell-derived cells often struggled with incomplete differentiation or insufficient insulin production in vivo.

What this Study Adds?

- It provides the first clinical proof-of-concept that stem cell-derived, fully differentiated islets (VX-880) can achieve insulin independence in humans.
- It demonstrates that these manufactured cells respond dynamically to glucose challenges, mirroring physiological pancreatic function.
- It shows that VX-880 effectively eliminates life-threatening severe hypoglycemic events

while maintaining glycated hemoglobin (HbA1c) within target ranges.

- It establishes a scalable alternative to cadaveric islets, potentially broadening the availability of cell replacement therapy for patients with unstable type 1 diabetes.

Major Strengths

- Use of fully differentiated, glucose-responsive islets rather than precursor cells
- Robust evidence of efficacy across multiple participants, including achieved insulin independence
- Detailed metabolic characterization using mixed-meal tolerance tests and continuous glucose monitoring (CGM) metrics

Limitations

- Small sample size and early-phase design lack a control group for comparative efficacy.
- Requirement for lifelong systemic immunosuppression limits the current candidate pool.
- Long-term durability of the stem cell-derived graft beyond the initial follow-up remains to be determined.

Clinical Implications

- Stem cell-derived islets offer a breakthrough for patients with "brittle" type 1 diabetes who have exhausted technological interventions.
- The elimination of severe hypoglycemia through biological replacement significantly reduces the risk of mortality and improves patient safety.
- If long-term safety and efficacy are confirmed, this could shift the treatment paradigm from mechanical insulin delivery to biological restoration of endocrine function.

Knowledge Gaps and Scope for Future Research

The immediate challenge remains the necessity for chronic immunosuppression, which carries significant long-term risks. Future research must investigate delivery methods such as macroencapsulation or gene-editing techniques (hypoimmunogenic cells) to protect islets from immune rejection without systemic drugs. Additionally, longer-term follow-up is essential to assess the functional longevity of stem cell-derived islets compared to cadaveric grafts. Expanding clinical trials to larger, more diverse cohorts will also be necessary to confirm safety and optimize dosing protocols for broader clinical adoption.

13. Corneal Confocal Microscopy Identifies Early and Definite Diabetic Cardiac Autonomic Neuropathy

Ref: Azmi S, Ferdousi M, Kalteniece A, Petropoulos IN, Alam U, Ponirakis G, et al. Corneal confocal microscopy identifies early and definite diabetic cardiac autonomic neuropathy. Diabetes Res Clin Pract. 2025;224:112172.

ABSTRACT

Objective: Diabetes patients who have advanced cardiac autonomic neuropathy (CAN) had higher mortality rates. The course of CAN can be slowed by early detection and mitigation of risk factors. However, cardiac autonomic reflex testing (CART), which is not commonly accessible, is necessary for the diagnosis of early CAN. In order to diagnose CAN, we have compared the diagnostic value of corneal confocal microscopy (CCM) and CART.

Methods and design of the research: CART and CCM were used to evaluate 238 people with type 1 and type 2 diabetes and 37 healthy controls.

Results: As the severity of CAN increased, there was a progressive and substantial decrease in DB-HRV (deep breathing heart rate variability), E:I (expiration to inspiration) ratio, 30:15 ratio, corneal nerve fiber density (CNFD), corneal nerve branch density (CNBD), and corneal nerve fiber length (CNFL). For detecting early and definitive CAN, CCM's sensitivity/specificity and receiver operating characteristic (ROC) area under the curve (AUC) were similar to those of CART.

Conclusion: CCM is a quick, noninvasive eye test that may be used to identify CAN in its early stages.

CRITICAL APPRAISAL

What was Known Prior to the Study?

- Advanced cardiac autonomic neuropathy is strongly linked to increased mortality rates in diabetic populations.
- Standard diagnosis depends on cardiac autonomic reflex testing (CART), which require specialized equipment and are often unavailable in clinical settings.
- Corneal confocal microscopy (CCM) had previously been established as a sensitive biomarker for identifying and stratifying the severity of diabetic peripheral neuropathy.

What this Study Adds?

- It provides robust evidence that CCM can detect early-stage cardiac autonomic neuropathy (CAN), which is often asymptomatic and difficult to diagnose using traditional methods.
- The study demonstrates that corneal nerve fiber loss directly mirrors the progressive deterioration of cardiac autonomic function.
- It validates CCM as having a sensitivity and specificity for CAN diagnosis that is equivalent to the established gold-standard CART.
- The research highlights CCM's advantage as a test unaffected by cardiovascular medications, such as beta-blockers, which can confound CART results.

Major Strengths

- Use of a large, well-characterized cohort including both type 1 and type 2 diabetes patients
- Comparative methodology against the gold-standard diagnostic criteria for CAN
- Masked analysis of corneal nerve morphology to ensure the objectivity of the results

Limitations

- The cross-sectional design limits the ability to determine the predictive value of CCM for future clinical events.
- Single-center study setting may affect the generalizability of findings to broader global populations.
- The manual quantification of corneal nerves is labor-intensive compared to automated systems.

Clinical Implications

- CCM can be utilized as a rapid, noninvasive screening tool to identify high-risk patients who require early intervention.
- Implementation of CCM in ophthalmic or diabetes clinics could improve the detection rates of undiagnosed CAN.
- The objective nature of CCM data allows for reliable monitoring of nerve health without the confounding effects of systemic medications.

Knowledge Gaps and Scope for Future Research

While this study establishes CCM's diagnostic accuracy, its ability to predict the long-term progression of CAN and associated mortality remains unconfirmed. Future research should prioritize longitudinal studies to evaluate whether changes in corneal nerve parameters can forecast major adverse cardiovascular events. Additionally, interventional trials are necessary to determine if therapeutic improvements in metabolic control are reflected in corneal nerve regeneration. Exploring the integration of fully automated artificial intelligence (AI)-driven CCM analysis could further enhance clinical throughput and reduce the subjectivity associated with manual quantification.

14. Prediction of the Risk of Diabetic Foot from Corneal Nerve Images Using Deep Learning Algorithms

Ref: Liu C, Zhu L, O'Donnell GP, Koh MH, Yu M, Lee IXY, et al. Prediction of the risk of diabetic foot from corneal nerve images using deep learning algorithms. Diabetes Res Clin Pract. 2025;230:112991.

ABSTRACT

Aims: Our goal was to create a deep learning algorithm (DLA) that uses corneal nerve pictures to predict the risk categories of diabetic foot.

Methods: A total of 23,550 photos from 471 participants' 942 eyes were used. Initially, we created a DLA using only corneal nerve pictures. To create hybrid DLAs, we then integrated quantitative corneal nerve characteristics with traditional clinical risk factors of diabetic peripheral neuropathy. The area under the receiver operating characteristic curve (AUC) was used to evaluate the model's performance.

Findings: The AUC for the DLA using corneal nerve pictures alone was 0.76 for identifying patients at high risk and 0.69 for predicting diabetic foot. The algorithm for the hybrid DLAs obtained an AUC of 0.94 for the prediction of diabetic foot with just the addition of HbA1c and an AUC of 0.93 for the identification of patients with high-risk diabetic foot with the addition of serum creatinine. When quantitative corneal nerve parameters were used instead of just corneal nerve images, there was no improvement in performance.

Conclusion: Our DLAs that combine corneal nerve pictures with blood creatinine or glycated hemoglobin (HbA1c) work well in predicting and classifying diabetic foot risk, offering a novel screening method.

CRITICAL APPRAISAL

What was Known Prior to the Study?

- Diabetic peripheral neuropathy (DPN) is a primary driver of foot ulcers and subsequent amputations.
- Subjective clinical assessments for diabetic foot risk often suffer from low repeatability and are time-intensive.
- Corneal nerve status, visible through in vivo confocal microscopy (IVCM), serves as a validated surrogate biomarker for peripheral nerve health and neurodegeneration.

What this Study Adds?

- It demonstrates the first application of deep learning for direct diabetic foot risk stratification using corneal nerve images.
- The study reveals that hybrid models combining images with single biomarkers [specifically glycated hemoglobin (HbA1c) or creatinine] are as effective as models using extensive clinical datasets.
- It establishes that automated deep learning analysis of raw images outperforms manual

or software-assisted quantitative nerve parameter extraction.
- The research provides a noninvasive, objective alternative to skin biopsies or time-consuming nerve conduction studies for foot risk assessment.

Major Strengths

- Large, high-quality dataset of over 23,000 IVCM images
- Robust methodology using ResNet-50 and XGBoost ensemble techniques to handle heterogeneous data
- Focus on clinical risk stratification rather than binary disease detection, enhancing practical utility

Limitations

- Retrospective, cross-sectional design limits the ability to establish temporal causality between nerve changes and ulcer development.
- Single-center study in Singapore may affect the generalizability of the findings to more diverse global populations.
- Reliance on IVCM technology, which requires specialized equipment and training

Clinical Implications

- The deep learning algorithm (DLA) offers a rapid, objective screening tool that could be integrated into routine ophthalmic or diabetic care.
- High-risk patients can be identified earlier, allowing for targeted preventative interventions and reduced healthcare costs.
- The technology simplifies assessment by requiring only a few key biomarkers alongside imaging, reducing the clinical burden of comprehensive foot examinations.

Knowledge Gaps and Scope for Future Research

The current study does not provide longitudinal data to confirm if these predictive models can forecast the exact timing of ulcer development. Future research should prioritize multicenter longitudinal trials to validate the DLA across different ethnicities and healthcare settings. Additionally, exploring the integration of these models with portable or more accessible corneal imaging technologies could expand their reach into primary care. Investigating whether improving corneal nerve health (through intensive metabolic control) directly corresponds to a reduced DLA-predicted risk score also remains a vital area for future clinical exploration.

---

15. Leveraging Artificial Intelligence and Machine Learning to Accelerate Discovery of Disease-modifying Therapies in Type 1 Diabetes (Review Article)

Ref: Shapiro MR, Tallon EM, Brown ME, Posgai AL, Clements MA, Brusko TM. Leveraging artificial intelligence and machine learning to accelerate discovery of disease-modifying therapies in type 1 diabetes (Review article). Diabetologia. 2025;68:477-94.

ABSTRACT

Limited animal models, the length and expense of clinical trials, challenges in identifying individuals who will progress more quickly to a clinical diagnosis of type 1 diabetes, and heterogeneous clinical responses in intervention trials have all impeded the development of therapies for the maintenance of endogenous insulin secretion in, or the prevention of, type 1 diabetes. Monotherapies, large participant groups, and long follow-up periods centered on clinical goals are common features of traditional placebo-controlled intervention trials. Although this method is still the "gold standard" for clinical research, new strategies that use machine learning and artificial intelligence (AI) to speed up drug development and efficacy testing are being developed. Here, we examine new strategies for choosing synergistic drug combinations to maximize therapeutic efficacy and repurposing medications used to treat conditions that share pathogenic pathways with type 1 diabetes. We talk about the potential for new biomarkers to be found and then translated into antigen-specific immunotherapies through the use of developing multiomics technologies, such as investigation of antigen processing and presentation to adaptive immune cells. We also talk about the possibility of employing AI to develop "digital twin" models that allow for quick in silico testing of customized medicines and dose calculation. In conclusion, we go over some of the drawbacks of machine learning and AI, such as problems with model interpretability and bias and the ongoing requirement for validation research using confirmatory intervention trials.

CRITICAL APPRAISAL

What was Known Prior to the Study?

- Type 1 diabetes is a heterogeneous disease, meaning patients respond differently to the same therapies.
- Developing disease-modifying therapies (DMTs) is hindered by high costs, long trial durations, and the lack of reliable animal models that mimic human disease.
- Traditional "gold standard" placebo-controlled trials often focus on single drugs, which may not be sufficient to halt the complex autoimmune destruction of beta cells.

What this Study Adds?

- It provides a comprehensive framework for using artificial intelligence (AI) to repurpose existing drugs from other autoimmune diseases (like lupus or psoriasis) for type 1 diabetes (T1D) based on shared molecular targets.
- The paper introduces the concept of "Digital Twins" and AI-simulated control groups to reduce the number of participants needed for clinical trials.
- It demonstrates how machine learning (ML) can integrate "multiomic" data (genetics, proteomics, etc.) to identify specific patient endotypes for personalized treatment.
- The authors propose AI-driven "adaptive" trial designs that allow for the simultaneous testing of multiple drug combinations, significantly increasing research efficiency.

Major Strengths

- It provides an interdisciplinary bridge between advanced computational science and clinical immunology.
- It offers a clear roadmap for transitioning from "one-size-fits-all" treatments to precision medicine.
- It critically addresses the high failure rate of traditional T1D intervention trials.

Limitations

- AI models depend heavily on the quality and diversity of input data, which may be biased or limited.
- The paper notes that many AI-derived insights currently lack rigorous prospective validation in human clinical trials.
- Ethical and regulatory frameworks for AI-designed trials are still in their infancy.

Clinical Implications

- *Precision screening*: ML can identify individuals at highest risk of rapid progression, allowing for earlier therapeutic intervention.
- *Combination therapies*: AI can predict which drug pairings will be most effective for an individual's specific disease profile, potentially improving success rates.
- *Reduced trial burden*: Using AI to optimize participant selection and trial duration could bring new therapies to market faster and at lower costs.

Knowledge Gaps and Scope for Future Research

A primary knowledge gap remains the "black box" nature of some ML algorithms, which can make it difficult for clinicians to interpret the biological rationale behind a prediction. Future research must focus on "Explainable AI" to ensure that computational findings are biologically plausible and clinically actionable. Additionally, there is a need for large-scale, open-access data repositories that allow researchers to train models on diverse global populations. Finally, prospective clinical trials must be conducted to prove that AI-optimized regimens actually outperform standard-of-care protocols.

Section 9: MISCELLANEOUS

Section Editor: Nisha Batra

1. The Fibrosis Investigating Navigator in Diabetes (FIND): A Tool to Predict Liver Fibrosis Risk in Subjects with Diabetes

Ref: Li M, Yu H, Wan S, Hu F, Luo Q, Gong W. The Fibrosis Investigating Navigator in Diabetes (FIND): A Tool to Predict Liver Fibrosis Risk in Subjects with Diabetes. Diabetes Obes Metab. 2025;27(3):1184-97.

ABSTRACT

Background: Liver cancer and cirrhosis are more common in those with type 2 diabetes. Early and noninvasive evaluation of liver fibrosis is crucial. Our goal was to create a score that would help with the preliminary evaluation of liver fibrosis in the diabetic population.

Techniques: The National Health and Nutrition Examination Survey (NHANES) dataset (2017–2020) was used to generate and validate the fibrosis investigating navigator in diabetes (FIND) score. A liver stiffness measurement (LSM) of ≥8.0 kPa was considered indicative of fibrosis. The diagnostic accuracies of fibrosis-4 (FIB-4), nonalcoholic fatty liver disease (NAFLD) fibrosis score (NFS), LiverRisk, steatosis-associated fibrosis estimator (SAFE) and metabolic dysfunction-associated fibrosis 5 (MAF-5) were compared. Between 2016 and 2020, FIND was also externally verified in an Asian center using biopsy as a reference for a variety of liver disorders. Lastly, we used data from the UK Biobank cohort (2006–2010) to investigate the prognostic implications of the FIND index.

Outcomes: For the prediction of an LSM ≥ 8 kPa in the validation set, the FIND score model produced an area under the receiver operating characteristic curve (AUROC) of 0.781, which was consistently higher than that of other models that were available (all $p < 0.05$). The 85% specificity cut-off of 0.31 was associated with a positive predictive value (PPV) of 50.6% and the 85% sensitivity cut-off of 0.16 with a negative predictive value (NPV) of 91.9% over the whole NHANES dataset. Using biopsy as a reference, FIND's overall accuracy in staging fibrosis stages was comparable to that of the other models. In the UK Biobank cohort, FIND > 0.31 was linked in adjusted models to a higher risk of liver-related and all-cause death in the diabetic population [hazard ratio (HR), 23.59; 95% confidence interval (CI) 13.67–40.69; HR 1.75; 95% CI 1.62–1.89].

Conclusion: The innovative FIND score does a good job of predicting all-cause and liver-related mortality in patients with diabetes as well as identifying individuals at risk of liver fibrosis.

CRITICAL APPRAISAL

Metabolic dysfunction-associated steatotic liver disease (MASLD) is highly prevalent and affects over half of individuals with type 2 diabetes mellitus (T2DM), in whom there is accelerated fibrosis progression and increased risk of cirrhosis and hepatocellular carcinoma.[1] Nearly 20% of diabetic patients have advanced fibrosis, highlighting the need for effective screening.[2] While liver biopsy is the reference standard, its invasive nature limits large-scale use and transient elastography, although validated, is constrained by availability and cost. Consequently, blood-based noninvasive tests are recommended as first-line tools; however, commonly used scores such as fibrosis-4 (FIB-4) and nonalcoholic fatty liver disease (NAFLD) fibrosis score (NFS) perform poorly in diabetic populations. Newer models including LiverRisk, steatosis-associated fibrosis estimator (SAFE), and metabolic dysfunction-associated fibrosis 5 (MAF-5) lack diabetes specificity or rely on biopsy-derived outcomes or metabolically variable parameters.[3,4] These limitations prompted the development of a simple, diabetes-specific noninvasive score to accurately identify patients at risk of liver fibrosis and guide referral pathways.

This study comprised three phases: Model development and internal validation, external validation, and prognostic assessment. The fibrosis investigating navigator in diabetes (FIND) score was developed using the National Health and Nutrition Examination Survey (NHANES) 2017–2020 data from adults with type 2 diabetes mellitus (T2DM) who underwent vibration-controlled transient elastography. Liver fibrosis risk was defined primarily as liver stiffness measurement (LSM) ≥ 8.0 kPa, with LSM ≥ 12.0 kPa assessed as a secondary endpoint. The NHANES cohort was randomly divided into training and validation sets. Candidate demographic, anthropometric, biochemical, and metabolic variables were evaluated, and least absolute shrinkage and selection operator (LASSO) regression was used to derive a parsimonious and clinically applicable model. Final FIND score included waist circumference, waist-to-height ratio, aspartate aminotransferase (AST), and gamma-glutamyl transferase (GGT), and was calculated using a weighted equation.

Diagnostic performance was assessed using area under the receiver operating characteristic curve (AUROC), calibration, and decision curve analysis, and compared with established fibrosis scores including FIB-4, NFS, LiverRisk, SAFE, and MAF-5. Predefined cut-offs were used for clinical risk stratification, with values <0.16 indicating low risk, 0.16–0.31 intermediate risk, and >0.31 high risk warranting specialist referral. External validation was performed in an independent Asian cohort of T2DM who underwent liver biopsy between 2016 and 2020, with fibrosis staged according to the Scheuer classification. Prognostic validity was evaluated in UK Biobank cohort by examining associations between FIND categories and all-cause and liver-related mortality using multivariable Cox proportional hazards models adjusted for relevant confounders.

A total of 1,200 participants from NHANES were included for model development and validation, among whom 21.6% had LSM ≥ 8 kPa and 7.7% had LSM ≥ 12 kPa. In the validation cohort, FIND achieved an AUROC of 0.781 for detecting LSM ≥ 8 kPa, outperforming all comparator models. Across the entire NHANES cohort, a cut-off of 0.16 yielded a sensitivity of 84.6% and a negative predictive value (NPV) of 91.9%, while a cut-off of 0.31 achieved a specificity of 85.0% and a positive predictive value (PPV) of 50.6%. FIND demonstrated stable performance across subgroups defined by age, sex, body mass index (BMI), alcohol use, hypertension, hepatic steatosis, and transaminase levels. In biopsy validation (n = 110), FIND increased progressively with fibrosis stage and showed diagnostic accuracy comparable to other models for significant (≥S2) and advanced fibrosis (≥S3), including in MASLD-only patients. In UK Biobank cohort (n = 24,430; median follow-up 155 months), higher FIND categories were strongly associated with increased all-cause mortality and liver-related mortality, with adjusted hazard ratios of 1.75 and 23.59 respectively for FIND > 0.31, and FIND demonstrated superior prognostic discrimination compared with existing scores.

This study presents the development and validation of FIND score, a simple, diabetes-specific noninvasive tool designed to identify patients at risk of clinically significant liver fibrosis and adverse outcomes. Unlike existing scores, FIND was derived using LSM as the primary screening reference, aligning with current guidelines for fibrosis assessment in diabetes. The model consistently outperformed FIB-4 and other established scores in identifying liver fibrosis and demonstrated robust prognostic value for all-cause and liver-related mortality. Compared with prior tools; SAFE, LiverRisk, and MAF-5; FIND score uses stable, routinely available variables, and avoids reliance on metabolically volatile measures like plasma glucose or lipid levels, which may fluctuate with therapy. Inclusion of waist-to-height ratio and gamma-glutamyl transferase (GGT) likely enhanced performance by capturing insulin resistance-driven metabolic risk and hepatic injury more accurately in diabetes. Key strengths of the study include its large population-based derivation cohort, external validation against biopsy-proven fibrosis, and long-term outcome assessment in an independent European cohort. However, there were some limitations as well, including relatively small single-center biopsy cohort, exclusion of patients with viral hepatitis, and moderate correlation with transient elastography. Future research is needed for multicenter validation across diverse ethnic groups, assessment of longitudinal changes in FIND over time, and integration into electronic health record-based referral algorithms to optimize early detection and management of liver fibrosis in patients with diabetes.

2. Benefits of Combining SGLT-2 Inhibitors and Pioglitazone on Risk of MASH in Type 2 Diabetes—A Real-world Study

Ref: Lee CH, Lui DT, Mak LY, Fong CH, Chan KS, Mak JH, et al. Benefits of Combining SGLT2 Inhibitors and Pioglitazone on Risk of MASH in Type 2 Diabetes—A Real-world Study. Diabetes Obes Metab. 2025;27(2):574-82.

ABSTRACT

Aim: In randomized clinical trials, pioglitazone and glucagon-like peptide 1 receptor agonists (GLP-1 RA) by themselves both ameliorate metabolic dysfunction-associated steatohepatitis (MASH); however, preclinical research indicated that MASH benefits with sodium-glucose cotransporter-2 inhibitors (SGLT-2i). In the real world, people with type 2 diabetes frequently need several medications to control their blood sugar levels. Here, we looked into how combining these agents could reduce the complications associated with MASH.

Supplies and procedures: 888 patients with type 2 diabetes had their FibroScan-aspartate aminotransferase (FAST) score assessed throughout time. Pioglitazone, GLP-1 RA, and/or SGLT-2i use was characterized as continuous prescriptions for at least 180 days before the last FibroScan reassessment. The relationships between the use of these drugs and changes in FAST scores were assessed using multivariable logistic regression analysis.

Results: Using more of these medications was substantially linked to higher FAST score reductions over a median follow-up of 3.9 years (p for trend <0.01). Compared to solo usage of any of these medicines, dual combination was independently linked to an increased chance of obtaining a poor FAST score at reassessment [odds ratio (OR) 2.84; $p = 0.01$]. After controlling for changes in body weight and glycemic control throughout the study, using SGLT-2i and pioglitazone (median dose 15 mg daily) together was linked to a higher likelihood of both low FAST score at reassessment (OR 6.51; $p = 0.008$) and FAST score regression (OR 12.52; $p = 0.009$).

Conclusion: SGLT-2i and pioglitazone together may be a preferred option for improving "at-risk" MASH in type 2 diabetic patients.

CRITICAL APPRAISAL

Metabolic dysfunction-associated steatotic liver disease (MASLD) is highly prevalent in type 2 diabetes,[5] with many patients progressing to at-risk metabolic dysfunction-associated steatohepatitis (MASH),[6] which is associated with increased liver-related and cardiovascular risk.[7] Although pioglitazone and glucagon-like peptide 1 receptor agonists (GLP-1 RA) have shown benefit in MASH, evidence for sodium-glucose cotransporter-2 inhibitors (SGLT-2i)—especially in combination regimens—remains limited. Given the multifactorial pathophysiology of MASH, combination metabolic therapy may provide additive benefit. This study aimed to evaluate the real-world impact of pioglitazone, GLP-1 receptor agonists, and SGLT-2i—alone and in combination—on MASH risk in patients with type 2 diabetes using noninvasive assessment.

This was a prospective, longitudinal, real-world observational study conducted within the Hong Kong West Diabetes nonalcoholic fatty liver disease (NAFLD) Cohort. Adult patients aged 21–80 years with type 2 diabetes mellitus (T2DM) who had undergone at least one reassessment vibration-controlled transient elastography (VCTE) between 2017 and 2023 were included, while those with other chronic liver diseases, significant alcohol intake, active malignancy, steatogenic drug use, or prior bariatric surgery were excluded. Liver assessment was performed using serial FibroScan examinations at 12–18-month intervals, and MASH risk was evaluated using the FibroScan–AST (FAST) score.

Use of pioglitazone, GLP-1 RA, and SGLT-2i was defined as continuous prescription for at least 180 days prior to the last FibroScan reassessment. Participants were categorized based on single, dual, or triple use of these agents. The primary outcomes were maintenance of a low FAST score (≤0.35) or regression of FAST score from >0.35 to ≤0.35 over follow-up. Multivariable logistic regression analyses were performed to assess independent associations between antidiabetic medication use and FAST score outcomes, adjusting for baseline FAST score, body mass index, platelet count, triglycerides, coronary heart disease, and changes in glycated hemoglobin (HbA1c) and body weight, with sensitivity analyses to test robustness.

A total of 888 patients with type 2 diabetes were followed for a median duration of 3.9 years. Increasing use of pioglitazone, GLP-1 receptor agonists, and SGLT-2i was associated with a greater likelihood of achieving and maintaining a low FAST score, indicating reduced risk of at-risk MASH (p for trend <0.01). Dual-agent therapy was superior to single-agent therapy, with the combination of SGLT-2i and pioglitazone showing the strongest association with both maintenance of a low FAST score [adjusted odds ratio (OR) 6.51] and regression from higher FAST categories to ≤0.35 (adjusted OR 12.52). These associations remained significant after adjustment for changes in HbA1c and body weight and were consistent across multiple sensitivity analyses.

The key finding of this study is the strong and consistent association between combined SGLT-2i and pioglitazone therapy and both maintenance and regression of low MASH risk. This association remained independent of changes in HbA1c and body weight, suggesting potential direct hepatic benefits beyond glycemic control and weight loss. The combination is biologically plausible, as pioglitazone improves insulin sensitivity via PPAR-γ activation, while SGLT-2i reduce hepatic inflammation and lipotoxicity and provide cardiorenal protection, potentially offsetting pioglitazone-related adverse effects.

However, important limitations need to be considered. The observational design precludes causal inference and is susceptible to confounding and treatment selection bias. Absence of liver histology limits definitive assessment of MASH, and reliance on the FAST score cannot fully substitute for biopsy-based outcomes. The relatively small number of GLP-1 RA users, modest drug doses, and absence of newer incretin agents such as high-dose semaglutide or tirzepatide restrict conclusions regarding incretin-based therapies. Additionally, the exclusively Chinese cohort may limit generalizability to other ethnic populations.

3. Diagnostic Accuracy of Agile-4 Score for Liver Cirrhosis in Patients with Metabolic Dysfunction-associated Steatotic Liver Disease. A Systematic Review and Meta-analysis of Diagnostic Test Accuracy Studies

Ref: Malandris K, Katsoula A, Liakos A, Karagiannis T, Sinakos E, Giouleme O, et al. Diagnostic Accuracy of Agile-4 Score for Liver Cirrhosis in Patients with Metabolic Dysfunction-associated Steatotic Liver Disease. A Systematic Review and Meta-analysis of Diagnostic Test Accuracy Studies. Diabetes Obes Metab. 2025;27(3):1406-14.

ABSTRACT

Aim: For the purpose of identifying cirrhosis in patients with metabolic dysfunction-associated steatotic liver disease (MASLD), a novel noninvasive score called the Agile-4 score has been developed. It combines liver stiffness measurements, aspartate aminotransferase/alanine aminotransferase, platelet count, diabetes status, and sex. We evaluated Agile-4's ability to rule out or rule in hepatic cirrhosis in patients with MASLD.

Materials and methods: Up until May 2024, we looked through the websites of Medline, the Cochrane Library, Web of Science, Scopus, and Echosens. Eligible studies investigated the accuracy of Agile-4 for ruling-in (≥0.565) and ruling-out (<0.251) liver cirrhosis, using biopsy as the reference standard, at predetermined criteria. For both Agile-4 thresholds, we computed pooled sensitivity and specificity values along with 95% confidence intervals using bivariate random-effect models. Using the Quality Assessment of Diagnostic Accuracy Studies-2 method, we evaluated the risk of bias.

Findings: Seven studies with 6,037 participants were included. A pooled specificity of 0.93 [95% confidence interval (CI) 0.86–0.97] was obtained with an Agile-4 score ≥0.565. Similarly, cirrhosis was ruled out with an Agile-4 score <0.251 and a summary sensitivity of 0.90 (0.80–0.95). The positive predictive value (PPV) for ruling-in cirrhosis was 80%, whereas the negative predictive value for ruling-out cirrhosis was 95%, assuming a 30% prevalence of cirrhosis. Because of issues with patient selection and the blinding of Agile-4 score interpretation in respect to biopsy results, the majority of studies had a high or unclear risk of bias.

Conclusion: In MASLD patients, the Agile-4 score does a good job of ruling out liver cirrhosis. Sequential use of the Agile-4 following fibrosis-4 (FIB-4) index testing may further improve its performance due to the comparatively low PPV.

CRITICAL APPRAISAL

Metabolic dysfunction-associated steatotic liver disease (MASLD) affects nearly 30% of the general population and up to 65% of individuals with type 2 diabetes mellitus (T2DM).[8] Its progressive form can lead to advanced fibrosis and cirrhosis, which can lead to liver-related complications and mortality, making early identification of patients with F3–F4 disease clinically critical. Although liver biopsy remains the reference standard, its invasiveness, cost, sampling error, and interobserver variability limit widespread use. Common noninvasive tools such as the fibrosis-4 (FIB-4) index and vibration-controlled transient elastography (VCTE) are effective for excluding advanced disease but have limited accuracy for confidently ruling in higher fibrosis stages.[9] To overcome these limitations, Agile scores were developed, with Agile-3+ targeting advanced fibrosis and Agile-4 specifically designed for cirrhosis.[10]

However, despite increasing clinical use of the Agile-4 score, its overall diagnostic accuracy for cirrhosis in MASLD had not been systematically evaluated. Therefore, this study was conducted to summarize and quantify the available evidence on the performance of Agile-4 for ruling in and ruling out liver cirrhosis using liver biopsy as the reference standard.

This systematic review and meta-analysis was conducted as per PRISMA-DTA guidelines and registered in PROSPERO. Medline, Scopus, Web of Science, Cochrane Library, and the Echosens website were searched up to May 2024. Cohort or cross-sectional studies in adults with MASLD that evaluated Agile-4 for diagnosing cirrhosis using liver biopsy as the reference standard were included. The Agile-4 score is a composite noninvasive index incorporating liver stiffness measurement, aspartate transaminase/alanine transaminase (AST/ALT) ratio, platelet count, diabetes status, and sex. Predefined cut-offs were used for ruling-in (≥0.565) and ruling-out (<0.251) cirrhosis. Sensitivity, specificity, likelihood ratios, and predictive values were pooled using bivariate random-effects models. Heterogeneity was explored visually and through meta-regression, while risk of bias and applicability were assessed using the QUADAS-2 tool.

Seven studies involving 6,037 participants were included, with most being multicenter, retrospective studies from tertiary care settings. Cirrhosis prevalence was 16.2%. For ruling-in cirrhosis, an Agile-4 score ≥0.565 showed a pooled specificity of 0.93 and a positive likelihood ratio of 9.5, indicating strong confirmatory ability. For ruling-out cirrhosis, a score <0.251 achieved a pooled sensitivity of 0.90 with a negative likelihood ratio of 0.12. Assuming a 30% cirrhosis prevalence, the positive predictive value was 80% and the negative predictive value was 95%. Considerable heterogeneity was observed, with age, body mass index (BMI), and diabetes prevalence identified as contributing factors. Many studies had high or unclear risk of bias, mainly related to patient selection and lack of blinding.

This meta-analysis demonstrates that the Agile-4 score performs well for both ruling-in and ruling-out cirrhosis in MASLD, with high specificity at the upper cut-off and high sensitivity at the lower cut-off. The strong performance is likely due to its composite nature, combining liver stiffness with clinical and biochemical variables. Findings align with the original derivation and validation studies by Sanyal et al.[10] and are consistent with external validation cohorts, while showing superior diagnostic accuracy compared with FIB-4 and performance comparable to VCTE. Strengths of this study include adherence to robust diagnostic meta-analysis methodology, use of standardized cut-offs, and clinically meaningful outcome measures. However, limited number of studies, heterogeneity, predominance of retrospective designs, and frequent risk of selection bias restrict generalizability. Additionally, a diagnostic "gray zone" remained for a proportion of patients. Future studies are needed regarding prospective validation, individual patient-level meta-analyses, evaluation across BMI and diabetes subgroups, or for assessment of sequential strategies such as FIB-4 followed by Agile-4, and exploration of Agile-4 as a predictor of liver-related clinical outcomes.

4. Efficacy and Safety of Survodutide on Glycemic Control and Weight Loss in Adults: A Systematic Review and Meta-analysis

Ref: Xiao YJ, Yu S, Zhang YL, Chen J, Liu YQ, Liu XL, et al. Efficacy and Safety of Survodutide on Glycemic Control and Weight Loss in Adults: A Systematic Review and Meta-analysis. Diabetes Obes Metab. 2025;27(12):7062-74.

ABSTRACT

Aim: The purpose of this meta-analysis was to assess the safety and effectiveness of survodutide on adult weight loss and glycemic management.

Techniques: Up until July 12, 2025, we thoroughly searched PubMed, Embase, the Cochrane Library, Scopus, Web of Science, and ClinicalTrials.gov for randomized controlled studies (RCTs) assessing the safety and effectiveness of survodutide. Changes in body weight, waist circumference, fasting glucagon levels, glycated hemoglobin (HbA1c), and the frequency of adverse events (AEs) were the main outcomes. Blood pressure, lipid profiles, and body mass index (BMI) were secondary outcomes.

Results: This meta-analysis includes six RCTs with 1,272 participants. Survodutide significantly lowered fasting glucagon levels [weighted mean difference (WMD): 7 pmol/L, 95% confidence interval (CI) (10.3, 3.69); $p = 0.016$] and HbA1c [WMD: 0.66%; 95% CI (1.08, 0.23); $p = 0.002$] when compared to placebo. The cohort receiving a total weekly dose of >2.4 mg showed larger decreases than the segment receiving ≤2.4 mg weekly. Additionally, survodutide significantly reduced waist circumference [WMD: 7.09 cm; 95% CI (9.44, 4.47); $p < 0.001$] and body weight [WMD: 6.7 kg; 95% CI (10.0, 3.4); $p < 0.001$], with greater benefits shown at larger total weekly doses (>2.4 mg) and longer treatment periods (>16 weeks). Significant drops in BMI were also seen, but blood pressure, triglycerides, and total cholesterol showed only slight drops. Although there was no discernible rise in the frequency of serious AEs, survodutide was linked to a higher risk of treatment discontinuation due to AEs, with gastrointestinal AEs being the most frequent.

Conclusion: Survodutide dramatically decreased waist circumference, body weight, and HbA1c. A larger total weekly dose (>2.4 mg) was specifically linked to a bigger reduction in HbA1c, and both higher doses and longer treatment durations (>16 weeks) were associated with more noticeable effects on body weight and waist circumference. Nonetheless, it is important to draw attention to the notable rise in gastrointestinal AEs and the corresponding risk of stopping treatment. To verify these findings across a variety of populations, more extensive, multicenter, long-term, high-quality RCTs are required.

CRITICAL APPRAISAL

Obesity and type 2 diabetes mellitus (T2DM) are major global health challenges,[11,12] and although glucagon-like peptide-1 (GLP-1) receptor agonists have improved glycemic control and promoted weight loss, their effects on energy expenditure and hepatic metabolism are limited. Dual activation of glucagon and GLP-1 receptors has emerged as a promising strategy to enhance metabolic outcomes by combining appetite suppression with increased energy expenditure while maintaining glycemic stability.[13]

Survodutide (BI 456906), a long-acting, once-weekly dual GLP-1/glucagon receptor agonist, has demonstrated encouraging results in preclinical studies and early clinical trials, including meaningful reductions in body weight and improvements in glycemic and cardiometabolic parameters.[14,15] However, existing clinical evidence is heterogeneous, with variability in study design, dosing, treatment duration, and reported outcomes, and its overall efficacy, dose–response relationships, and safety profile remain incompletely defined. Therefore, a systematic review and meta-analysis were conducted to evaluate the drug's efficacy and safety in randomized controlled studies (RCTs) and to clarify its role in managing obesity and metabolic disorders.

This systematic review and meta-analysis was conducted as per Preferred Reporting Items for Systematic Reviews and Meta-Analyses (PRISMA) guidelines. PubMed, Embase, the Cochrane Library, Scopus, Web of Science, and ClinicalTrials.gov were searched from inception to 12 July 2025 for randomized controlled trials evaluating survodutide in adults. Eligible studies included adult participants who received survodutide and reported at least one predefined efficacy or safety outcome, with placebo or comparator arms. The primary outcomes were changes in glycated hemoglobin (HbA1c), fasting glucagon levels, body weight, waist circumference, and adverse events (AEs) while secondary outcomes included body mass index (BMI), lipid parameters and blood pressure. Prespecified subgroup analyses were performed based on weekly dose (≤2.4 mg vs. >2.4 mg) and treatment duration (≤16 vs. >16 weeks). Study quality was assessed using the Cochrane Risk of Bias tool. Pooled estimates were calculated as weighted mean differences with 95% confidence intervals using random-effects models, with heterogeneity assessed by the I^2 statistic.

The search found six RCTs with 1,272 participants which were included in the quantitative synthesis. Across pooled analyses, survodutide treatment resulted in a statistically significant reduction in HbA1c compared with placebo (WMD –0.66%; 95% CI –1.08 to –0.23), with subgroup analyses demonstrating greater HbA1c lowering in studies using total weekly doses >2.4 mg. Fasting glucagon concentrations were also significantly reduced (WMD –7 pmol/L; 95% CI –10.3 to –3.69). With respect to anthropometric outcomes, survodutide was associated with significant decreases in body weight (WMD –6.7 kg) and waist circumference (WMD –7.09 cm), with larger effect sizes observed in trials with longer treatment duration (>16 weeks) and higher doses (>2.4 mg/week).

Reductions in BMI were consistent with changes in body weight. Secondary metabolic outcomes showed modest but significant improvements in total cholesterol, triglycerides, and blood pressure. Treatment discontinuation rates were higher in the survodutide groups, largely driven by gastrointestinal events; however, the rate of serious AEs did not differ significantly between survodutide and placebo arms.

This meta-analysis shows that survodutide produces clinically meaningful reductions in body weight and waist circumference, along with modest improvements in glycemic control, with greater effects at higher weekly doses and longer treatment durations. These benefits are biologically plausible given its dual GLP-1 and glucagon receptor agonism, combining appetite suppression with increased energy expenditure while maintaining glycemic stability, and the observed reduction in fasting glucagon supports effective receptor engagement and metabolic adaptation.

Compared with conventional GLP-1 receptor agonists, survodutide appears to achieve greater weight loss but less pronounced HbA1c reduction, and its efficacy is lower than that reported with newer multi-agonists such as tirzepatide or retatrutide, reflecting differences in receptor targeting and study populations. Strengths of this analysis include the inclusion of randomized controlled trials, dose- and duration-based subgroup analyses, and comprehensive evaluation of efficacy and safety.

However, certain limitations need to be considered, including heterogeneity in trial design, relatively short follow-up, limited data in advanced diabetes. In addition, gastrointestinal AEs leading to treatment discontinuation remain a concern and may influence real-world adherence. Future large-scale, long-term randomized trials are therefore required to define the durability of weight loss, optimize dosing and titration strategies, evaluate cardiovascular and hepatic outcomes, and clarify the most appropriate clinical positioning of survodutide within the expanding landscape of incretin-based and multiagonist therapies.

5. Impact of Bodyweight Loss on Type 2 Diabetes Remission: A Systematic Review and Meta-regression Analysis of Randomized Controlled Trials

Ref: Kanbour S, Ageeb RA, Malik RA, Abu-Raddad LJ. Impact of Bodyweight Loss on Type 2 Diabetes Remission: A Systematic Review and Meta-Regression Analysis of Randomised Controlled Trials. Lancet Diabetes Endocrinol. 2025;13(4):294-306.

ABSTRACT

Background: Type 2 diabetes remission is linked to bodyweight loss; however, the quantitative association between the degree of bodyweight loss and the chance of remission, after adjusting for confounding variables, is yet unknown. After adjusting for a number of confounding variables, we sought to analyze the association between the degree of bodyweight reduction and diabetes remission and to estimate the impact of these variables on diabetes remission.

Techniques: In order to systematically examine, synthesize, and present global data from randomized controlled trials conducted in people with type 2 diabetes who are overweight or obese, this meta-regression analysis and systematic review adhered to Cochrane and PRISMA criteria. At least 1 year following a bodyweight loss intervention, the percentage of participants with complete diabetes remission [glycated hemoglobin (HbA1c) < 6.0% (42 mmol/mol) or fasting plasma glucose (FPG) <100 mg/dL (5.6 mmol/L), or both, without the use of glucose-lowering medications] or partial diabetes remission [HbA1c < 6.5% (48 mmol/mol) or FPG < 126 mg/dL (7.0 mmol/L), or both, without the use of glucose-lowering medications]. From the database's creation until July 30, 2024, we searched PubMed, Embase, and trial registries. Information was taken from reports that had been published. The data was analyzed using meta-regressions and meta-analyses. PROSPERO has registered the study protocol (CRD42024497878).

Findings: We found 22 pertinent publications that included 33 outcome measures of partial remission and 29 outcome measures of complete diabetic remission. One year after the intervention, the pooled mean percentage of participants who experienced complete remission was 0.7% (95% CI 0.1–4.6) for those who lost <10% of their body weight, 49.6% (40.4–58.9) for those who lost 20–29% of their body weight, and 79.1% (68.6–88.1) for those who lost 30% or more. No studies that reported complete remission with 10–19% body weight loss. One year after the intervention, the pooled mean percentage of participants who experienced partial remission was 5.4% (95% CI 2.9–8.4) for those who lost <10% of their body weight, 48.4% (36.1–60.8) for those who lost 10–19%, 69.3% (55.8–81.3) for those who lost 20–29%, and 89.5% (80.0–96%) for those who lost 30% or more. Remission and bodyweight decrease were strongly positively correlated. The likelihood of achieving complete remission improved by 2.17 percentage points (95% CI 1.94–2.40) and the likelihood of achieving partial remission increased by 2.74 percentage points (2.48–3.00) for every percentage point drop in bodyweight. Age, sex, race, length of diabetes, baseline body mass index (BMI), HbA1c, insulin use, or type of bodyweight loss intervention did not significantly or appreciably correlate with remission. In all quality domains, the data came from randomized controlled trials that had a low risk of bias.

Interpretation: Regardless of age, length of diabetes, HbA1c, BMI, or kind of intervention, a strong dose-response connection between bodyweight loss and diabetes remission was found. These results demonstrate how important bodyweight loss is for controlling type 2 diabetes and lowering the likelihood of complications from the disease.

CRITICAL APPRAISAL

Type 2 diabetes mellitus (T2DM) affects over 537 million adults globally and is projected to rise substantially, contributing significantly to morbidity, mortality, and healthcare costs.[16] More than 85% of individuals with T2DM are overweight or obese.[11] Diabetes remission—defined as achieving normoglycemia without glucose-lowering therapy—has emerged as an important therapeutic goal and is biologically linked to improvements in insulin sensitivity and β-cell function following reduction in ectopic fat.[17] While multiple trials suggest that greater weight loss, younger age, shorter diabetes duration, better glycemic control, absence of insulin use, and intervention type may influence remission, the independent quantitative contribution of bodyweight loss after adjusting for these factors has remained unclear.[18]

This study aimed to define the dose-response relationship between bodyweight loss and diabetes remission and to estimate the effect sizes of other potential predictors using pooled randomized controlled trial data.

This systematic review and meta-regression followed Cochrane and PRISMA guidelines and included randomized controlled trials in adults with T2DM and overweight or obesity [body mass index (BMI) ≥25 kg/m^2, or ≥23 kg/m^2 in Asian populations]. PubMed, Embase, ClinicalTrials.gov, and the WHO International Clinical Trials Registry Platform were searched from inception to July 30, 2024. Trials were required to report mean bodyweight loss and diabetes remission at ≥1 year following lifestyle, pharmacological, or surgical weight-loss interventions. Studies using glucose-lowering drugs with weight-loss effects were excluded unless remission was assessed ≥3 months after discontinuation. Bariatric procedures accounted for nearly all interventions achieving ≥20% bodyweight loss. Complete remission was defined as glycated hemoglobin (HbA1c) < 6.0% or fasting plasma glucose <100 mg/dL without therapy, and partial remission as HbA1c < 6.5% or fasting plasma glucose <126 mg/dL without therapy. Intention-to-treat estimates were used. Random-effects meta-analyses and meta-regressions assessed associations between remission and bodyweight loss while adjusting for age, sex, race, diabetes duration, HbA1c, insulin use, BMI, intervention type, and risk of bias.

About 22 publications were included, contributing 29 outcome measures for complete remission and 33 for partial remission across diverse global regions. One year after intervention, complete remission occurred in 0.7% of participants with <10% weight loss, 49.6% with 20–29% loss, and 79.1% with ≥30% loss; no studies reported complete remission with 10–19% loss. Partial remission occurred in 5.4%, 48.4%, 69.3%, and 89.5% of participants with <10%, 10–19%, 20–29%, and ≥30% weight loss, respectively. Meta-regression showed a strong, independent dose–response relationship: Each 1% reduction in bodyweight increased the probability of complete remission by 2.17% points and partial remission by 2.74% points. After adjustment, no significant or clinically meaningful associations were observed for age, sex, race, diabetes duration, baseline HbA1c, BMI, insulin use, or intervention type.

This analysis demonstrates a strong, independent dose–response relationship between weight loss and T2DM remission, with each 1% reduction in weight increasing the probability of complete and partial remission by 2% and 3%, respectively. These findings support weight loss as the primary determinant of remission, likely via reduction in ectopic fat, improved insulin sensitivity, and partial recovery of β-cell function. Partial remission occurred at lower levels of weight loss than complete remission.

Although bariatric surgery showed higher remission rates in unadjusted analyses, this effect was fully explained by magnitude of weight loss, confirming that remission is driven by weight reduction rather than intervention type. Lack of significant associations with age, diabetes duration, baseline HbA1c, BMI, insulin use, or sex suggests that sufficient weight loss can induce remission across diverse patient profiles, though smaller effects might not have been detectable.

Overall, the findings reinforce bodyweight loss as a central, scalable strategy for altering the trajectory of T2DM and reducing its long-term complications. Inclusion of overweight or obese individuals limits generalizability to those with near-normal BMI, and the number of included trials was insufficient to precisely estimate small effects of some covariates. Additionally, long-term outcomes beyond one year were sparsely reported.

Future research is needed to evaluate the durability of remission with newer pharmacotherapies, particularly after treatment discontinuation, and for direct comparison of pharmacological and surgical strategies at equivalent levels of weight loss.

6. Effect of Gastric Bypass versus Sleeve Gastrectomy on the Remission of Type 2 Diabetes, Weight Loss, and Cardiovascular Risk Factors at 5 Years (Oseberg): Secondary Outcomes of a Single-centre, Triple-blind, Randomized Controlled Trial

Ref: Wågen Hauge J, Borgeraas H, Birkeland KI, Johnson LK, Hertel JK, Hagen M. Effect of Gastric Bypass versus Sleeve Gastrectomy on the Remission of Type 2 Diabetes, Weight Loss, and Cardiovascular Risk Factors at 5 Years (Oseberg): Secondary Outcomes of a Single-Centre, Triple-Blind, Randomised Controlled Trial. Lancet Diabetes Endocrinol. 2025;13(5):397-409.

ABSTRACT

Background: Losing weight can help people with type 2 diabetes and obesity achieve remission by improving their β-cell function and insulin sensitivity. However, it is yet unknown how well sleeve gastrectomy and regular gastric bypass work in the long run to induce type 2 diabetes remission. 5 years following surgery, we sought to assess the effects of sleeve gastrectomy and gastric bypass on cardiovascular risk factors, weight loss, and type 2 diabetes remission.

Methods: A two-armed, single-center, triple-blind, randomized controlled trial carried out in a public tertiary obesity center in Norway is the subject of our secondary analysis. A computerized random number generator was used to randomly assign (1:1) adults (i.e., age ≥18 years) with type 2 diabetes and obesity to either laparoscopic gastric bypass or sleeve gastrectomy, with balanced block sizes of 10. Up until a year following surgery, study staff, participants, and the primary outcome assessor were all blind to the allocation; after that, follow-up was open label. 5 years following surgery, changes in important secondary outcomes such as weight loss, remission of type 2 diabetes, and cardiovascular risk variables were evaluated. All randomized individuals' treatment effects were evaluated via the trial technique estimand, with data obtained following conversional surgery excluded from analysis. The study was finished in December 2022 and was filed with ClinicalTrials.gov (NCT01778738).

Findings: After 319 patients were evaluated for eligibility between October 15, 2012, and September 1, 2017, 109 individuals were randomly randomized to either sleeve gastrectomy (n = 55) or gastric bypass (n = 54). At baseline, the mean age was 47.7 years [standard deviation (SD) 9.6], the mean body mass index (BMI) was 42.3 kg/m^2 (SD 5.3), and there were 37 (34%) men and 72 (66%) women. The 5-year follow-up was completed by 93 (85%) participants [47 (85%) in the sleeve gastrectomy group and 46 (85%) in the gastric bypass group]. Type 2 diabetes remission rates were higher following gastric bypass than following sleeve gastrectomy [glycated hemoglobin (HbA1c) ≤6.0% 23 (50%) of 46 vs. 9 (20%) of 44, risk difference 29 5% (95% CI 10.8 to 48.3); HbA1c < 6.5%]. Risk difference: 33.5% (14.1 to 52.9), 29 (63%) vs. 13 (30%). Gastric bypass reduced low-density lipoprotein (LDL) cholesterol [treatment difference −0.5 mmol/L (−0.8 to −0.1)] and increased bodyweight reduction [mean 22.2% (95% CI 20.3 to 24.1) vs. 17.2% (15.3 to 19.1), treatment difference 5.0% (2.4 to 7.7)]. While Barrett's esophagus and erosive esophagitis were equally common in both groups, pathological acid reflux was more common following sleeve gastrectomy [risk difference 51.1% (28.0 to 74.2)]. Following gastric bypass as opposed to sleeve gastrectomy, more patients experienced symptomatic postprandial hypoglycemia [15 (28%) vs. 1 (2%)].

Interpretation: Although there was a greater incidence of symptomatic postprandial hypoglycemia, gastric bypass was superior to sleeve gastrectomy in terms of long-term remission of type 2 diabetes, weight loss, and LDL cholesterol concentrations. These results may influence future recommendations and clinical practice concerning the best surgical technique for individuals with type 2 diabetes.

CRITICAL APPRAISAL

Metabolic bariatric surgery provides major benefits for patients with type 2 diabetes, including improved glycemic control, weight reduction, favorable effects on cardiovascular risk factors, and better quality of life, but it is also associated with surgical and metabolic complications.[19] Current guidelines recommend bariatric surgery for patients with type 2 diabetes mellitus (T2DM) and severe obesity but do not specify the preferred surgical procedure. Roux-en-Y gastric bypass and sleeve gastrectomy together account for the vast majority of bariatric surgeries performed worldwide, yet their long-term comparative effectiveness remains uncertain.[20]

Existing evidence from long-term randomized trials is limited and inconsistent. While some studies suggest greater weight loss or diabetes remission with gastric bypass, others report comparable outcomes, often due to limited power, heterogeneous populations, or diabetes being a secondary outcome.[21,22] Prior results from the Oseberg trial at shorter follow-up showed superior diabetes remission and weight-related quality of life after gastric bypass.

Therefore, this study aimed to compare the 5-year outcomes of gastric bypass and sleeve gastrectomy, focusing on diabetes remission, weight loss, cardiovascular risk factors, and patient-reported outcomes.

The Oseberg trial was a two-arm, single-center, triple-blind randomized controlled study conducted at a public tertiary obesity center in Norway. Adults aged 18 years or older with type 2 diabetes and obesity—defined as a previously documented body mass index (BMI) ≥ 35.0 kg/m^2 and a current BMI ≥ 33.0 kg/m^2 at enrolment—were eligible. Participants were randomly assigned in a 1:1 ratio to laparoscopic Roux-en-Y gastric bypass or sleeve gastrectomy using a computer-generated sequence with balanced block sizes.

Blinding was maintained for the first year, after which follow-up was open label. Both groups received identical perioperative care, including a preoperative low-calorie diet, standardized surgical procedures, and predefined postoperative medication and supplementation protocols, with follow-up visits continuing for 5 years.

This analysis assessed prespecified secondary outcomes at 5 years, including diabetes remission, glycemic control, weight and body composition, cardiovascular risk factors, gastroesophageal reflux, adverse events, and patient-reported outcomes.

A total of 109 participants were randomized (54 gastric bypass and 55 sleeve gastrectomy), and 93 (85%) completed 5-year follow-up. Mean baseline age was 47.7 years and mean BMI 42.3 kg/m^2, with comparable groups. Diabetes remission at 5 years was significantly higher after gastric bypass than sleeve gastrectomy using both glycated hemoglobin (HbA1c) criteria (≤6.0%: 50% vs. 20%; <6.5%: 63% vs. 30%), although overall HbA1c reduction was similar.

Gastric bypass produced greater weight loss (22.2% vs. 17.2%) with larger reductions in BMI, waist circumference, and fat mass, while fat-free mass loss was comparable. Fewer participants required antidiabetic medications after gastric bypass, with no difference in insulin use.

Both procedures improved cardiovascular risk factors; however, gastric bypass resulted in lower total and low-density lipoprotein (LDL) cholesterol and a higher rate of achieving the American Diabetes Association (ADA) composite metabolic target. Blood pressure and triglyceride changes were similar, with a small additional reduction in diastolic blood pressure after gastric bypass.

Pathological acid reflux was more frequent after sleeve gastrectomy, whereas rates of erosive esophagitis and Barrett's esophagus were similar. Symptomatic postprandial hypoglycemia occurred more often after gastric bypass. Quality of life improved after both surgeries, with greater gains in weight-related quality of life after gastric bypass, and overall late adverse event rates were comparable.

This 5-year randomized trial shows that Roux-en-Y gastric bypass is more effective than sleeve gastrectomy in achieving long-term remission of T2DM, greater weight loss, and more favorable lipid outcomes. The results are consistent with previous randomized trials and observational studies suggesting stronger weight-independent metabolic effects of gastric bypass. Both procedures improved overall glycemic control and cardiovascular risk factors, but important trade-offs were observed: Gastric bypass was associated with a higher risk of postprandial hypoglycemia, whereas sleeve gastrectomy led to significantly more pathological acid reflux, in line with earlier physiological and endoscopic studies.

The study's strengths include its randomized design, long-term follow-up, high retention rate, and standardized perioperative care, with diabetes remission as a prespecified outcome. However, there were certain limitations of the study, including the single-center setting, modest sample size, and lack of power to assess hard cardiovascular endpoints. Despite these facts, the findings provide robust long-term comparative data to support procedure selection and shared decision-making in patients with T2DM and obesity.

---

7. Effects of Choline Alfoscerate on Cognitive Function and Quality of Life in Type 2 Diabetes: A Double-blind, Randomized, Placebo-controlled Trial

Ref: Sohn M, Park YH, Lim S. Effects of Choline Alfoscerate on Cognitive Function and Quality of Life in Type 2 Diabetes: A Double-Blind, Randomized, Placebo-Controlled Trial. Diabetes Obes Metab. 2025;27(3):1350-8.

ABSTRACT

Aim: In type 2 diabetes mellitus (T2DM) patients with modest cognitive decline, the effects of choline alfoscerate on cognitive performance and quality of life were assessed.

Supplies and procedures: We enrolled 36 people with T2DM with mild cognitive impairment [measured by the Mini-Mental State Examination (MMSE) score of 25–28] for a double-blind, randomized, and placebo-controlled experiment. They were then randomly assigned to receive either 1,200 mg/day of choline alfoscerate or a placebo. The Korean version of activities of daily living (ADL), the 36-Item Short Form Survey, the modified Informant Questionnaire on Cognitive Decline in the Elderly, and the Patient Health Questionnaire were all examined at 6 and 12 months and analyzed using mixed-effects models for repeated measures.

Results: Participants in the study were 69.4% female and had an average age of 71.8 ± 5.3 years. The MMSE score increased non-significantly from 26.2 ± 1.3 to 26.9 ± 2.0 after 6 months of choline alfoscerate treatment, whereas the placebo group's score decreased nonsignificantly from 26.6 ± 1.3 to 25.9 ± 2.3. The mean difference between the two groups was +1.4 ($p = 0.059$). At 12 months, there was a statistically significant rise in the mean difference to +1.7 ($p < 0.001$). The SF-36 assessment revealed that the choline alfoscerate group's physical health was much better than that of the placebo group.

Conclusion: In T2DM patients with mild cognitive impairment, choline alfoscerate 1,200 mg once daily treatment showed a slight improvement in cognitive function at 6 months, but it became significant at 12 months when compared to placebo, indicating its potential as an adjuvant therapy for managing early cognitive decline.

CRITICAL APPRAISAL

Type 2 diabetes mellitus (T2DM) is highly prevalent in older adults and is strongly associated with accelerated cognitive decline, dementia, and reduced quality of life.[23] The postulated mechanisms include chronic hyperglycemia, insulin resistance, oxidative stress, neuroinflammation, endothelial dysfunction, and cerebral microvascular disease, all of which contribute to neuronal injury.[24] Cognitive impairment in T2DM is often subtle and progressive, making early intervention critical, yet effective pharmacological options for mild cognitive impairment (MCI) in diabetes are limited.

Choline alfoscerate (α-glycerylphosphorylcholine), a choline-containing phospholipid precursor of acetylcholine, has demonstrated cognitive benefits in Alzheimer's disease and vascular cognitive impairment, but its effects in diabetes-related cognitive decline have not been studied.[25] Given the mixed vascular and neurodegenerative pathophysiology of cognitive impairment in T2DM, this trial aimed to evaluate the efficacy and safety of choline alfoscerate on cognitive function and quality of life in older patients with T2DM and mild cognitive decline.

This double-blind, randomized, placebo-controlled trial was conducted at a tertiary hospital in Korea. 36 adults aged ≥60 years with T2DM and MCI [Mini-Mental State Examination (MMSE) score 25–28) were enrolled and randomly assigned in a 1:1 ratio to receive either choline alfoscerate 1,200 mg/day or matching placebo. Individuals with conditions or treatments that could influence cognitive function—such as poorly controlled diabetes, vitamin B12 deficiency, thyroid dysfunction, major neurological disease, recent hospitalization, or alcoholism—were excluded. Cognitive function and quality of life were evaluated at baseline, 6 months, and 12 months using the MMSE (primary outcome), SF-36, modified IQCODE, Korean activities of daily living (ADL), and PHQ-9. Analyses followed the intention-to-treat principle and used mixed-effects models for repeated measures, adjusting for baseline values, time, and treatment-by-time interaction.

Of the 36 randomized patients (mean age 71.8 years; 69.4% women), 28 completed the 6-month study and entered the 12-month extension. Baseline demographics, diabetes control, comorbidities, and medication use were comparable between groups. At 6 months, MMSE scores increased modestly in the choline alfoscerate group and declined slightly in the placebo group, yielding a between-group difference of +1.4 points, however, not significant ($p = 0.059$). At 12 months, the difference increased to +1.7 points and became statistically significant ($p < 0.001$), with improvements mainly in orientation and language domains. Physical health scores on the SF-36 improved significantly with choline alfoscerate at 6 months and remained superior to placebo at 12 months, whereas mental health domains, ADL, depressive symptoms, and IQCODE scores did not differ between groups. Adverse events were infrequent, mild, and similar between groups, with no serious adverse events reported.

This study trial demonstrates that long-term choline alfoscerate therapy leads to a modest but statistically significant improvement in global cognitive function and physical quality of life in older patients with T2DM and early cognitive decline. The delayed emergence of statistical significance at 12 months suggests that sustained treatment might be needed to counteract the slow progression of diabetes-related cognitive impairment. The observed benefits are biologically plausible, as choline alfoscerate enhances acetylcholine synthesis, supports neuronal membrane integrity, and exerts neuroprotective and endothelial-stabilizing effects, which are particularly relevant in the mixed vascular–neurodegenerative cognitive phenotype seen in T2DM. Compared with prior studies conducted in Alzheimer's disease, where larger cognitive gains were observed in individuals with more advanced impairment, the smaller effect size in this study aligns with the milder baseline deficits present in the participants. Additionally, expected age-related variability in MMSE scores may also contribute to these findings. The improvement in physical health may reflect enhanced neuromuscular function and acetylcholine-mediated motor performance, aligning with previous reports of improved physical capacity with choline supplementation.

The study was well designed and did a comprehensive multidimensional assessment of cognition and quality of life. However, the sample size was small, and the study included a single-center, relatively homogeneous and well-controlled diabetic population limiting the generalizability of the findings. Lack of any biomarker or neuroimaging data to clarify underlying mechanisms is the other limitation. Future larger, multicenter trials with longer follow-up, mechanistic endpoints, and broader diabetic populations are needed to confirm these findings and define the role of choline alfoscerate in early cognitive management in T2DM.

8. Increased Risk of Dementia in Type 1 Diabetes: A Systematic Review with Meta-analysis

Ref: Li L, Wong D, Fisher CA, Conn JJ, Wraight PR, Davies A, et al. Increased Risk of Dementia in Type 1 Diabetes: A Systematic Review with Meta-analysis. Diabetes Res Clin Pract. 2025;222:112043.

ABSTRACT

The goal of this systematic review and meta-analysis was to compile data regarding the relationship between dementia risk and type 1 diabetes mellitus. 19 pertinent studies were found for inclusion after a thorough search of the CINAHL, EMBASE, MEDLINE, PSYCINFO, and Web of Science databases. The QUADAS-2 tool was used to evaluate the quality of English-language studies, and data was taken for synthesis. Six studies that reported hazard ratios (HRs) for dementia risk in people with type 1 diabetes compared to controls were meta-analyzed. People with type 1 diabetes had a 50% higher risk of dementia than controls, according to the pooled HR for all-cause dementia, which was 1.50 [95% confidence interval (CI) 1.25–1.80; $p < 0.001$]. This review emphasizes the need for focused screening and preventative measures for this population and offers solid evidence connecting type 1 diabetes to an increased risk of dementia. The factors underlying the link between type 1 diabetes and dementia require more investigation.

CRITICAL APPRAISAL

Dementia is a growing global health burden, and diabetes has emerged as an important risk factor for cognitive decline. While the association between type 2 diabetes mellitus (T2DM) and dementia is well established, the same for type 1 diabetes mellitus (T1DM) and dementia remains less clear.[26] T1DM is characterized by lifelong exposure to hyperglycemia, frequent hypoglycemic episodes, and an increased burden of microvascular and macrovascular complications, all of which might lead to neurodegenerative and vascular brain injury.[27]

Several biological mechanisms have been proposed to explain a potential link between T1DM and dementia, including chronic glucose toxicity, cerebral microvascular disease, oxidative stress, inflammation, and repeated hypoglycemia. However, individual observational studies in this regard have reported inconsistent results, often limited by small sample sizes and methodological differences.[28] Given the increasing life expectancy of T1DM patients, clarifying long-term cognitive risks is clinically very important.

Therefore, this study aimed to systematically review and quantitatively synthesize existing evidence to determine whether T1DM is associated with an increased risk of dementia and its major subtypes, including Alzheimer's disease and vascular dementia.

This systematic review and meta-analysis was conducted as per the Preferred Reporting Items for Systematic Reviews and Meta-Analyses (PRISMA) guidelines. Electronic databases were searched up to the prespecified date to identify observational studies examining the association between T1DM and dementia. Six observational studies (cohort and case-control designs) involving over 1.2 million participants were included. Studies compared T1DM patients with nondiabetic controls and reported risk estimates for dementia outcomes.

The primary outcome was all-cause dementia, with secondary outcomes including Alzheimer's disease and vascular dementia. Dementia outcomes were ascertained from routinely collected clinical data, including national health or hospital registers and medical records, using standard diagnostic codes, with analyses performed for all-cause dementia and major subtypes. Pooled relative risks were calculated using random-effects models. Statistical heterogeneity was assessed using the I^2 statistic, and sensitivity analyses were conducted to test the robustness of findings.

As compared with individuals without diabetes, T1DM patients had a significantly higher risk of all-cause dementia, with a pooled relative risk of approximately 1.5–1.6. Subgroup analyses showed an increased risk of Alzheimer's disease (pooled relative risk around 1.3–1.4) and a more pronounced association with vascular dementia (pooled relative risk close to 2.0). Moderate heterogeneity was observed across studies, but sensitivity analyses confirmed the robustness of the associations.

The study concluded that T1DM is associated with a significantly increased risk of dementia, particularly vascular dementia, highlighting an important but under-recognized long-term complication of the disease. The findings are broadly consistent with earlier individual cohort studies and align with the well-established association between T2DM and cognitive decline, although the magnitude and mechanisms may differ. The stronger association with vascular dementia supports the role of chronic microvascular and macrovascular injury, while the increased risk of Alzheimer's disease suggests additional contributions from long-term hyperglycemia, oxidative stress, inflammation, and recurrent hypoglycemia. As compared to previous narrative reviews, this study provides quantitative pooled estimates, strengthening the evidence base. Key strengths include systematic study identification, large combined sample size, use of random-effects modeling, and evaluation of dementia subtypes. However, the study relied on observational data and was subject to potential misclassification of diabetes type and dementia diagnoses, residual confounding, and heterogeneity in study design, follow-up duration, and covariate adjustment. Despite these limitations, the consistency of results across analyses supports a true association and underscores the need for long-term cognitive surveillance and preventive strategies in individuals with type 1 diabetes.

9. Use of Sodium-glucose Cotransporter-2 Inhibitors and Risk of Dementia: A Population-based Cohort Study

Ref: Zhuo L, Zhang B, Yin Y, Sun Y, Shen P, Jiang Z, et al. Use of Sodium-glucose Cotransporter-2 Inhibitors and Risk of Dementia: A Population-based Cohort Study. Diabetes Obes Metab. 2025;27(5):2430-41.

ABSTRACT

Background and aim: In the Chinese population, the impact of sodium-glucose cotransporter-2 inhibitor (SGLT-2i) on dementia risk has not been evaluated. Our objective was to evaluate the relationship between SGLT-2i use and dementia incidence in a Chinese population living on the mainland.

Materials and methods: The Yinzhou Regional Health Care Database was used to create cohorts of type 2 diabetes mellitus patients who were new users of either SGLT-2i or dipeptidyl peptidase 4 inhibitor (DPP-4i) in order to simulate a target trial. The hazard ratio (HR) of the relationship between the usage of SGLT-2i and incident dementia was estimated using a Cox model after potential confounding was controlled using inverse probability of treatment weighting (IPTW).

Results: There were 47,335 new DPP-4i or SGLT-2i users in the final cohort. According to the primary study, the incidence of dementia among DPP-4i and SGLT-2i users was 500.2 and 347.5 per 100,000 person years, respectively. After controlling for potential confounding using IPTW, SGLT-2i use was linked to a lower incidence of incident dementia, with an HR of 0.74 [95% confidence interval (CI), 0.60–0.93]. Sensitivity analyses and other subgroup analyses often yielded consistent results.

Conclusion: In the mainland Chinese study population, the use of SGLT-2i is linked to a lower risk of dementia occurrence.

CRITICAL APPRAISAL

Type 2 diabetes mellitus (T2DM) is associated with a substantially increased risk of cognitive impairment and dementia, with epidemiological studies showing a *~1.5–2-fold higher risk* of dementia compared with individuals without diabetes.[29] Dementia affects > *55 million people worldwide*, and its burden is expected to rise sharply[30] with aging populations and the increasing prevalence of diabetes, particularly in Asia. The mechanisms linking T2DM to dementia include chronic hyperglycemia, insulin resistance, cerebrovascular disease, oxidative stress, and neuroinflammation.[24] While some glucose-lowering agents may influence dementia risk, comparative evidence between drug classes is limited. Sodium-glucose cotransporter-2 inhibitor (SGLT-2i), which provide cardiovascular and metabolic benefits beyond glucose lowering, have been hypothesized to confer neuroprotective effects.[31] This study therefore aimed to compare the risk of incident dementia among new users of SGLT-2i versus dipeptidyl peptidase 4 inhibitor (DPP-4i) using large-scale real-world data from mainland China.

This study emulated a target trial using population-based observational data from the Yinzhou Regional Health Care Database in mainland China. Adults aged 50 years or older with T2DM who were new users of either SGLT-2i or DPP-4i were included, while patients with a prior diagnosis of dementia were excluded. An active-comparator, new-user design was employed to minimize confounding by indication and immortal time bias. To further control for measured confounders, inverse probability of treatment weighting (IPTW) based on propensity scores was applied to balance baseline demographic characteristics, diabetes-related variables, comorbidities, and concomitant medications between treatment groups.

Participants were followed from the time of drug initiation until the occurrence of incident dementia, death, loss to follow-up, or end of the study period. Incident dementia was identified using diagnostic codes based on ICD 10 codes F00-F03 and G30. The association between SGLT-2i use and dementia risk was evaluated using Cox proportional hazards regression, with results expressed as hazard ratios (HRs) and 95% confidence intervals (CIs). Prespecified subgroup analyses and multiple sensitivity analyses were conducted to assess the robustness and consistency of the findings.

The final study cohort comprised 47,335 new users of either SGLT-2i or DPP-4i (27,404 for DPP-4i and 19,931 for SGLT-2i with a median follow-up time of 2.8 and1.6 years, respectively. During follow-up, the incidence rate of dementia was 500.2 per 100,000 person-years among DPP-4i users and 347.5 per 100,000 person-years among SGLT-2i users. In the primary analysis, after adjustment for baseline differences using IPTW, initiation of SGLT-2i was associated with a 26% lower risk of incident dementia compared with DPP-4i (HR 0.74; 95% CI 0.60–0.93). This protective association remained consistent across multiple subgroup analyses and sensitivity analyses, supporting the robustness of the findings.

This study shows that initiation of SGLT-2i is associated with a significantly lower risk of incident dementia compared with DPP-4i in patients with T2DM (HR 0.74). This clinically meaningful reduction supports the concept that SGLT-2i has pleiotropic benefits beyond glycemic control. Proposed mechanisms include improved glycemic variability and insulin sensitivity, reduced vascular inflammation, better endothelial function, and favorable cerebral energy metabolism. The findings are consistent with previous observational studies and post-hoc analyses suggesting lower dementia risk with SGLT-2i.[31,32] The use of an active comparator, target trial emulation, and IPTW, along with a large real-world cohort of over 47,000 patients, strengthens the validity and clinical relevance of the results.

However, the observational design limits causal inference, and residual confounding from unmeasured factors such as lifestyle, education, hypoglycemia burden, and diabetes severity cannot be excluded. Dementia diagnoses were based on administrative codes rather than standardized testing, and follow-up duration and detailed cognitive trajectories were not fully assessed. Future prospective studies and randomized trials with dedicated cognitive endpoints and longer follow-up are needed to confirm a causal neuroprotective role of SGLT-2i and to identify patients most likely to benefit.

10. Repeated Fecal Microbiota Transplantation for Individuals with Type 1 Diabetes and Gastroenteropathy

Ref: Høyer KL, Kornum DS, Baunwall SMD, Klinge MW, Drewes AM, Yderstræde KB, et al. Repeated Faecal Microbiota Transplantation for Individuals with Type 1 Diabetes and Gastroenteropathy. Diabetologia. 2025;68(12):2795-806.

ABSTRACT

Aim/hypothesis: A recent placebo-controlled trial showed that fecal microbiota transplantation (FMT) may reduce gastrointestinal symptoms in people with diabetic gastroenteropathy. The majority of individuals experienced temporary symptom alleviation, necessitating more treatments. The long-term effectiveness, safety, and viability of repeated, on-demand FMT as a maintenance treatment in this patient population were evaluated in this study.

Methods: Extended open-label treatment with FMT was made available to all 20 participants in the randomized clinical trial. The Gastrointestinal Symptom Rating Scale for Irritable Bowel Syndrome (GSRS-IBS) was used to conduct telephone symptom evaluations every 2–3 months. Bowel movement frequency, stool consistency measured with the Bristol Stool Scale, perceived treatment benefit on a seven-point Likert scale, and adverse events (AEs) were secondary variables. For those who were unable to take the capsules, colonoscopy was utilized. FMT was mainly administered orally.

Results: From September 2021 to December 2024, 17 of the initial 20 individuals were enrolled in the current study. The median follow-up period was 33.2 months (range 14.7–39.1 months). A total of 95 FMT treatments were administered to the participants, with a median of five treatments per participant and a median interval of 5.3 months between treatments. Throughout several treatments, FMT consistently reduced GSRS-IBS scores and relieved symptoms. The mean GSRS-IBS score dropped from 60 [95% confidence interval (CI) 54, 66] at baseline to 35 (95% CI 29, 40) at the end of the most recent FMT therapy, with a mean difference of −25 (95% CI −18, −33). 2 weeks following therapy, the frequency of bowel motions (>7 per day) dropped from 19% (95% CI 10%, 28%) to 3% (95% CI 0%, 7%). Following treatment, the frequency of normal stool types (Bristol Stool Scale score 3–5) rose from 28% (95% CI 18%, 39%) to 76% (95% CI 66%, 86%). Additionally, stool consistency improved. 86% of participants reported significant advantages, indicating high participant satisfaction (Likert scores 5–7). The majority of AEs were moderate and self-limiting, and repeated FMT was generally well tolerated. Only one of the fifteen identified major AEs was thought to be potentially connected to FMT.

Conclusion and interpretation: For the long-term treatment of people with type 1 diabetes and severe diabetic gastroenteropathy, repeated, on-demand FMT is safe and effective.

CRITICAL APPRAISAL

Diabetic gastroenteropathy is a disabling complication of diabetes, primarily driven by irreversible autonomic and enteric neuropathy, resulting in symptoms such as bloating, abdominal pain, diarrhea, constipation, and early satiety, with substantial impairment of quality of life.[33] Available therapies are largely symptomatic, have limited efficacy, and are often associated with adverse effects. Growing evidence implicates gut microbiota dysbiosis in gastrointestinal dysmotility and inflammation, prompting interest in microbiota-based therapies.[34]

Fecal microbiota transplantation (FMT) is well established for recurrent *Clostridioides difficile* infection, but its benefits in other gastrointestinal disorders have been inconsistent, likely due to disease heterogeneity, donor variability, and host factors.[35] The FADIGAS randomized controlled trial previously demonstrated that FMT significantly improved gastrointestinal symptoms in individuals with type 1 diabetes and severe gastroenteropathy; however, symptom relief was transient, necessitating repeated treatments.[36] This extension study was therefore designed to assess whether repeated, on-demand FMT could provide sustained symptom control and be feasible and safe as a long-term management strategy.

This open-label extension study enrolled adults who had completed the placebo-controlled FADIGAS trial, including individuals with type 1 diabetes mellitus (T1DM) of >5 years' duration and severe gastrointestinal symptoms [Gastrointestinal Symptom Rating Scale for Irritable Bowel Syndrome (GSRS-IBS) ≥40]. Participants were followed for 3 years (2021–2024) with structured telephone assessments every 2–3 months using the validated GSRS-IBS questionnaire. Symptom recurrence, defined as a GSRS-IBS score >40 combined with clinical assessment, triggered on-demand retreatment, with a mandatory minimum interval of 2 months between FMTs. Secondary outcomes included stool frequency, stool consistency assessed by the Bristol Stool Scale, patient-reported treatment benefit measured on a 7-point Likert scale, and adverse events (AEs) graded using CTCAE version 5.0. FMT was primarily administered as oral capsules, with colonoscopic delivery used when capsules could not be swallowed. Donors were rigorously screened according to international guidelines; each treatment used a single donor, with different donors employed across treatments.

About 17 of original 20 participants (85%) entered the extension study and were followed for a median of 33.2 months, receiving a total of 95 FMTs, with a median of 5 treatments per participant and a median intertreatment interval of 5.3 months. Repeated FMT produced consistent and clinically meaningful improvement in gastrointestinal symptoms across all GSRS-IBS domains. Mean GSRS-IBS scores decreased from 60 [95% confidence interval (CI) 54–66] before treatment to 35 (95% CI 29–40) after the final FMT, corresponding to a mean reduction of –25 points. Significant improvements were observed in diarrhea, early satiety, abdominal pain, bloating, and constipation. Stool frequency normalized, with the proportion reporting >7 stools/day decreasing from 19 to 3% and mean stool frequency declining from 4.6 to 2.1 stools/day. Stool consistency improved substantially, with normal stool types (Bristol 3–5) increasing from 28 to 76%. Patient-reported benefit was high, with 86% of responses indicating meaningful symptom improvement. FMT was generally well tolerated; most AEs were mild and self-limiting. 15 serious AEs occurred during follow-up, of which only one was considered possibly related to FMT, with no evidence of cumulative toxicity across repeated treatments.

This open-label extension study demonstrated that repeated, on-demand FMT provides sustained and clinically meaningful symptom relief and is generally safe in T1DM patients with severe diabetic gastroenteropathy. Patients needed repeated treatments, supporting the concept of FMT as a maintenance rather than curative therapy, likely due to persistent autonomic neuropathy and altered gut motility that predispose to recurrent dysbiosis. The magnitude and consistency of GSRS-IBS improvement across multiple treatment cycles were comparable to those observed in the original placebo-controlled FADIGAS trial, where FMT produced significantly greater symptom relief than placebo, suggesting effects beyond natural symptom fluctuation or placebo response. As compared with mixed results of FMT in conditions such as irritable bowel syndrome and inflammatory bowel disease, these data suggest that individuals with severe diabetic gastroenteropathy may be particularly responsive to microbiota-based therapy.

The study's strengths include long-term follow-up, objective symptom assessments, real-world retreatment, screened single donors, and safety monitoring. However, the study had certain limitations including its open-label design, small sample size, reliance on self-reported outcomes, and lack of microbiome analyses. Safety data indicated most AEs were mild, with no cumulative toxicity and one serious event possibly linked to FMT. Future studies should focus on placebo-controlled maintenance, response predictors, donor selection, microbiome profiling, and adjunctive methods like dietary interventions or scheduled oral FMT.

11. Effect of Fenofibrate on Residual Beta Cell Function in Adults and Adolescents with Newly Diagnosed Type 1 Diabetes: A Randomized Clinical Trial

Ref: Hostrup PE, Schmidt T, Hellsten SB, Gerwig RH, Størling J, Johannesen J, et al. Effect of Fenofibrate on Residual Beta Cell Function in Adults and Adolescents with Newly Diagnosed Type 1 Diabetes: A Randomised Clinical Trial. Diabetologia. 2025;68(1):29-40.

ABSTRACT

Aim/hypothesis: In preclinical research on type 1 diabetes, fenofibrate, a peroxisome proliferator-activated receptor alpha agonist, shows some promise in reducing beta cell stress and maintaining beta cell function. This phase 2, placebo-controlled, double-blind, randomized clinical trial sought to determine fenofibrate's safety and effectiveness in adults and adolescents with recently diagnosed type 1 diabetes.

Techniques: For 52 weeks, we randomly assigned 58 people (aged 16 to 40 years) with newly diagnosed type 1 diabetes to receive daily oral therapy with fenofibrate 160 mg or a placebo (in a block design with a block size of 4, assigned in a 1:1 ratio). After 52 weeks of treatment, we measured the change in beta cell function using the area under the curve (AUC) for C-peptide levels after a 2-hour mixed-meal tolerance test. Proinsulin/C-peptide (PI/C) ratio as a sign of beta cell stress, daily insulin use, and glycemic management [measured by glycated hemoglobin (HbA1c) and continuous glucose monitoring] were secondary outcomes. Prior to and following 4, 12, 26, and 52 weeks of treatment, we evaluated outcome measures. All personnel involved in handling outcome samples and assessment, as well as participants and their healthcare professionals, were kept blind.

Results: 56 participants were included in the statistical analysis for the primary outcome (n = 29 in the placebo group and n = 27 in the fenofibrate group following two withdrawals). After 52 weeks of treatment, we did not find any significant changes between the groups in glycemic control, insulin use, or 2-hour C-peptide levels {mean difference of 0.08 nmol/L [95% confidence interval (CI) –0.05, 0.23]}. Conversely, at week 52, the fenofibrate group had a higher PI/C ratio than the placebo group [mean difference of 0.024 (95% CI 0.000 0.048); $p < 0.05$]. When compared to a placebo, fenofibrate suppressed pathways related to sphingolipid metabolism and signaling at week 52, according to blood lipidome analysis. There were few adverse events and no significant adverse events over the 52-week intervention. Subsequent in vitro studies in human pancreatic islets showed that fenofibrate had a stress-inducing effect.

Conclusion and interpretation: This long-term, randomized, placebo-controlled trial did not support the use of fenofibrate for maintaining beta cell activity in people with recently diagnosed type 1 diabetes, despite the positive effects of fenofibrate observed in preclinical research.

CRITICAL APPRAISAL

Type 1 diabetes (T1D) is an autoimmune disorder requiring lifelong insulin therapy. The treatment is effective, but quite burdensome and associated with hypoglycemia, highlighting the need for therapies that preserve residual beta cell function. Experimental evidence suggests that altered sphingolipid metabolism, particularly reduced sulfatide levels, contributes to beta cell stress and dysfunction in early T1D.[37] Fenofibrate, a PPARα agonist which regulates lipid and sphingolipid metabolism, has shown protective effects in preclinical models, including prevention and reversal of diabetes in nonobese diabetic (NOD) mice.[38] Postulated mechanisms include alleviation of beta cell stress and decreased islet inflammation. A case report also suggested preserved insulin independence with early fenofibrate use in T1D.[39] However, robust clinical evidence in humans is lacking in this regards and therefore, this trial was planned to evaluate the efficacy and safety of fenofibrate in preserving beta cell function in newly diagnosed T1D.

This was a phase 2, double-blind, randomized, placebo-controlled trial conducted in Denmark, enrolling adolescents and adults aged 16–40 years with newly diagnosed stage 3 T1D within 6 weeks of diagnosis. 58 participants were randomized 1:1 to receive fenofibrate 160 mg daily or placebo for 52 weeks. The primary outcome was change in endogenous insulin secretion assessed by 2-hour C-peptide area under the curve (AUC) during a mixed-meal tolerance test (MMTT). Secondary outcomes included peak C-peptide, glycated hemoglobin (HbA1c), continuous glucose monitoring (CGM) metrics, daily insulin dose, partial remission status, and the proinsulin/C-peptide (PI/C) ratio as a marker of beta cell stress. Safety outcomes were assessed by adverse event reporting. Lipidomic profiling was performed to evaluate systemic lipid pathway changes. Additionally, mechanistic in vitro experiments were conducted using human pancreatic islets exposed to inflammatory cytokines with and without fenofibrate.

About 56 participants were included in the primary analysis (27 fenofibrate and 29 placebo). After 52 weeks, fenofibrate did not significantly improve beta cell function as compared to placebo, as reflected by similar changes in C-peptide AUC, peak C-peptide levels, insulin requirements, HbA1c, CGM-derived glycemic control, and remission rates. However, the PI/C ratio was significantly higher in the fenofibrate group at week 52, indicating increased beta cell stress. Lipidomic analysis demonstrated significant downregulation of sphingolipid metabolism and signaling pathways by fenofibrate. The drug was well tolerated, with no serious adverse events and safety profile comparable to placebo. In vitro human islet studies showed that fenofibrate reduced cytokine-induced insulin hypersecretion but paradoxically increased beta cell death under inflammatory and hyperglycemic conditions.

This study demonstrates that fenofibrate does not preserve beta cell function in adolescents and adults with newly diagnosed T1D, despite being safe and well tolerated. This lack of clinical benefit contrasts with promising preclinical findings and may reflect fundamental differences between animal models and human disease. Although fenofibrate inhibited insulin secretion in inflamed human islets, this did not translate into reduced beta cell stress; instead, it was associated with a higher PI/C ratio and increased cytokine-induced beta cell death, suggesting potential harm with prolonged exposure. Unlike immunomodulatory agents or calcium-channel blockers such as verapamil that have shown modest beta cell preservation in clinical trials, fenofibrate failed to demonstrate functional benefit.

The study was well-designed, conducted a comprehensive metabolic phenotyping, and integrated lipidomics and mechanistic human islet data as well. However, the sample size was small, and a higher-than-expected remission rate was seen in the placebo group that might have masked small treatment effects. Future research needed to focus on therapies directly targeting immune-mediated beta cell destruction or stress pathways, potentially in combination regimens, rather than repurposing lipid-lowering agents like fenofibrate for beta cell preservation in early T1D.

12. Effect of Alirocumab on Postprandial Hyperlipidemia in Patients with Type 2 Diabetes: A Randomized, Double-blind, Placebo-controlled, Cross-over Trial

Ref: Cariou B, Thys A, Oliveira AR, Letertre MPM, Guyomarch B, Carpentier M, et al. Effect of Alirocumab on Postprandial Hyperlipidaemia in Patients with Type 2 Diabetes: A Randomized, Double-Blind, Placebo-Controlled, Cross-Over Trial. Diabetes Obes Metab. 2025;27(6):3006-16.

ABSTRACT

Aim: Type 2 diabetes (T2D) is frequently associated with postprandial hyperlipidemia (PPL), which is defined by high triglyceride (TG) concentrations following a meal and is frequently acknowledged as an independent cardiovascular risk factor. Here, we sought to evaluate the impact of alirocumab-induced proprotein convertase subtilisin/kexin type 9 (PCSK9) inhibition on PPL in T2D patients.

Supplies and procedures: Male T2D patients participated in the randomized, double-blind, placebo-controlled cross-over study EUTERPE. Two consecutive 10-week treatment sequences (alirocumab 75 mg Q2W or placebo s/c) were administered to the participants, followed by a 10-week washout period. The percentage decrease in plasma TG response following an oral fat load [incremental area under the curve $(iAUC)_{0-8h}$ TG) was the main outcome. Apolipoprotein assays using mass spectrometry and lipoprotein profiling using nuclear magnetic resonance (NMR) were secondary endpoints.

Outcomes: Fourteen people were included: age 59 ± 9 years, body mass index (BMI) 32.8 ± 5.5 kg/m^2, glycated hemoglobin (HbA1c) 6.7 ± 0.5%. Alirocumab did not lower PPL in comparison to placebo [$iAUC_{0-8h}$ TG: –5% {confidence interval (CI) 95% 28, +25}, $p = 0.68$]. Alirocumab reduced the levels of apoB100 (21.2 ± 6.4%; $p = 0.004$), apoE (15.3 ± 6.6%; $p = 0.02$), residual cholesterol (20.0 ± 13.3%; $p = 0.04$), and fasting non-high-density lipoprotein (HDL) cholesterol (38.5 ± 5.6%; $p = 0.0003$). Alirocumab reduced postprandial $VLDL_2$ cholesterol [42% (55, 25); $p < 0.001$] and low-density lipoprotein (LDL) cholesterol [26% (38, 12); $p = 0.0007$], but had no effect on TG or $VLDL_1$ cholesterol concentrations, according to NMR studies.

Conclusion: PPL in T2D was not decreased by alirocumab-induced PCSK9 inhibition, indicating that PCSK9 regulates residual cholesterol catabolism rather than intestine chylomicron formation.

CRITICAL APPRAISAL

Despite substantial low-density lipoprotein (LDL) cholesterol reduction with statins and other lipid-lowering therapies, people with type 2 diabetes (T2D) continue to carry a high residual risk of cardiovascular disease. Postprandial hyperlipidemia (PPL), characterized by exaggerated and prolonged postmeal elevations of triglycerides (TGs) and TG-rich lipoproteins, is increasingly recognized as a driver of atherosclerosis, particularly in insulin-resistant states.[40,41] Cholesterol-rich remnant lipoproteins, which readily accumulate within the arterial wall, play a central role in this process. Although proprotein convertase subtilisin/kexin type 9 (PCSK9) inhibitors provide robust LDL cholesterol lowering and cardiovascular benefit, their effects on postprandial lipoprotein metabolism in humans remain uncertain, with inconsistent findings across genetic, experimental, and clinical studies.[42] Considering the clinical relevance of PPL in T2D, this study investigated the impact of PCSK9 inhibition with alirocumab on postprandial lipid and lipoprotein responses after a standardized fat load in patients with T2D.

The EUTERPE was a single-center, randomized, double-blind, placebo-controlled, cross-over trial conducted in male patients with T2D. Eligible participants were aged 18–75 years, had glycated hemoglobin (HbA1c) <9%, body mass index (BMI) 20–45 kg/m^2, fasting TGs between 150 and 500 mg/dL, and stable glucose-lowering and lipid-lowering therapies while those receiving insulin, fibrates, or omega-3 fatty acids were excluded. All the participants received two 10-week treatment periods of subcutaneous alirocumab 75 mg every 2 weeks or placebo, separated by a 10-week washout. At the end of each treatment period, a standardized high-fat meal test was performed, with serial blood sampling over 8 hours. Primary endpoint was relative difference in postprandial TG response, assessed as incremental area under the curve ($iAUC_{0-8h}$ TG). Secondary endpoints included fasting and postprandial lipids, apolipoproteins measured by liquid chromatography tandem mass spectrometry (LC-MS/MS), and lipoprotein subclass composition assessed by nuclear magnetic resonance.

About 14 male patients completed the study and were included in the analysis, with a mean age of 59 ± 9 years, BMI 32.8 ± 5.5 kg/m^2, and HbA1c 6.7 ± 0.5%. Most participants were receiving statins and metformin-based antidiabetic therapy. Alirocumab did not significantly reduce postprandial hyperlipidemia compared with placebo, as reflected by a nonsignificant change in TG $iAUC_{0-8h}$ (–5%, 95% CI –28 to +25; $p = 0.68$), nor did it significantly affect postprandial apoB48 responses. However, the drug significantly reduced fasting non-high-density lipoprotein (HDL) cholesterol (–38.5 ± 5.6%), remnant cholesterol (–20.0 ± 13.3%), measured LDL cholesterol (–43.2 ± 5.7%), apoB100 (–21.2 ± 6.4%), apoE (–15.3 ± 6.6%), and lipoprotein(a). Nuclear magnetic resonance (NMR) analyses demonstrated significant reductions in $VLDL_2$ and LDL particle numbers and cholesterol content, without significant effects on larger $VLDL_1$ particles or TG concentrations, indicating preferential enhancement of remnant lipoprotein clearance. Alirocumab was well tolerated and did not adversely affect glycemic parameters.

This study shows that PCSK9 inhibition with alirocumab does not reduce postprandial hyperlipidemia in men with T2D, despite marked lowering of fasting atherogenic lipoproteins. The findings suggest that the lipid-lowering action of PCSK9 inhibition is driven predominantly by enhanced clearance of apoB-containing remnant particles rather than by inhibition of intestinal chylomicron production. Although earlier animal studies and small clinical trials implied a role for PCSK9 in postprandial TG and apoB48 metabolism, the present results are consistent with human kinetic studies demonstrating unchanged chylomicron production but accelerated catabolism of smaller VLDL and LDL particles. Variability across studies may reflect differences in patient characteristics, insulin use, glycemic control, meal composition, duration of postprandial assessment, and higher PCSK9 inhibitor doses used previously. Key strengths include the randomized double-blind cross-over design, limiting interindividual variability, and comprehensive NMR-based lipoprotein profiling supporting mechanistic conclusions. However, the sample size was quite small, and all participants were males limiting the generalizability. Lowest dose of Alirocumab was used in the study and use of background statins might have attenuated postprandial effects.

Further studies are warranted to evaluate intensified dosing strategies, include women, explore the influence of contemporary glucose-lowering therapies, and determine the cardiovascular implications of sustained remnant cholesterol reduction in T2D.

13. Effectiveness of Probiotic Therapy as an Adjunct in the Management of Periodontal Disease in Type 2 Diabetics: A Systematic Review and Meta-analysis

Ref: Yuqi W, Hangying X, Ruyi Y, Xiaolan Z, Yajing C. Effectiveness of probiotic therapy as an adjunct in the management of periodontal disease in type 2 diabetics: A systematic review and meta-analysis. Diabetes Res Clin Pract. 2025;226:112358.

ABSTRACT

Background: Diabetes mellitus and periodontal disease are closely related chronic conditions that are highly prevalent worldwide. In the treatment of type-2 diabetes mellitus (T2DM) with periodontal disease, adjunctive probiotic therapy has drawn more and more interest.

Objective: The purpose of this review is to clarify how probiotic therapy affects glycated hemoglobin (HbA1c), periodontal parameters, and inflammatory markers in individuals with both T2DM and periodontal disease.

Techniques: From the time of their creation until June 8, 2025, a thorough literature search was carried out in seven electronic databases. Nonsurgical periodontal treatment (NSPT) monotherapy and adjuvant probiotic therapy were compared in randomized controlled trials (RCTs) and quasi-experimental studies (QERs). Using the Joanna Briggs Institute (JBI) critical appraisal tool for QERs and the Cochrane Risk of Bias 2 (RoB 2) tool for RCTs, two reviewers independently selected papers, retrieved data, and evaluated the risk of bias.

Findings: There were seven studies with 514 people (two QERs and five RCTs). Adjunctive probiotic therapy increased interleukin-6 (IL-6) levels [standardized mean difference (SMD) –1.07; 95% confidence interval (CI) –1.91 to –0.24; $p = 0.01$) and probing depth (SMD –1.13; 95% CI –2.19 to –0.07; $p = 0.04$) when compared with NSPT monotherapy.

Conclusion: In individuals with T2DM accompanied by periodontal disease, adjunctive probiotic therapy successfully lowers IL-6 levels and probing depth.

CRITICAL APPRAISAL

Type-2 diabetes mellitus (T2DM) and periodontal disease are common chronic conditions with a well-established bidirectional relationship.[43] Periodontal disease can worsen glycemic control and increase the risk of diabetic complications through chronic systemic inflammation, while hyperglycemia in T2DM promotes a proinflammatory state and alters the oral microbiota, increasing susceptibility to periodontal disease. Elevated inflammatory mediators such as interleukin-6 (IL-6), tumor necrosis factor-alpha (TNF-α), and C-reactive protein (CRP) play a central role in this interaction.[44]

Probiotics, defined as beneficial live microorganisms can modulate oral and gut microbiota, inhibit pathogenic bacteria, and regulate inflammatory responses.[45] Emerging studies suggest that probiotic supplementation, when used as an adjunct to nonsurgical periodontal therapy, may improve periodontal inflammation and metabolic parameters in patients with T2DM; however, findings are inconsistent due to heterogeneity in study design, probiotic formulations, and sample sizes.[46,47]

Therefore, this systematic review was undertaken to evaluate the effects of adjunctive probiotic therapy on inflammatory markers, periodontal outcomes, and glycemic control in patients with coexisting T2DM and periodontal disease.

This systematic review and meta-analysis was conducted in accordance with PRISMA guidelines and registered in PROSPERO (CRD42025630407). Seven electronic databases (PubMed, Cochrane Library, EMBASE, Web of Science, China National Knowledge Infrastructure, WanFang, and Chinese Biomedical Literature Database) were searched from inception to June 8, 2025. Randomized controlled trials and quasi-experimental studies involving adults (≥18 years) with both T2DM and periodontal disease were included. All participants received nonsurgical periodontal treatment comprising oral hygiene instruction, full-mouth scaling, and root planing. The intervention group additionally received probiotic therapy. Probiotic interventions varied across studies and included *Lactobacillus reuteri* alone or multi-strain probiotic/synbiotic formulations containing *Lactobacillus* and *Bifidobacterium* species. Outcomes assessed were inflammatory markers (hs-CRP, IL-6, and TNF-α), periodontal parameters (probing depth and clinical attachment loss), and glycemic control [glycated hemoglobin (HbA1c)]. Pregnant women and studies lacking usable data, conference abstracts, protocols, reviews, and secondary analyses were excluded. Intervention duration ranged from 21 to 90 days, with follow-up periods of 8 weeks, 3 months, or up to 6 months.

Seven studies (five randomized controlled trials and two quasi-experimental studies) involving 514 participants met the inclusion criteria, with 256 receiving adjunctive probiotic therapy and 258 receiving NSPT alone. Age of participants ranged from 35 to 78 years and 58.2% were males. Adjunctive probiotic therapy significantly reduced IL-6 levels compared with NSPT alone (5 studies, $n = 427$; SMD −1.07; 95% CI −1.91 to −0.24; $p = 0.01$; $I^2 = 93\%$), with subgroup differences observed by country but not probiotic type. No significant overall differences were observed for hs-CRP or TNF-α; although sensitivity analyses indicated that exclusion of individual studies reduced heterogeneity and, for hs-CRP, revealed a significant reduction. Periodontal outcomes showed a significant reduction in probing depth with probiotic therapy (six studies, $n = 467$; SMD −1.13; 95% CI −2.19 to −0.07; $p = 0.04$; $I^2 = 96\%$), with heterogeneity partly explained by country-level differences, while no significant effect was observed for clinical attachment loss. Glycemic control was not significantly improved, as HbA1c levels did not differ between groups, even after sensitivity analyses.

This systematic review shows that adjunctive probiotic therapy in patients with T2DM and periodontal disease leads to significant reductions in IL-6 levels and probing depth, indicating improvement in inflammatory burden and periodontal health, while consistent benefits were not observed for hs-CRP, TNF-α, clinical attachment loss, or glycemic control assessed by HbA1c. These findings suggest that probiotics may primarily act through modulation of local and systemic inflammatory pathways rather than direct metabolic effects. The results are in keeping with earlier clinical and experimental studies demonstrating improvements in periodontal parameters with probiotic supplementation, while also reflecting prior evidence of inconsistent effects on systemic inflammation and glycemic outcomes in diabetes.

The reliability of earlier-mentioned findings is supported by the use of rigorous systematic review methodology, prospective protocol registration, and evaluation of clinically relevant inflammatory, periodontal, and metabolic outcomes. At the same time, the interpretation of results requires caution due to the limited number of studies, marked heterogeneity, short intervention and follow-up durations, and variable reporting of probiotic dose, viability, and adherence. The predominance of studies from limited geographic regions may restrict generalizability, and several potential confounders—including antidiabetic therapies, dietary patterns, oral hygiene practices, and antibiotic exposure—were inconsistently controlled. In addition, the short follow-up and reliance on surrogate markers may have limited the ability to detect sustained improvements in glycemic control or periodontal tissue regeneration.

Future research should focus on adequately powered randomized trials using standardized probiotic preparations with longer follow-up and careful control of confounding variables. Incorporation of microbiome profiling and mechanistic biomarkers may further clarify how probiotics influence inflammatory pathways and translate into metabolic improvements in patients with coexisting T2DM and periodontal disorders.

14. Metformin Lowers Risk of Hearing Loss and Mortality in Type 2 Diabetes

Ref: Huang CC, Hsu RF, Chen WM, Shia BC, Wu SY, Huang CC. Metformin lowers risk of hearing loss and mortality in type 2 diabetes. Diabetes Obes Metab. 2025;27(3):1327-36.

ABSTRACT

Aim: To evaluate the relationship between metformin use and the risk of sudden sensorineural hearing loss (SSNHL) in individuals with type 2 diabetes (T2D), a group that is more susceptible to SSNHL.

Supplies and procedures: Using data from Taiwan's National Health Insurance Research Database, this cohort study tracked T2D patients from the database's baseline in 2008 to 2019. Achieving ≥80% of the medication possession ratio (MPR) and ≥28 cumulative defined daily doses (cDDD) in three months was considered metformin usage. To ensure active treatment comparability, individuals with ≥80% MPR from different antidiabetic medications were included in the control group. Covariates were balanced using propensity score matching, and mortality was taken into consideration by competing risk models. Calculations were made for incidence rates (IRs), hazard ratios (HRs), and incidence rate ratios (IRRs).

Results: With an IRR of 0.73 (95% CI 0.66–0.82; $p < 0.0001$), metformin users showed a lower incidence of SSNHL (IR: 11.48 per 10,000 person-years) than nonusers (IR 15.66 per 10,000 person-years). A 27% decrease in SSNHL risk was shown by adjusted HRs (HR 0.73; 95% CI 0.66–0.82). Additional risk reductions were associated with higher cumulative doses (Q4: HR 0.36; 95% CI 0.29–0.46) and daily doses ≥1 DDD (HR 0.78; 95% CI 0.69–0.87). Lower overall mortality was also linked to metformin use.

Conclusion: Metformin treatment is linked to a dose-dependent decrease in the risk of SSNHL and decreased mortality in people with T2D. These results highlight the potential relevance of metformin in preventing SSNHL and improving survival due to the strict definitions of metformin exposure and an actively treated comparison group.

CRITICAL APPRAISAL

Sudden sensorineural hearing loss (SSNHL) is a rapidly developing condition that can lead to significant and sometimes permanent hearing impairment, impairing quality of life.[48] The incidence is higher in individuals with metabolic and autoimmune disorders, particularly type-2 diabetes (T2D). Diabetes is believed to increase SSNHL risk through vascular, metabolic, inflammatory, and immune-mediated mechanisms, and a considerable proportion of affected individuals develop permanent hearing loss, underscoring the need for effective preventive strategies.[49]

Metformin, a widely used antidiabetic agent, exhibits anti-inflammatory, antioxidant, endothelial-protective, and adenosine monophosphate (AMP)-activated protein kinase-mediated effects that may confer protection against cochlear injury. Although prior observational studies have suggested a potential association between metformin use and reduced SSNHL risk, the available evidence has been limited by small sample sizes, insufficient adjustment for confounders, and the use of untreated comparator groups.[50] In view of these limitations, the present study was planned to evaluate the association between metformin use and the risk of SSNHL in patients with T2D using a large, real-world database with an actively treated comparator group and robust analytical methods.

This nationwide, population-based cohort study used data from Taiwan's National Health Insurance Research Database. Adult patients with T2D who received at least one antidiabetic medication between the years 2008 and 2019 were included and followed until 2022. Participants were classified into a metformin group and an active comparator group based on medication possession ratio (MPR) (≥80%) and cumulative defined daily doses (cDDD) (≥28 cDDDs within 3 months), ensuring comparable treatment exposure.

Patients with prior SSNHL, conditions or medications associated with hearing loss, autoimmune diseases, or early mortality were excluded. Propensity score matching was applied to balance demographic characteristics, diabetes duration and severity, comorbidities, medication use, and lifestyle-related variables between groups.

The primary outcome was incident SSNHL, confirmed using standardized diagnostic criteria by certified otolaryngologists. All-cause mortality was included as a competing risk. Hazard ratios were estimated using Cox proportional hazards models, time-dependent exposure analyses, and Fine–Gray competing risk models.

After propensity score matching, 161,400 patients with T2D were analyzed (80,700 metformin users and 80,700 non-metformin users), with well-balanced baseline characteristics. Metformin use was associated with a lower incidence of SSNHL compared with nonuse (11.48 vs. 15.66 per 10,000 person-years), yielding an incidence rate ratio of 0.73 [95% confidence interval (CI) 0.66–0.82; $p < 0.0001$]. Multivariable Cox regression demonstrated a consistent 27% reduction in SSNHL risk with metformin use [adjusted hazard ratio (HR) 0.73; 95% CI 0.66–0.82], which remained significant after competing risk analysis for mortality.

A dose–response relationship was observed, with greater risk reduction at higher cumulative metformin exposure (Q4: adjusted HR 0.36; 95% CI 0.29–0.46; $p < 0.0001$). All-cause mortality was significantly lower in metformin users (11.5%) than in nonusers (19.8%), with adjusted HRs of approximately 0.50 across fully adjusted models ($p < 0.0001$), and survival benefits increased with higher cumulative metformin exposure.

The study offers novel insights into the long-term incidence and prevention of SSNHL in T2D, filling a key gap in literature. This is the largest study to date to quantify SSNHL risk in T2D and demonstrates a reduced risk associated with metformin use. A 27% overall reduction in SSNHL risk was observed, with progressively greater protection at higher cumulative and daily metformin doses. These findings are consistent with, but extend beyond, earlier observational studies that suggested a protective association between metformin and SSNHL, which were limited by small sample sizes, inadequate adjustment for confounding, absence of competing mortality risk analyses, and use of untreated comparator groups. The present study addressed these, thereby providing more robust and generalizable evidence. The observed dose–response relationship further supports a biologically plausible effect of metformin, in line with experimental data implicating AMP-activated protein kinase activation, reduced oxidative stress, improved endothelial function, and anti-inflammatory mechanisms in cochlear protection.[51]

Key strengths of this study include its large sample size, long-term follow-up, and rigorous analytical approach including propensity score matching and use of an active comparator group with time-varying exposure analysis. However, there are certain limitations to be noted. The reliance on administrative data precluded access to detailed audiometric measurements, and SSNHL diagnoses were based on International Classification of Diseases (ICD) codes rather than direct hearing assessments, although diagnoses were made by certified otolaryngologists, reducing misclassification risk. Residual confounding from unmeasured factors such as lifestyle behaviors cannot be excluded, and the observational design does not allow causal inference. Finally, as the study was conducted within Taiwanese population, this limits the generalizability to other ethnic groups.

15. Treatment Outcomes with Oral Anti-hyperglycemic Therapies in People with Diabetes Secondary to a Pancreatic Condition (Type-3c Diabetes): A Population-based Cohort Study

Ref: Hopkins R, Young KG, Thomas NJ, Jones AG, Hattersley AT, Shields BM, et al.; MASTERMIND consortium. Treatment outcomes with oral anti-hyperglycaemic therapies in people with diabetes secondary to a pancreatic condition (type 3c diabetes): A population-based cohort study. Diabetes Obes Metab. 2025;27(3):1544-53.

ABSTRACT

Aim: To evaluate the effectiveness of oral antihyperglycemic medications in patients with type 3c diabetes, a pancreas disease for which there is little particular therapeutic advice.

Supplies and procedures: We identified 7,084 individuals with a pancreatic condition (acute pancreatitis, chronic pancreatitis, pancreatic cancer, and hemochromatosis) prior to diabetes diagnosis (type 3c cohort), starting oral glucose-lowering therapy [metformin, sulfonylureas, sodium-glucose cotransporter-2 (SGLT-2)-inhibitors, dipeptidyl peptidase-4 (DPP4)-inhibitors, or thiazolidinediones), and not receiving concurrent insulin treatment using hospital-linked UK primary care records (Clinical Practice Research Datalink; 2004–2020). We matched 97,227 type-2 diabetes mellitus (T2DM) controls after stratifying by pancreatic exocrine insufficiency (PEI) ($n = 5,917$ without PEI, 1,167 with PEI). Type 3c and T2D were compared in terms of 12-month glycated hemoglobin (HbA1c) response, weight change, and 6-month treatment discontinuation.

Findings: Oral treatments significantly reduced the mean HbA1c in those with type-3c diabetes, both with and without PEI {12.2 [95% confidence interval (CI) 12.0–12.4] mmol/mol and 9.4 (8.9–10.0) mmol/mol, respectively}. People with type 3c without PEI had comparable odds of cessation [odds ratio (OR): 1.08 (0.98–1.19)] and mean HbA1c reduction [0.7 (0.4–1.0) mmol/mol difference) to T2D controls. Compared to T2D controls, those with type 3c and PEI had higher discontinuation [OR 2.03 (1.73–2.36)] and a lower mean HbA1c response [3.5 (2.9–4.1) mmol/mol smaller decrease]. Type 3c's weight change was comparable to that of T2DM. Across drug classes and underlying pancreatic diseases, the results were generally consistent.

Conclusion: People with type-3c diabetes benefit from oral antihyperglycemic medications, which may play a significant role in glycemic control. People with type-3c who need more careful treatment response monitoring may be identified by PEI.

CRITICAL APPRAISAL

Type-3c diabetes, also known as pancreatogenic diabetes results from pancreatic damage due to conditions such as acute or chronic pancreatitis, pancreatic cancer, or hemochromatosis.[52] It comprises 5-10% of people with diabetes in Western populations but is frequently misclassified as type 2 diabetes mellitus (T2DM), resulting in poor treatment response and more complications.[53,54] Guidance for the management of type-3c diabetes remains limited. Current treatment approaches are largely extrapolated from type 1 diabetes mellitus (T1DM) or T2DM, with recommendations including early insulin initiation and avoiding incretin-based therapies because of concerns regarding pancreatitis.[55] There is a lack of evidence evaluating the effectiveness of oral glucose-lowering therapies in this population, as these patients are usually excluded from major clinical trials, raising concerns about suboptimal treatment in routine care.

Treatment response in Type-3c diabetes may vary as per the extent of pancreatic damage. Pancreatic exocrine insufficiency (PEI), a feature reflecting impaired exocrine function, may act as a marker of disease severity and influence response to oral anti-hyperglycemic therapies. This study therefore aimed to evaluate outcomes of oral glucose-lowering treatment in type-3c diabetes, assess heterogeneity by PEI status and underlying pancreatic disease, and compare findings with those in T2DM.

This population-based cohort study used UK primary care data from the Clinical Practice Research Datalink linked to Hospital Episode Statistics and deprivation data (2004–2020). Diabetes was identified using clinical codes, glucose-lowering prescriptions, or glycated hemoglobin (HbA1c) ≥48 mmol/mol. Type-3c diabetes was defined by diabetes following acute pancreatitis, chronic pancreatitis, pancreatic cancer, or hemochromatosis, excluding cystic fibrosis and isolated pancreatic resection. PEI was defined by a diagnosis code, fecal elastase-1 <200 μg/g, or pancreatic enzyme replacement therapy before diabetes diagnosis.

A total of 7,084 individuals with type-3c diabetes initiating oral therapy without insulin were included (5,917 without PEI and 1,167 with PEI) and matched to 97,227 T2DM controls by sex, ethnicity, deprivation, age, calendar year, and prior therapy use. Oral therapies included metformin, sulfonylureas, thiazolidinediones, dipeptidyl peptidase-4 (DPP-4) inhibitors, and sodium-glucose cotransporter-2 (SGLT-2) inhibitors. Outcomes were 12-month change in HbA1c and weight on unchanged therapy and 6-month treatment discontinuation. HbA1c and weight were analyzed using adjusted linear regression and discontinuation using logistic regression. Analyses were conducted overall, by pancreatic subtype and drug class, with sensitivity analyses for alcohol use, PEI definition, and timing of acute pancreatitis.

Substantial reductions in HbA1c were observed in type 3c diabetes without PEI {12.2 mmol/mol [95% confidence interval (CI) 12.0–12.4]} and with PEI [9.4 mmol/mol (95% CI 8.9–10.0)]. Compared with T2DM, HbA1c reduction was similar in those without PEI [difference 0.7 mmol/mol (95% CI 0.4–1.0)] but was significantly lower in those with PEI [3.5 mmol/mol (95% CI 2.9–4.1) less reduction]. 6-month treatment discontinuation was comparable between type-3c diabetes without PEI and T2DM [odds ratio (OR) 1.08 (95% CI 0.98–1.19)] but was higher in those with PEI [OR 2.03 (95% CI 1.73–2.36)] with the greatest increase observed for metformin. Early insulin initiation was substantially higher in type-3c diabetes than T2DM, particularly in those with PEI (43.7% at 3 years). Glycemic response across drug classes was generally preserved, although reduced responses to metformin and sulfonylureas were noted in PEI, while SGLT-2 inhibitors and thiazolidinediones showed no reduction. Weight change was largely similar to T2DM, with greater weight loss on SGLT-2 inhibitors and less weight gain on sulfonylureas in PEI. Findings were consistent across pancreatic disease subtypes and remained robust in sensitivity analyses.

The findings indicate that oral glucose-lowering therapies can produce meaningful improvements in glycemic control in individuals with type-3c diabetes, particularly in those without PEI. Conversely, the presence of PEI was associated with a diminished HbA1c response and a markedly higher likelihood of treatment discontinuation, most notably with metformin, underscoring the clinical heterogeneity of type-3c diabetes and the importance of disease severity in shaping treatment outcomes.

Several mechanisms may explain these observations. Advanced pancreatic damage in individuals with PEI is likely to result in more profound β-cell dysfunction, impaired enteroinsular signaling, and gastrointestinal disturbances related to malabsorption and nutritional compromise, all of which may reduce both the effectiveness and tolerability of oral agents. The relatively preserved efficacy of SGLT-2 inhibitors and thiazolidinediones suggests that therapies acting through insulin-independent or peripheral pathways may retain effectiveness despite advanced pancreatic dysfunction.

Evidence for pharmacological management of type-3c diabetes has been limited and has largely favored early insulin therapy. This large real-world study adds to the existing literature by demonstrating the effectiveness of oral glucose-lowering agents in a substantial proportion of individuals with type-3c diabetes, while confirming poorer control and higher insulin needs in advanced disease.

The study is strengthened by its large, nationally representative cohort, linkage of primary and secondary care datasets, inclusion of diverse pancreatic disease etiologies, and stratification by PEI as a clinically relevant indicator of disease severity, supported by robust matching to a large T2DM comparator group and multiple sensitivity analyses. However, the observational design introduces the potential for residual confounding, misclassification of both type-3c diabetes and PEI remains possible, and reliance on prescribing records precluded identification of specific clinical reasons for treatment discontinuation.

The study findings highlight the need for prospective studies to define optimal, phenotype-specific treatment strategies in type-3c diabetes, particularly stratified by pancreatic exocrine insufficiency.

16. Risk Acceleration by Gout on Major Adverse Cardiovascular Events and All-cause Death in Patients with Diabetes and Chronic Kidney Disease

Ref: Lee DY, Moon JS, Jung I, Chung SM, Park SY, Yu JH, et al. Risk acceleration by gout on major adverse cardiovascular events and all-cause death in patients with diabetes and chronic kidney disease. Diabetes Obes Metab. 2025;27(3):1554-63.

ABSTRACT

Aim: Our goal was to investigate how gout affects the risk of cardiovascular disease (CVD) and death in individuals with type 2 diabetes, as well as whether chronic kidney disease (CKD) influences this relationship.

Supplies and procedures: 757,378 people with type 2 diabetes were categorized into the CKDGout, CKDGout+, CKD+Gout, and CKD+Gout+ groups using the Korean National Health Insurance Service database. After controlling for cardiometabolic variables, the risk of myocardial infarction (MI), ischemic stroke, and mortality was evaluated using Cox proportional hazard models.

Results: 25,618, 38,691, and 78,628 people had MI, stroke, and death over a median follow-up of 9.3 years, respectively. With the highest adjusted hazard ratio (HR) in the CKD+Gout+ group [HR 1.57; 95% confidence interval (CI) 1.46–1.69] and the CKD + Gout – group (HR 1.23; 95% CI 1.20–1.26), the risk of MI or stroke gradually increased across the categories. The highest risks for MI (HR 1.71), stroke (HR 1.46), and death (HR 1.78) were found in the CKD+Gout+group. When compared to people without gout or CKD, individuals with gout alone did not show a statistically significant increase in risk. Gout had a greater impact on the outcomes in patients with CKD, according to interaction analyses. Consistent results across a range of clinical and demographic factors were obtained from subgroup analysis.

Conclusion: Gout and CKD both raised the risk of CVD and death, with the CKD+Gout+ group showing the highest risk. These results were greatly impacted by the relationship between gout and CKD.

CRITICAL APPRAISAL

Gout is increasingly prevalent worldwide and is closely linked with cardiometabolic comorbidities, including type 2 diabetes mellitus (T2DM) and chronic kidney disease (CKD), as well as higher cardiovascular and mortality risk.[56,57] However, whether gout independently contributes to cardiovascular disease (CVD) remains uncertain due to confounding by shared risk factors and the strong interrelationship between serum urate levels and kidney function. CKD both predisposes to gout and markedly increases CVD and mortality risk, making causal interpretation difficult, particularly in patients with diabetes who commonly have overlapping metabolic and renal disease. The combined and interactive effects of gout and CKD on cardiovascular outcomes in patients with T2DM have not been clearly defined. Therefore, this study aimed to examine the impact of gout on CVD and all-cause mortality in individuals with T2DM and to determine whether these associations differ according to CKD status using a nationwide cohort.

This nationwide cohort study used data from the Korean National Health Insurance Service, including adults with T2DM who underwent health examinations in 2009. After excluding those <20 year of age and with prior myocardial infarction (MI), stroke, incomplete data, or uncertain gout diagnosis, total 757,378 participants were analyzed. Participants were classified into four groups based on the presence or absence of CKD and gout: (1) CKD–/Gout–, (2) CKD–/Gout+, (3) CKD+/Gout–, and (4) CKD+/Gout+. CKD was defined by estimated glomerular filtration rate (eGFR) (<60 mL/min/1.73 m^2) or renal replacement therapy, while gout was identified using repeated or inpatient International Classification of Diseases-10 (ICD-10) diagnostic codes. Participants were followed until incident MI, ischemic stroke, death, or end of follow-up (2018). Cox proportional hazards models were used to estimate adjusted risks for cardiovascular outcomes and mortality, accounting for demographic factors, lifestyle behaviors, cardiometabolic comorbidities, and diabetes-related variables, with additional interaction and subgroup analyses to assess effect modification by CKD status.

Of 757,378 patients with T2DM, 672,649 had neither CKD nor gout, 17,921 had gout alone, 62,607 had CKD alone, and 4,201 had both CKD and gout. Over a median 9.3-year follow-up, 25,618 MIs, 38,691 ischemic strokes, and 78,628 deaths occurred. Incidence rates for MI or stroke increased stepwise across groups (8.40, 9.81, 17.31, and 22.93 per 1,000 person-years, respectively; log-rank p <0.001).

In fully adjusted analyses, compared with CKD–/Gout–, risk of MI or stroke was highest in CKD+/Gout+ [hazard ratio (HR) 1.57; 95% confidence interval (CI) 1.46–1.69], followed by CKD+/Gout– (HR 1.23; 95% CI 1.20–1.26), while gout without CKD was not significant (HR 1.05; 95% CI 1.00–1.11). CKD+/Gout+ also had the greatest risks for MI (HR 1.71), stroke (HR 1.46), and all-cause mortality (HR 1.78). Among patients with CKD, gout further increased risks of MI or stroke (HR: 1.29), MI (HR 1.30), stroke (HR 1.26), and death (HR 1.27), with significant CKD–gout interaction and strongest effects at eGFR <30 mL/min/1.73 m^2.

This large nationwide cohort study demonstrates that, among patients with T2DM, gout alone does not independently increase the risk of CVD or all-cause mortality, whereas CKD is a strong determinant of both outcomes, and the coexistence of gout with CKD confers the highest risk. Notably, the presence of gout significantly amplified CV mortality risk only in patients with CKD, with a clear interaction between the two conditions and a graded effect according to CKD severity, strongest at eGFR <30 mL/min/1.73 m^2. These findings help reconcile inconsistencies in prior epidemiological studies that reported associations between gout and cardiovascular outcomes by highlighting the critical confounding and modifying role of kidney function. Earlier population-based studies in the general population reported higher CV mortality risks in patients with gout,[58] while Mendelian randomization analyses largely failed to support a causal role for gout itself.[59] The results from this study align with this interpretation, showing no excess risk attributable to gout in the absence of CKD, while supporting a synergistic effect when gout coexists with renal dysfunction, potentially mediated through heightened inflammation, oxidative stress, endothelial dysfunction, insulin resistance, and the accumulation of traditional cardiovascular risk factors common to both conditions.

The study had certain limitations, including retrospective observational design, reliance on ICD-10 codes for gout diagnosis with possible misclassification, lack of data on urate-lowering therapy and newer glucose-lowering agents with cardiovascular benefit, and inability to account for medication adherence or changes over time. Despite all these limitations, this study provides robust evidence that gout meaningfully increases cardiovascular (CV) and mortality risk primarily in the presence of CKD, underscoring the need for CV risk assessment and targeted management in patients with diabetes who have both conditions.

17. Overweight and Obesity—Capturing the Whole Picture

Ref: Aroda VR, Perreault L. Overweight and Obesity—Capturing the Whole Picture. N Engl J Med. 2025;392(22):2269-71.

ABSTRACT

Obesity and overweight are treatable proximal causes of chronic illness. Overweight and obesity are becoming more commonplace worldwide; estimates suggest that by 2050, over half of all adults will be overweight or obese, with China accounting for the largest share at 627 million. Over the past 40 years, China has seen a sharp rise in the number of overweight and obese people, which has significantly raised the risk of noncommunicable diseases such as type 2 diabetes, cancer, and cardiovascular disease as well as premature mortality. The multifaceted approach to improve evidence-based obesity management in China includes focused interventional trials in Chinese populations. The effectiveness and safety of mazdutide, a once-weekly dual glucagon-like peptide-1 (GLP-1) and glucagon receptor agonist, in 610 Chinese people with overweight or obesity are currently reported by Ji and colleagues in the Journal. The potential impacts of multihormonal incretin-based therapy, which uses GLP-1's capacity to limit the glycolytic effects of glucagon while exerting its influence on weight reduction in a method that may particularly mobilize liver fat, were investigated in this phase 3, double blind, placebo-controlled experiment. Although it is becoming more and more clear that glucagon agonism has quite different effects when administered in conjunction with GLP-1 than when administered alone, it is impossible to separate the impact of glucagon receptor agonism from that of GLP-1 receptor agonism in the current trial.

CRITICAL APPRAISAL

This editorial discusses the growing global burden of overweight and obesity, which are major, preventable causes of chronic diseases. Current projections suggest that by 2050 > 50% of the world's adult population will have overweight or obesity, with the largest numbers in China (≈627 million people).[12] This rise has contributed to sharp increases in type 2 diabetes, cardiovascular disease, cancer, and premature mortality. The authors highlight that obesity should be viewed as a multisystem disease, not merely excess body weight.

This editorial focuses on the GLORY-1 trial,[60] a phase 3, randomized, double-blind, placebo-controlled study of mazdutide, once-weekly dual glucagon-like peptide-1 (GLP-1) and glucagon receptor agonist, conducted in 610 Chinese adults with overweight or obesity.

At 32 weeks, placebo-adjusted mean weight loss was –13.0% [95% confidence interval (CI) –14.31 to –11.70] with mazdutide 6 mg and –10.54% (95% CI –11.83 to –9.26) with 4 mg, from a mean baseline weight of 87.2 kg. A greater proportion of participants receiving mazdutide achieved clinically meaningful weight loss, including ≥15% weight reduction in 44% of those receiving the 6-mg dose.

Importantly, the trial assessed outcomes beyond body weight. The drug improved other measures of adiposity—total fat mass on dual-energy X-ray absorptiometry (DXA), waist, hip, and neck circumference, glycemic parameters [glycated hemoglobin (HbA1c), fasting glucose, fasting insulin, and Homeostatic Model Assessment 2–Insulin Resistance (HOMA2-IR)], cardiovascular risk markers (systolic and diastolic blood pressure, high-sensitivity C-reactive protein, uric acid, and urinary albumin), liver markers [alanine aminotransferase (ALT) and aspartate transaminase (AST) in the full cohort and liver fat content in those with steatosis], and physical function and quality of life (SF-36 and QOL-Lite questionnaires). This comprehensive assessment supports a whole-body, risk-focused approach to obesity treatment.

The editorial also discusses the key differences in the phenotype of obesity in GLORY-1 as compared to western counterparts. Participants in this trial were younger (mean age 34.2 years) and had a lower mean body mass index (BMI) (31.1 kg/m^2) compared with Western obesity trials. Despite this, prevalence of obesity-related conditions was high: 48.9% had metabolic dysfunction-associated fatty liver disease, 62.3% had dyslipidemia, and 88.9% had at least one weight-related comorbidity, while prediabetes (10.7%) and hypertension (22.8%) were less common. These findings highlight that metabolic risk in Asian populations occurs at lower BMI and younger ages.

The authors have mentioned important limitations of GLORY-1 trial, including short duration of follow-up, inability to separate the specific contribution of glucagon receptor agonism from GLP-1 effects, and uncertainty about long-term safety and outcomes, particularly in younger individuals. The authors argue that reliance on BMI-based treatment algorithms is insufficient and emphasize the need for individualized risk assessment when managing obesity.

To conclude, the editorial underscores the newer agents like mazdutide can produce meaningful weight loss and broad metabolic benefits. However, pharmacotherapy is only one component of obesity care, which must combine early identification, individualized treatment, and public health strategies to address the global obesity epidemic.

18. Redefining End Points in MASH Cirrhosis

Ref: Garcia-Tsao G. Redefining End Points in MASH Cirrhosis. N Engl J Med. 2025;392(24):2475-7.

ABSTRACT

The final stage of chronic liver disease, cirrhosis, is characterized by progressive liver fibrosis from stage 1 (portal fibrosis) to stage 4 (cirrhosis). A patient is only at danger of dying from chronic liver disease when cirrhosis appears. Patients with hepatic decompensation (decompensated cirrhosis), which is characterized by the development of ascites, variceal bleeding, hepatic encephalopathy, or all three symptoms, are most at risk. Cirrhosis is most commonly caused by alcohol-induced liver disease and metabolic dysfunction-associated steatohepatitis (MASH). Preventing the development of cirrhosis from a noncirrhotic stage (1, 2, or 3) would be the optimum course of treatment for MASH.

CRITICAL APPRAISAL

This editorial focused on the challenges of developing effective therapies for metabolic dysfunction-associated steatohepatitis (MASH)-related cirrhosis, the stage of chronic liver disease with high risk of mortality. Risk is particularly high once hepatic decompensation occurs, manifesting as ascites, variceal bleeding, or hepatic encephalopathy. Along with alcohol-related liver disease, MASH is now one of the leading causes of cirrhosis worldwide.

In noncirrhotic MASH, recent phase 3 trials of semaglutide and resmetirom have shown benefits in terms of MASH resolution and improvement in fibrosis by at least one stage, supporting early intervention. However, up to 25% of patients already have cirrhosis at first diagnosis, shifting therapeutic goals toward preventing decompensation or ideally achieving regression to a noncirrhotic stage, which is very difficult to accomplish.

This editorial discussed a phase 2b, randomized, placebo-controlled trial by Noureddin et al,[61] which evaluated efruxifermin, FGF21 analog, in patients with biopsy-proven compensated MASH cirrhosis. Primary endpoint was improvement of fibrosis by at least one stage without worsening of MASH at 36 weeks. This endpoint was achieved in 13% of placebo-treated patients, 18% of those receiving 28 mg, and 19% of those receiving 50 mg of efruxifermin, with no statistically significant difference between treatment and placebo groups. Importantly, no meaningful weight loss was observed, suggesting limited impact on the underlying primary driver of disease.

The main argument of this editorial was that histologic fibrosis regression may be an inappropriate or insufficient endpoint in trials of cirrhosis. Liver biopsy samples represent only a very small fraction of the liver and do not capture the heterogeneity of cirrhosis.[62] Moreover, compensated cirrhosis is not a uniform condition. It consists of at least two biologically and clinically distinct stages, defined by the presence or absence of clinically significant portal hypertension (CSPH).

Portal hypertension arises as progressive fibrosis thickens and distorts the hepatic architecture, increasing intrahepatic vascular resistance and ultimately producing a hyperdynamic circulatory state.[63] Once CSPH develops, risk of hepatic decompensation increases markedly. At this stage, fibrosis regression is unlikely or occurs very slowly; therefore, preventing decompensation becomes a more clinically relevant goal than achieving short-term histologic improvement.

The editorial also highlighted that CSPH can be assessed invasively by measuring the hepatic venous pressure gradient, but can also be estimated noninvasively using liver stiffness measurements combined with platelet count, with improved predictive models in patients with obesity. In the efruxifermin trial, median liver stiffness values suggested that at least half of the enrolled patients already had CSPH, which explains the lack of treatment response and the heterogeneity of outcomes. Notably, clinical decompensation occurred in three patients receiving efruxifermin and in none of the placebo group, raising concerns about endpoint selection rather than definitive drug failure.

In conclusion, the editorial stressed upon the fact that negative primary outcome of this trial should not be interpreted as lack of therapeutic promise, but rather to be taken as evidence that clinical trial design in MASH cirrhosis needs to be changed. Future trials are needed which stratify patients by CSPH status and use clinically meaningful endpoints, like prevention of decompensation, rather than relying only on histologic fibrosis regression. Redefining endpoints is essential to understand effective therapies for patients with MASH cirrhosis, for whom treatment options are limited and urgently needed.

19. Expanding the Treat-to-Target Toolbox for Obesity and Diabetes Care

Ref: Hales CM. Expanding the Treat-to-Target Toolbox for Obesity and Diabetes Care. N Engl J Med. 2025;393(7):712-4.

ABSTRACT

Tirzepatide and semaglutide are effective medicinal treatments for clinical obesity, a chronic illness caused by impaired organ or physical functioning due to excess body fat. These medications provide concurrent treatment of type 2 diabetes and obesity for the 90% of people who have both conditions. Similar to algorithms developed for the treatment of other chronic diseases such as diabetes and hypertension, algorithms to guide personalized treatment intensity are required since the many metabolic and physical signs and consequences of obesity respond differently to treatment. Additional options would improve the capacity of both physicians and patients to find customized strategies for each patient's unique health needs, given the varying individual efficacy and adverse effects of the existing treatments. Garvey et al. and Davies et al. present findings from two phase 3 clinical studies evaluating a combination of medications with different but complementary modes of action. The combination of semaglutide, a glucagon-like peptide-1 (GLP-1) receptor agonist, and cagrilintide, a long-acting amylin analog, given as a single weekly injection for the treatment of individuals with obesity or overweight without type 2 diabetes (REDEFINE 1) or with type 2 diabetes (REDEFINE 2) has also promising results.

CRITICAL APPRAISAL

This New England Journal of Medicine (NEJM) editorial discusses the evolving concept of a treat-to-target strategy for obesity and type 2 diabetes care, highlighting the limitations of a one-size-fits-all, body mass index (BMI)-centric approach. Obesity is a chronic and heterogeneous disease that commonly coexists with type 2 diabetes mellitus (T2DM), with nearly 90% of patients with diabetes being overweight or obese.[64] As the metabolic and functional consequences of obesity vary widely among individuals, the author argues for individualized treatment goals, rather than focusing only on weight loss.

The editorial discusses about REDEFINE-1[65] and REDEFINE-2[66] phase 3 trials evaluating the fixed-dose combination of cagrilintide, a long-acting amylin analog, and semaglutide, a glucagon-like peptide-1 (GLP-1) receptor agonist. REDEFINE-1 enrolled obese/overweight adults without T2DM and demonstrated a mean body-weight reduction of 20.4% at 68 weeks with combination therapy, substantially greater than placebo and superior to either agent used alone. This degree of weight loss was accompanied by clinically meaningful reductions in systolic and diastolic blood pressure, improvements in lipid profiles and physical functioning, and a high rate of reversion from prediabetes to normoglycemia, indicating broad metabolic benefits beyond weight reduction alone.

The REDEFINE-2 extended these findings to overweight or obese T2DM adults. In this trial, combination therapy produced a mean weight loss of 13.7% over 68 weeks and resulted in marked glycemic improvement, with nearly three-quarters of participants achieving a glycated hemoglobin (HbA1c) of 6.5% or lower. Cardiovascular risk factors and measures of physical function improved in parallel, reinforcing the multiple benefits of the intervention.

Safety findings showed that gastrointestinal side effects and injection-site reactions occurred more often with the combination therapy than with semaglutide alone, resulting in higher treatment discontinuation rates.

Serious adverse events were also reported more frequently in the combination group, and the occurrence of suicides raised concern, although a definite causal link to treatment was not established. Importantly, the trials demonstrated that flexible dosing strategies, such as slower dose escalation or dose reduction, helped many participants remain on therapy while still achieving meaningful clinical benefits.

The authors interpret these results as supporting the expansion of available drug options for obesity and diabetes treatment, especially because individual responses to any single medication are variable and difficult to predict. The editorial challenges the use of BMI as the primary treatment target, noting its limitations as a surrogate for adiposity and health risk, especially in older adults where muscle and bone loss are critical concerns. The fact that metabolic improvements often occur earlier than maximal weight loss further supports the use of biomarker-based and functional targets rather than weight alone.

In conclusion, the editorial emphasizes that obesity treatment should prioritize long-term health outcomes, functional status, and sustained benefits rather than focusing only on greater weight loss. Although combination therapies such as cagrilintide–semaglutide are an important advance, longer-term safety data, clearer treatment targets, and better access are needed to achieve meaningful population-level health benefits.

REFERENCES (Miscellaneous)

1. Younossi ZM, Golabi P, de Avila L, Paik JM, Srishord M, Fukui N, et al. The global epidemiology of NAFLD and NASH in patients with type 2 diabetes: a systematic review and meta-analysis. J Hepatol. 2019;71(4):793-801.
2. Wongtrakul W, Niltwat S, Charatcharoenwitthaya N, Karaketklang K, Charatcharoenwitthaya P. Global prevalence of advanced fibrosis in patients with type 2 diabetes mellitus: a systematic review and meta-analysis. J Gastroenterol Hepatol. 2024;39:2299-307.
3. European Association for the Study of the Liver. EASL clinical practice guidelines on non-invasive tests for evaluation of liver disease severity and prognosis—2021 update. J Hepatol. 2021;75(3):659-89.
4. Graupera I, Thiele M, Serra-Burriel M, Caballeria L, Roulot D, Wong GL, et al. Low accuracy of FIB-4 and NAFLD fibrosis scores for screening for liver fibrosis in the population. Clin Gastroenterol Hepatol. 2022;20(11):2567-76.e6.
5. En Li Cho E, Ang CZ, Quek J, Fu CE, Lim LKE, Heng ZEQ, et al. Global prevalence of non-alcoholic fatty liver disease in type 2 diabetes mellitus: an updated systematic review and meta-analysis. Gut. 2023;72(11):2138-48.
6. Castera L, Laouenan C, Vallet-Pichard A, Vidal-Trécan T, Manchon P, Paradis V, et al. High prevalence of NASH and advanced fibrosis in type 2 diabetes: a prospective study of 330 outpatients undergoing liver biopsies for elevated ALT, using a low threshold. Diabetes Care. 2023;46(7):1354-62.
7. Dulai PS, Singh S, Patel J, Soni M, Prokop LJ, Younossi Z, et al. Increased risk of mortality by fibrosis stage in non-alcoholic fatty liver disease: systematic review and meta-analysis. Hepatology. 2017;65(5):1557-65.
8. Younossi ZM, Golabi P, Paik JM, Henry A, Van Dongen C, Henry L. The global epidemiology of nonalcoholic fatty liver disease (NAFLD) and nonalcoholic steatohepatitis (NASH): a systematic review. Hepatology. 2023;77:1335-47.
9. Xiao G, Zhu S, Xiao X, Yan L, Yang J, Wu G. Comparison of laboratory tests, ultrasound, or magnetic resonance elastography to detect fibro sis in patients with nonalcoholic fatty liver disease: a meta-analysis. Hepatology. 2017;66: 1486-501.
10. Sanyal AJ, Foucquier J, Younossi ZM, Harrison SA, Newsome PN, Chan WK, et al. Enhanced diagnosis of advanced fibrosis and cirrhosis in individuals with NAFLD using FibroScan-based agile scores. J Hepatol. 2023;78: 247-59.
11. GBD 2021 Diabetes Collaborators. Global, regional, and national bur den of diabetes from 1990 to 2021, with projections of prevalence to 2050: a systematic analysis for the global burden of disease study 2021. Lancet. 2023; 402(10397):203-34.
12. GBD 2021 Adult BMI Collaborators. Global, regional, and national prevalence of adult overweight and obesity, 1990–2021, with forecasts to 2050: a forecasting study for the global burden of disease study 2021. Lancet. 2025; 405(10481):813-38.
13. Salem V, Izzi-Engbeaya C, Coello C, Thomas DB, Chambers ES, Comninos AN, et al. Glucagon increases energy expenditure independently of brown adipose tissue activation in humans. Diabetes Obes Metab. 2016;18(1):72-81.
14. Sanyal AJ, Bedossa P, Fraessdorf M, Neff GW, Lawitz E, Bugianesi E, et al. A phase 2 randomized trial of Survodutide in MASH and fibrosis. N Engl J Med. 2024;391(4): 311-9.
15. le Roux CW, Steen O, Lucas KJ, Startseva E, Unseld A, Hennige AM. Glucagon and GLP-1 receptor dual agonist survodutide for obesity: a randomised, double-blind, placebo-

controlled, dose-finding phase 2 trial. Lancet Diabetes Endocrinol. 2024;12(3):162-73.
16. International Diabetes Federation. IDF Diabetes Atlas, 10th Edition. Brussels: International Diabetes Federation; 2021.
17. Riddle MC, Cefalu WT, Evans PH, Gerstein HC, Nauck MA, Oh WK, et al. Consensus report: definition and interpretation of remission in type 2 diabetes. Diabet Med. 2022;39: e14669.
18. Sattar N, Welsh P, Leslie WS, Thom G, McCombie L, Brosnahan N, et al. Dietary weight-management for type 2 diabetes remissions in South Asians: the South Asian diabetes remission randomised trial for proof-of-concept and feasibility (STANDby). Lancet Reg Health Southeast Asia. 2023;9:100111.
19. Murphy R, Plank LD, Clarke MG, Evennett NJ, Tan J, Kim DDW, et al. Effect of banded Roux-en-Y gastric bypass versus sleeve gastrectomy on diabetes remission at 5 years among patients with obesity and type 2 diabetes: a blinded randomized clinical trial. Diabetes Care. 2022;45:1503-11.
20. Aminian A, Wilson R, Zajichek A, Tu C, Wolski KE, Schauer PR, et al. Cardiovascular outcomes in patients with type 2 diabetes and obesity: comparison of gastric bypass, sleeve gastrectomy, and usual care. Diabetes Care. 2021;44: 2552-63.
21. Biter LU, 't Hart JWH, Noordman BJ, Smulders JF, Nienhuijs S, Dunkelgrün M, et al. Long-term effect of sleeve gastrectomy vs Roux-en-Y gastric bypass in people living with severe obesity: a phase III multicentre randomised controlled trial (SleeveBypass). Lancet Reg Health Eur. 2024;38:100836.
22. Peterli R, Wölnerhanssen BK, Peters T, Vetter D, Kröll D, Borbély Y, et al. Effect of laparoscopic sleeve gastrectomy vs laparoscopic Roux-en-Y Gastric bypass on weight loss in patients with morbid obesity: the SM-BOSS randomized clinical trial. JAMA. 2018;319:255-65.
23. Xu WL, von Strauss E, Qiu CX, Winblad B, Fratiglioni L. Uncontrolled diabetes increases the risk of Alzheimer's disease: a population-based cohort study. Diabetologia. 2009;52(6):1031-9.
24. Singh DD, Shati AA, Alfaifi MY, Elbehairi SEI, Han I, Choi EH, et al. Development of dementia in type 2 diabetes patients: mechanisms of insulin resistance and antidiabetic drug development. Cells. 2022;11(23):3767.
25. De Jesus Moreno Moreno M. Cognitive improvement in mild to moderate Alzheimer's dementia after treatment with the acetylcholine precursor choline alfoscerate: a multicenter, double-blind, randomized, placebo-controlled trial. Clin Ther. 2003;25(1):178-93.
26. Biessels GJ, Staekenborg S, Brunner E, Brayne C, Scheltens P. Risk of dementia in diabetes mellitus: a systematic review. Lancet Neurol. 2006;5:64-74.
27. Li W, Huang E, Gao S. Type 1 diabetes mellitus and cognitive impairments: a systematic review. J Alzheimers Dis. 2017;57:29-36.
28. De la Monte SM. Insulin resistance and neurodegeneration: progress towards the development of new therapeutics for Alzheimer's disease. Drugs. 2017;77:47-65.
29. Chatterjee S, Peters SAE, Woodward M, Mejia Arango S, Batty GD, Beckett N, et al. Type 2 diabetes as a risk factor for dementia in women compared with men: a pooled analysis of 2.3 million people comprising more than 100,000 cases of dementia. Diabetes Care. 2016;39(2):300-7.
30. GBD 2019 Dementia Forecasting Collaborators. Estimation of the global prevalence of dementia in 2019 and forecasted prevalence in 2050: an analysis for the global burden of disease study 2019. Lancet Public Health. 2022;7(2): e105-25.
31. Kim HK, Biessels GJ, Yu MH, Hong N, Lee YH, Lee BW, et al. SGLT2 inhibitor use and risk of dementia and Parkinson disease among patients with type 2 diabetes. Neurology. 2024;103(8):e209805.
32. Youn YJ, Kim S, Jeong HJ, Ah YM, Yu YM. Sodium-glucose cotransporter-2 inhibitors and their potential role in dementia onset and cognitive function in patients with diabetes mellitus: a systematic review and meta-analysis. Front Neuroendocrinol. 2024;73:101131.
33. Meldgaard T, Keller J, Olesen AE, Olesen SS, Krogh K, Borre M, et al. Pathophysiology and management of diabetic gastroenteropathy. Therap Adv Gastroenterol. 2019; 12:1756284819852047.
34. Kornum DS, Krogh K, Keller J, Malagelada C, Drewes AM, Brock C. Diabetic gastroenteropathy: a pan-alimentary complication. Diabetologia. 2025;68(5):905-19.
35. Porcari S, Baunwall SMD, Occhionero AS , Ingrosso MR, Ford AC, Hvas CL, et al. Fecal microbiota transplantation for recurrent C. difficile infection in patients with inflammatory bowel disease: a systematic review and meta-analysis. J Autoimmun. 2023;141:103036.
36. Høyer KL, Dahl Baunwall SM, Kornum DS, Klinge MW, Drewes AM, Yderstræde KB, et al. Faecal microbiota transplantation for patients with diabetes type 1 and severe gastrointestinal neuropathy (FADIGAS): a randomised, double-blinded, placebo-controlled trial. EClinicalMedicine.2024;79:10030.
37. Gurgul-Convey E. Sphingolipids in type 1 diabetes: focus on beta-cells. Cells. 2020;9(8):1835.
38. Holm LJ, Krogvold L, Hasselby JP, Kaur S, Claessens LA, Russell MA, et al. Abnormal islet sphingolipid metabolism in type 1 diabetes. Diabetologia. 2018;61(7):1650-61.
39. Buschard K, Holm LJ, Feldt-Rasmussen U. Insulin independence in newly diagnosed type 1 diabetes patient following fenofibrate treatment. Case Rep Med.2020:2020: 6865190.
40. Nordestgaard BG, Benn M, Schnohr P, Tybjærg-Hansen A. Nonfasting triglycerides and risk of myocardial infarction, ischemic heart disease, and death in men and women. JAMA. 2007;298(3):299.
41. Björnson E, Adiels M, Taskinen MR, Burgess S, Rawshani A, Borén J, et al. Triglyceride-rich lipoprotein remnants, low-density lipoproteins, and risk of coronary heart disease: a UK biobank study. Eur Heart J. 2023;44(39):4186-95.
42. Burggraaf B, Pouw NMC, Fernández-Arroyo S, van Vark-van der Zee LC, van de Geijn GM, Birnie E, et al. A placebo controlled proof-of-concept study of alirocumab on postprandial lipids and vascular elasticity in insulin-treated

patients with type 2 diabetes mellitus. Diabetes Obes Metab. 2020;22(5):807-16.
43. Stöhr J, Barbaresko J, Neuenschwander M, Schlesinger S. Bidirectional association between periodontal disease and diabetes mellitus: A systematic review and meta- analysis of cohort studies. Sci Rep. 2021;11:13686.
44. Wu CZ, Yuan YH, Liu HH, Li SS, Zhang BW, Chen W, et al. Epidemiologic relationship between periodontitis and type 2 diabetes mellitus. BMC Oral Health. 2020;20(1):204.
45. Ince G, Gürsoy H, Ipçi SD, Cakar G, Emekli-Alturfan E, Yılmaz S. Clinical and biochemical evaluation of lozenges containing *Lactobacillus reuteri* as an adjunct to non-surgical periodontal therapy in chronic periodontitis. J Periodontol. 2015;86:746-54.
46. Kassaian N, Feizi A, Aminorroaya A, Amini M. Probiotic and synbiotic supplementation could improve metabolic syndrome in prediabetic adults: A randomized controlled trial. Diabetes Metab Syndr. 2019;13(5):2991-6.
47. Hu B, Qu J, Han T, Leng J. Effect of basic periodontal therapy combined with probiotics on oral microecology and blood sugar control in patients with diabetes and periodontitis. Pak. J. Zool. 2023;55:1109-14.
48. Alexander TH, Harris JP. Incidence of sudden sensorineural hearing loss. Otol Neurotol. 2013;34(9):1586-9.
49. Chien CY, Tai SY, Wang LF, Hsi E, Chang NC, Wu MT, et al. Metabolic syndrome increases the risk of sudden sensorineural hearing loss in Taiwan: A case-control study. Otolaryngol Head Neck Surg. 2015;153(1):105-11.
50. Chen HC, Chung CH, Lu CH, Chien WC. Metformin decreases the risk of sudden sensorineural hearing loss in patients with diabetes mellitus: A 14-year follow-up study. Diab Vasc Dis Res. 2019;16(4):324-7.
51. Föller M, Jaumann M, Dettling J, Saxena A, Pakladok T, Munoz C, et al. AMP-activated protein kinase in BK-channel regulation and protection against hearing loss following acoustic overstimulation. FASEB J. 2012;26(10):4243-53.
52. Andersen DK, Korc M, Petersen GM, Eibl G, Li D, Rickels MR, et al. Diabetes, pancreatogenic diabetes, and pancreatic cancer. Diabetes. 2017;66(5):1103-10.
53. Cui Y, Andersen DK. Pancreatogenic diabetes: Special considerations for management. Pancreatology. 2011; 11(3):279-94.
54. Olesen SS, Svane HML, Nicolaisen SK, Kristensen JK, Drewes AM, Brandslund I, et al. Clinical and biochemical characteristics of postpancreatitis diabetes mellitus: A cross-sectional study from the Danish nationwide DD2 cohort. J Diabetes. 2021;13(12):960-74.
55. American Diabetes Association Professional Practice Committee. Diagnosis and classification of diabetes: Standards of Care in Diabetes-2024. Diabetes Care. 2024; 47(Suppl 1):S20-42.
56. Choi HK, McCormick N, Yokose C. Excess comorbidities in gout: The causal paradigm and pleiotropic approaches to care. Nat Rev Rheumatol. 2022;18:97-111.
57. Zhu Y, Pandya BJ, Choi HK. Comorbidities of gout and hyperuricemia in the US general population: NHANES 2007-2008. Am J Med. 2012;125:679-87.e1.
58. Kuo CF, See LC, Luo SF, Ko YS, Lin YS, Hwang JS, et al. Gout: An independent risk factor for all cause and cardiovascular mortality. Rheumatology (Oxford). 2010;49:141-6.
59. Zhu J, Zeng Y, Zhang H, Qu Y, Ying Z, Sun Y, et al. The association of hyperuricemia and gout with the risk of cardiovascular diseases: A cohort and mendelian randomization study in UK biobank. Front Med (Lausanne). 2021;8:817150.
60. Ji L, Jiang H, Bi Y, Li H, Tian J, Liu D, et al. Once-weekly mazdutide in Chinese adults with obesity or overweight. N Engl J Med. 2025;392:2215-25.
61. Noureddin M, Rinella ME, Chalasani NP, Neff GW, Lucas KJ, Rodriguez ME, et al. Efruxifermin in compensated liver cirrhosis caused by MASH. N Engl J Med. 2025;392:2413-24.
62. Harrison SA, Dubourg J. Liver biopsy evaluation in MASH drug development: think thrice, act wise. J Hepatol. 2024; 81:886-94.
63. de Franchis R, Bosch J, Garcia-Tsao G, Reiberger T, Ripoll C; Baveno VII Faculty. Baveno VII—renewing consensus in portal hypertension. J Hepatol. 2022;76:959-74.
64. Centers for Disease Control and Prevention. (2026). National Diabetes Statistics Report. [online] Available from https://www.cdc.gov/diabetes/php/data-research/index.html. [Last accessed January, 2026].
65. Garvey WT, Blüher M, Osorto Contreras CK, Davies MJ, Winning Lehmann E, Pietiläinen KH, et al. Coadministered cagrilintide and semaglutide in adults with overweight or obesity. N Engl J Med. 2025;393:635-47.
66. Davies MJ, Bajaj HS, Broholm C, Eliasen A, Garvey WT, le Roux CW, et al. Cagrilintide-semaglutide in adults with overweight or obesity and type 2 diabetes. N Engl J Med. 2025;393:648-59.

Index

D

E

F

G

H

I

K

L

M

N

O

P

Q

R

S

T

U

V

W